Lecture Notes in Computer Science 16473

The series Lecture Notes in Computer Science (LNCS), including its subseries Lecture Notes in Artificial Intelligence (LNAI) and Lecture Notes in Bioinformatics (LNBI), has established itself as a medium for the publication of new developments in computer science and information technology research, teaching, and education.

LNCS enjoys close cooperation with the computer science R & D community, the series counts many renowned academics among its volume editors and paper authors, and collaborates with prestigious societies. Its mission is to serve this international community by providing an invaluable service, mainly focused on the publication of conference and workshop proceedings and postproceedings. LNCS commenced publication in 1973.

Federico Bolelli · Achraf Ben-Hamadou ·
Yaqi Wang · Luca Lumetti · Sergi Pujades ·
Shuai Wang · Kevin Marchesini ·
Costantino Grana
Editors

Oral and Dental Image Analysis

First International Workshop, ODIN 2025, and MICCAI Challenges, ToothFairy 2025 and STSR 2025, Held in Conjunction with MICCAI 2025
Daejeon, South Korea, September 27, 2025
Proceedings

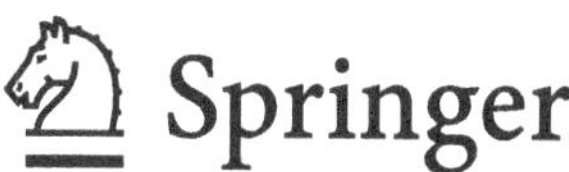

Editors
Federico Bolelli
University of Modena and Reggio Emilia
Modena, Italy

Achraf Ben-Hamadou
Digital Research Center of Sfax
Sfax, Tunisia

Yaqi Wang
University of Hangzhou
Hangzhou, China

Luca Lumetti
University of Modena and Reggio Emilia
Modena, Italy

Sergi Pujades
Université Grenoble Alpes
Montbonnot Saint Martin, France

Shuai Wang
Hangzhou Dianzi University
Hangzhou, China

Kevin Marchesini
University of Modena and Reggio Emilia
Modena, Italy

Costantino Grana
University of Modena and Reggio Emilia
Modena, Italy

ISSN 0302-9743 ISSN 1611-3349 (electronic)
Lecture Notes in Computer Science
ISBN 978-3-032-20710-4 ISBN 978-3-032-20711-1 (eBook)
https://doi.org/10.1007/978-3-032-20711-1

This Springer imprint is published by the registered company Springer Nature Switzerland AG
The registered company address is: Gewerbestrasse 11, 6330 Cham, Switzerland

ODIN 2025 Workshop Preface

The *Oral and Dental Image aNalysis* workshop, ODIN 2025, an international workshop on multi-structure and multi-modal learning for 3D dental image analysis, was organized as a satellite event of the 28th International Conference on Medical Image Computing and Computer Assisted Intervention (MICCAI 2025) in Daejeon, South Korea. The workshop was held on September 27, 2025 at the Daejeon Convention Center, in conjunction with MICCAI 2025, and brought together researchers and practitioners working at the intersection of medical imaging, computer vision, dentistry, and maxillofacial surgery.

Computer-aided diagnosis and planning tools are increasingly adopted in modern dental practice, supported by the growing availability of 3D imaging modalities such as Cone Beam Computed Tomography (CBCT) and Intra-oral Scans (IOS). CBCT provides volumetric information on dental and maxillofacial anatomy, while IOS delivers highly accurate surface reconstructions of tooth crowns and gingiva. Accurate segmentation, instance delineation, landmark detection, and registration across these modalities are essential prerequisites for a wide range of clinical workflows, including implant planning, orthognathic surgery, orthodontics, and post-operative assessment. However, compared to natural-image benchmarks, dental imaging tasks pose unique challenges: 3D voxel data, acquisition artifacts, strong anatomical variability, domain shifts across scanners and protocols, and a persistent scarcity of large-scale, publicly available annotated datasets.

The ODIN workshop was designed to foster a focused and engaged community by promoting rigorous evaluation, encouraging reproducibility, and stimulating discussion on both methodological advances and clinically grounded constraints. In addition to contributed papers, the program included invited talks and dedicated sessions aimed at bridging the gap between established medical image analysis approaches and emerging techniques from the broader vision and learning communities. A key emphasis of ODIN 2025 was to move beyond "what is known to work" and to cultivate exploration of alternative modeling paradigms, data-centric strategies, and efficiency-aware solutions that can accelerate translation into clinical practice.

The workshop was closely connected to the ODIN 2025 challenge cluster, which provided a complementary benchmarking ecosystem and an additional venue for sharing competitive insights. This synergy enabled participants to discuss datasets, metrics, evaluation protocols, and practical deployment constraints with many experts gathered in the same place, stimulating conversations that continued beyond the formal sessions.

The ODIN 2025 proceedings include the workshop track contributions selected through a rigorous peer-review process. In total, the workshop track received 13 submissions, of which 9 papers were accepted for publication in this LNCS volume. Each manuscript was evaluated in a single-blind review process involving 3 reviewers and a meta-reviewer from the Program Committee, composed of experts in medical image analysis and dental imaging. The accepted papers span a broad range of topics, including (but not limited to) CBCT and IOS registration, multi-instance and multi-structure segmentation, landmark detection, learning with limited supervision, trustworthy and interpretable AI, and efficient methods suitable for constrained computational environments.

We wish to thank all authors for their submissions and their willingness to share methods and results, the Program Committee members and reviewers for their time and careful evaluations, the invited speakers for their insightful contributions, and all attendees for creating an engaging environment for discussion and collaboration. We are also grateful to the workshop sponsors for their support.

January 2026

Federico Bolelli
Achraf Ben-Hamadou
Yaqi Wang
Luca Lumetti
Dahong Qian
Kevin Marchesini
Jun Liu
Niels van Nistelrooij
Sergi Pujades
Lan Feng
Yifan Zhang
Shankeeth Vinayahalingam
Costantino Grana

ToothFairy3 Preface

The third edition of the ToothFairy challenge series, *ToothFairy3: Fast Multi-Structure Segmentation in CBCT Volumes*, was organized as part of the ODIN 2025 challenge cluster and presented as a satellite event of the 28th International Conference on Medical Image Computing and Computer Assisted Intervention (MICCAI 2025) in Daejeon, South Korea. The results of the challenge were presented during the associated ODIN 2025 workshop held on September 27, 2025, at the Daejeon Convention Center, in conjunction with MICCAI 2025. The challenge was hosted on the Grand Challenge platform, which supports standardized evaluation and, beyond the official competition timeline, enables post-challenge submissions through a live leaderboard designed to facilitate fair comparison of new methods on the internal test set.

The use of Cone Beam Computed Tomography (CBCT) continues to expand not only in dentistry, but across head and neck and maxillofacial surgery. Its key advantages are short acquisition time and relatively low radiation exposure, while preserving excellent visualization of hard tissues and clinically relevant anatomical structures. In the first ToothFairy edition (MICCAI 2023), we addressed the segmentation of the Inferior Alveolar Canal (IAC), a critical mandibular structure whose identification and preservation are essential in many surgical interventions. In ToothFairy2 (MICCAI 2024), we broadened the scope by extending segmentation to a larger set of anatomical structures relevant for cross-disciplinary clinical practice and surgical planning. Building on this trajectory, ToothFairy3 further advanced CBCT segmentation by expanding the set of target structures and emphasizing practical constraints that matter for real-world adoption.

ToothFairy3 was designed to promote the development of deep learning frameworks that can accurately and efficiently segment multiple anatomical structures in CBCT volumes. In addition to improving segmentation quality, the 2025 edition explicitly prioritized computational efficiency, reflecting the growing need for methods that can be integrated into clinical workflows where runtime and resource constraints are paramount. The challenge included two complementary tracks: (i) a *fast multi-structure segmentation* task targeting an expanded set of anatomical classes (including, among others, pulp chamber, root canals, incisive nerves, and the lingual foramen, for a total of 77 classes), and (ii) an *interactive segmentation* task focused on the Inferior Alveolar Canal (IAC), where participants developed click-based approaches to refine predictions with minimal user input, aligning with emerging clinical and dataset-creation scenarios where human-in-the-loop interaction can substantially improve quality.

The competition timeline included the release of training data on May 9, 2025, followed by a debugging submission phase running from July 1, 2025 to August 24, 2025, and a final test submission phase running from August 8, 2025 to August 24, 2025. The official results were released on September 27, 2025, and top-performing teams were invited to present their approaches at the ODIN workshop. Beyond the formal presentations, the in-person setting fostered lively discussion and knowledge exchange, with many researchers working on dental image analysis gathered together in the same room, enabling detailed conversations about model design choices, data-centric strategies, evaluation pitfalls, and efficiency-accuracy trade-offs.

The ToothFairy3 proceedings present the contributions associated with the challenge, summarizing key methodological insights and lessons learned from the competition. In total, the challenge attracted 185 teams and received 18 valid submissions in the final test phase. Participants who completed the final phase were invited to submit manuscripts for inclusion in this LNCS volume. All submissions underwent a rigorous single-blind peer-review process involving 3 reviewers and one meta-reviewer from the Program Committee. The six accepted papers (from seven submissions) cover a wide range of approaches, including novel training strategies, architectural innovations, post-processing and interaction mechanisms for fine structures, and efficiency-aware pipelines designed to meet the runtime constraints emphasized by this edition. To ensure transparency, reproducibility, and a long-term fair evaluation, we have made the evaluation scripts and the code for the submissions publicly available on GitHub (https://github.com/AImageLab-zip/ToothFairy) and configured the Grand Challenge platform to accept post-challenge submissions.

We wish to thank all ToothFairy3 participants for their interest and effort, the authors of the proceedings for sharing their methods and insights, the Program Committee members and reviewers for their thorough evaluations, and the annotators and collaborators who contributed to the creation and curation of the ToothFairy datasets. We also acknowledge the support of the ODIN 2025 workshop and challenge sponsors and all collaborators who helped make the event possible. Further material related to the challenge, including rules, updates, and public resources, is available through the official ToothFairy3 Grand Challenge website.

January 2026

Federico Bolelli
Luca Lumetti
Zdravko Marinov
Shankeeth Vinayahalingam
Niels van Nistelrooij
Mattia Di Bartolomeo
Kevin Marchesini
Torkan Gholamalizadeh
Laura Montesdeoca Fenoy
Natasha Hallberg
Rainer Stiefelhagen
Alexandre Anesi
Costantino Grana

STSR 2025 Preface

The third international challenge on Semi-supervised Teeth Segmentation, now expanded to *Semi-supervised Teeth Segmentation and Registration (STSR 2025)*, was organized as a satellite event of the 28th International Conference on Medical Image Computing and Computer Assisted Intervention (MICCAI 2025). Building on the success of the previous editions, STSR 2025 was held in conjunction with other dental-focused challenges, fostering a collaborative environment for advancing digital dentistry. The challenge was hosted online with a live leaderboard to ensure transparency and continuous evaluation.

Computer-aided diagnosis tools are increasingly pivotal in modern dental practice, particularly for complex procedures such as root canal therapy, orthodontics, and implantology. While 2D panoramic X-rays remain efficient for screening, 3D Cone-Beam Computed Tomography (CBCT) has become indispensable for visualizing volumetric structures. However, the precise delineation of fine-grained anatomical structures (such as root pulp canals) and the fusion of multi-modal data (CBCT and Intraoral Scans) remain bottlenecks due to the labor-intensive nature of manual annotation. Consequently, the scarcity of high-quality labeled data limits the development of fully supervised deep learning algorithms. As a potent alternative, semi-supervised learning (SSL) offers the ability to explore and leverage vast amounts of useful information from unlabeled cases.

With this challenge, we aimed to benchmark and advance SSL algorithms for advanced dental tasks. We extended the scope from the previous instance-level segmentation to two distinct and more challenging tasks: (1) Semi-supervised segmentation of teeth and root pulp canals in 3D CBCT, and (2) Semi-supervised rigid registration of CBCT and IOS data. The dataset for STSR 2025 was significantly expanded, comprising a total of 859 CBCT scans curated from clinical practice, alongside 129 paired IOS data. This large-scale resource supports the training of robust models capable of handling real-world anatomical variability.

The challenge attracted significant community interest, with 78 teams participating in the segmentation task and 52 teams in the registration task. Top teams submitted open-source solutions that were rigorously evaluated for algorithmic excellence. All successful submissions leveraged deep learning-based SSL methods. To ensure transparency and reproducibility, both the challenge dataset and the participants' submitted code have been made publicly available on GitHub (https://github.com/ricoleehduu/STS-Challenge-2025).

The top participants were invited to share their insights during the ODIN workshop event organized at MICCAI. Speakers presented their submissions in detail, covering data filtering, model training, hyperparameter tuning, and final results on the internal validation and official test sets. These proceedings present the state-of-the-art methods selected through a rigorous single-blind peer-review process. Each of the six submitted manuscripts received reviews from three to five experts in the field. The five accepted papers explore hybrid SSL frameworks, innovative network architectures, and advanced techniques for multi-modal fusion.

We wish to thank all the participants for their interest, the authors for their contributions, the members of the Program Committee, and the reviewers for their invaluable work. In addition to the papers presented within this volume, further comprehensive details and updates are available on the official STSR 2025 main website (https://songhen15.github.io/STSdevelop.github.io/miccai2025).

September 2025

Yaqi Wang
Dahong Qian
Shuai Wang
Yifan Zhang
Huiyu Zhou
Jun Liu
Zhi Li
Chengyu Wu

Organization

General Chair—ODIN 2025

Federico Bolelli	University of Modena and Reggio Emilia, Italy

Program Committee Chairs—ODIN 2025

Achraf Ben-Hamadou	Digital Research Center of Sfax, Tunisia
Yaqi Wang	Hangzhou Dianzi University, China
Luca Lumetti	University of Modena and Reggio Emilia, Italy
Sergi Pujades	Inria, University of Grenoble Alpes, France
Kevin Marchesini	University of Modena and Reggio Emilia, Italy
Costantino Grana	University of Modena and Reggio Emilia, Italy

Program Committee—ODIN 2025

Dahong Qian	Shanghai Jiao Tong University, China
Niels van Nistelrooij	Radboud University, Netherlands
Lan Feng	Zhejiang University, China
Yifan Zhang	Hangzhou Dental Group, China
S. Vinayahalingam	Radboud University, Netherlands

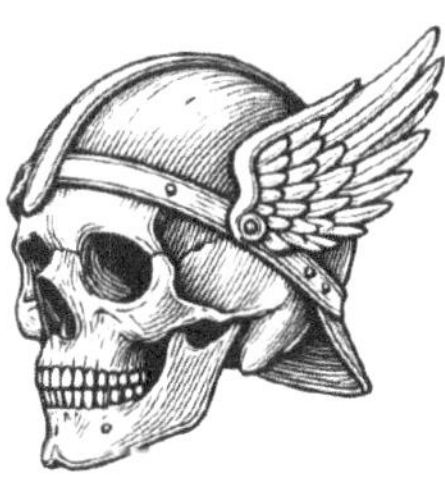

General Chair—ToothFairy3

Federico Bolelli	University of Modena and Reggio Emilia, Italy

Program Committee Chairs—ToothFairy3

Luca Lumetti	University of Modena and Reggio Emilia, Italy
Zdravko Marinov	Karlsruhe Institute of Technology, Germany
Costantino Grana	University of Modena and Reggio Emilia, Italy

Program Committee—ToothFairy3

Alexandre Anesi	University of Modena and Reggio Emilia, Italy
Mattia Di Bartolomeo	Sapienza University of Rome, Italy
Kevin Marchesini	University of Modena and Reggio Emilia, Italy
Niels van Nistelrooij	Radboud University, Netherlands
T. Gholamalizadeh	3Shape A/S, Denmark
Laura M. Fenoy	3Shape A/S, Denmark
Natasha Hallberg	3Shape A/S, Denmark
Rainer Stiefelhagen	Karlsruhe Institute of Technology, Germany
S. Vinayahalingam	Radboud University, Netherlands

Sponsor—ToothFairy3

We are very grateful to our sponsor, See Through S.r.l, for their invaluable support in organizing the ToothFairy3 Challenge and awarding the prizes.

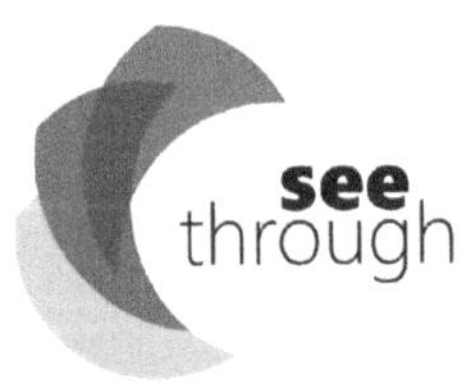

General Chair—STSR 2025

Yaqi Wang	Hangzhou Dianzi University, China

Program Committee Chairs—STSR 2025

Dahong Qian	Shanghai Jiao Tong University, China
Shuai Wang	Hangzhou Dianzi University, China
Jun Liu	Hangzhou Dianzi University, China
Yifan Zhang	Hangzhou Dental Group, China

Program Committee—STSR 2025

Zhi Li	Hangzhou Dianzi University, China
Chengyu Wu	Shandong University, China

Sponsor—STSR 2025

We would like to express our sincere appreciation to our sponsor, Hangzhou Association for Artificial Intelligence, for their essential support in organizing the STSR 2025 challenge.

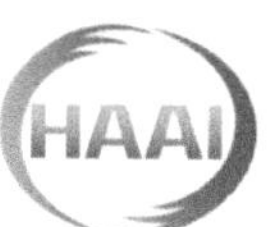

Hangzhou Association for
Artificial Intelligence

Additional Workshop and Challenge Reviewers

Abhi Desai
Adham Bekhit
Chenfan Xu
Claudio Landi
Donghang Lyu
Jaehwan Han
Jialuo Chen
Lisheng Wang
Mahmoud Gamal
Marek Wodzinski
Mattia Di Bartolomeo
Ni Jiaxue

Nicola Morelli
Qianni Zhang
Qun Jing
Shuai Wang
Taijero Tomas
Tomasz Szczepański
Vicent Caselles-Ballester
Xuan Yang
Yannick Kirchhoff
Yunxiang Li
Zhi Li
Zhi Qin Tan

Contents

ToothFairy3 Challenge

STSR 2025 Challenge

ODIN 2025 – Oral and Dental Image aNalysis Workshop

3D Dental Arch Curve Detection from CBCT Images and Its Applications to Tooth Segmentation

Benxiang Jiang[1,2], Songze Zhang[1,2], Jingyi Lyu[1,2], and Hongjian Shi[1,2](✉)

[1] Beijing Normal-Hong Kong Baptist University, Zhuhai, China
[2] Hong Kong Baptist University, Hong Kong, China
shihj@bnbu.edu.cn

Abstract. The three-dimensional (3D) dental arch curve, representing the spatial trajectory of dentition in either the maxilla or mandible, exhibits systematic alignment of tightly and orderly arranged teeth along its path. This structural configuration underscores its critical role as comprehensive anatomical guidance in digital dentistry, enabling high-precision tooth segmentation. In this study, we present a novel method for 3D dental arch curve detection from the volumetric cone beam computed tomography (CBCT) image, which, to our knowledge, represents the first successful implementation of 3D dental arch curve detection from the volumetric data. Specifically, we: (1) formulates and validates a dental arch curve fitting function, (2) identifies 3D uniformly distributed feature points proximal to the true dental arch curve through a feature point network framework, and (3) optimizes model parameters of the fitting function through a modified Expectation-Maximization (EM) algorithm with gradient descent. The proposed detection is then used to guide tooth segmentation through the curvilinear volume parameterization that unwind the vicinity of the dental arch curve. Experimental results demonstrate the accuracy for 3D dental arch curve detection and performance enhancements in the downstream task of tooth segmentation, improving segmentation precision compared to conventional approaches.

Keywords: CBCT · 3D Dental Arch Curve · Tooth Segmentation · EM Algorithm · Digital Dentistry

1 Introduction

The dental arch constitutes the curved arrangement of teeth within the maxilla or mandible, with its morphology typically characterized through parametric curve representations [5,16,17]. Along this critical anatomical feature, teeth exhibit precise spatial organization and are systematically and tightly aligned. For volumetric data processing, this anatomical feature enables the extraction

F. Bolelli et al. (Eds.): ODIN 2025, LNCS 16473, pp. 3–12, 2026.
https://doi.org/10.1007/978-3-032-20711-1_1

of dentition region-of-interest (ROI) since the dental arch curve's vicinity works as a filter to preserve diagnostically relevant dentition regions as illustrated in Fig. 1.

The dental arch in the volumetric data set is three-dimensional (3D) that preserves authentic spatial inter-tooth relationships. However, current researches reveal an absence of robust algorithms for the detection of the 3D dental arch curve. Existing algorithms have succeeded in detecting dental arch curves with two-dimensional (2D) cone beam computed tomography (CBCT) projections [14, 16,29] or three-dimensional (3D) dental mesh surfaces [19,22,30] through arch point detection and subsequent curve interpolation. In 3D volumetric space, on the other side, the critical challenge lies in reliably detecting arch points within the 3D CBCT image. This detection challenge hindering progress in detecting true 3D dental arch from the 3D CBCT image.

A specific curve can be described either by interpolation [11] or fitting [2] from given points. Interpolation defines the curve by passing through all given points and so require high accurate and reliable point detection. Fitting, on the other hand, utilizes given points to estimate parameters of a function. The function with estimated parameters fits a curve. In 3D dental arch curve detection from the volumetric data, detecting feature points uniformly distributed around the true 3D dental arch is practicable. Thus, fitting presents a more sensible strategy for 3D dental arch curve detection. Fitting based 3D dental arch curve detection involves three main challenges: 1. Formulation of a fitting function for the dental arch curve that suits the dental arch arrangement; 2. Automated detection of uniformly distributed feature points along the dental arch trajectory; and 3. Robust parameter estimation with latent variables that connect the feature points and the fitting function.

To resolve these challenges, this study proposes a three-stage fitting-based method for 3D dental arch curve detection in the 3D CBCT image as shown in Fig. 1. The method comprises: 1. A parametric curve equation to fit the dental arch curve; 2. A feature point network framework to identify uniformly distributed feature points proximal to the true dental arch curve; 3. A modified Expectation-Maximization (EM) algorithm [8] with the gradient descent [3] to optimize parameters and latent variables.

The clinical applications of 3D dental arch curves are primarily in guiding tooth segmentation, the task that segments and numbers individual tooth within the 3D CBCT image. Therefore, we also propose a curvilinear volume parameterization method based on the 3D dental arch curve in this study, as illustrated in Fig. 1. Through this parameterization, the dentition region within the CBCT image can be transformed into two curvilinear volumes as two narrow cuboid volumes specifically designed to localize the maxillary and mandibular dentitions, respectively. Within each curvilinear volume, all maxillary or mandibular tooth are closely and orderly arranged from left to right and constitute the dominant region of the space. In contrast, within the original CBCT image, teeth exhibit an arch-shaped arrangement, and the dentition occupies only a minor portion of the overall volume. Consequently, compared to performing segmentation directly within the CBCT space, our proposed curvilinear volume parameterization method, based on the 3D dental arch curve, serves as an effective plug-and-play tool to enhance the accuracy of existing tooth segmentation methods. To validate the efficacy of the curvilinear volume parameterization method based on the 3D dental arch curve, we conducted comprehensive tests using several baseline segmentation methods, including nnUNet 2D [12], nnUNet 3D [13], SegResNet [21], and MedNext [23]. The experimental results demonstrate that curvilinear volume parameterization, functioning as a plug-and-play tool, effectively improves tooth segmentation accuracy.

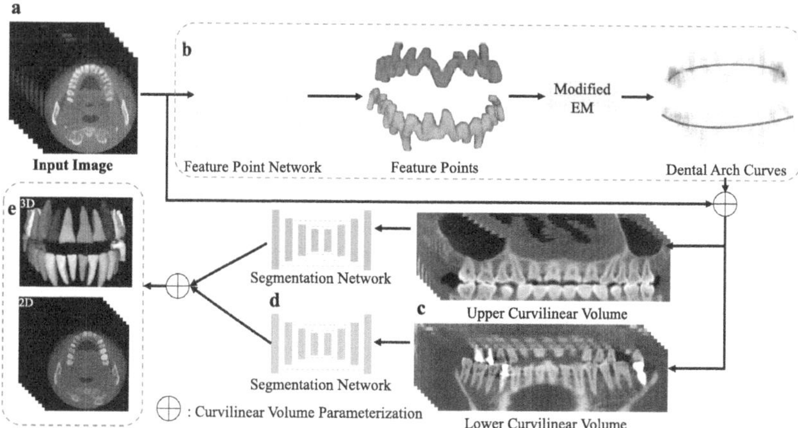

Fig. 1. Overview of the proposed method for fitting 3D dental arch curves, and serving as a plug-and-play tool for segmenting individual teeth from a 3D CBCT image. a. The input 3D CBCT image. b. Proposed 3D dental arch curve detection. c. Curvilinear volume parameterization to transform the CBCT image into two narrow cuboid volumes where teeth are closely and orderly arranged from left to right. d. Tooth segmentation implementation in the curvilinear volumes. e. Curvilinear volume parameterization to transform the segmented teeth into the CBCT image.

2 Methods

2.1 Dental Arch Curve Fitting Function

Contemporary orthodontic research emphasizes that any plan of dental arch determination must be flexible enough to produce arches varying in form through a parabola, cubic parabola, etc. [5]. Therefore, our 3D dental arch curve fitting function is a parametric curve that combines two cubic parabolas and a linear polynomial to capture both anatomical curvature and alveolar bone orientation:

$$\boldsymbol{C}(u) = (x(u), y(u), z(u)) = \begin{pmatrix} \theta_1 u + \theta_2 u^2 + \theta_3 u^3 + \theta_4 \\ \theta_5 u + \theta_6 u^2 + \theta_7 u^3 + \theta_8 \\ \theta_9 u^2 + \theta_{10} u + \theta_{11} \end{pmatrix} \tag{1}$$

where $u \in [0, 1]$ parameterizes the dental arch trajectory in the DICOM coordinate system (x-axis: Left to Right, y-axis: Anterior to Posterior, z-axis: Inferior to Superior) [28] and $\{\theta_1, ..., \theta_1 1\}$are unobserved parameters for curve fitting. The parametric curve in Eq. (1) achieves both anatomical fidelity and computational efficiency. The cubic parabola terms describe the natural variations and smooth transitions of the arch-shaped structure of the dental arch curve. The parabola term approximates the orientation of the alveolar bone. The 11 parameters in Eq. (1) balances complexity of the fitting function and the optimization feasibility. The three polynomial expressions in Eq. (1) enable derivatives for parameter estimation.

2.2 Feature Point Network Framework

Our feature point network framework processes a 3D CBCT image to uniformly distributed feature points along the maxillary and mandibular dental arch trajectories, as illustrated in Fig. 1. The critical component of the framework is ground truth generation. After collecting ground truths, we employ a 3D residual encoder U-Net [1,13] implemented within the nnU-Net framework [12]. The nnU-Net framework automatically configures hyperparameters verified in segmentation tasks [9,13]. This approach transforms the feature point detection task into a simpler binary volume segmentation problem. All segmented foreground voxels within the network output can subsequently be utilized as feature points for dental arch curve detection.

We propose an algorithm to generate ground truth feature points from manual tooth segmentation masks [7,15], addressing the labor-intensive challenges of manual feature point annotation along 3D dental arches. The procedure initiates by fitting a parabolic curve to the axial projection of tooth centroids:

$$\xi(x) = \beta_1 x + \beta_2 x^2 + \beta_3 \tag{2}$$

where parameters $\beta_1, \beta_2, \beta_3$ are optimized through least squares estimation [27] from the axial coordinates of all maxillary/mandibular tooth voxels. To ensure uniform feature point distribution, the parabola in Eq. (2.2) undergoes uniform discrete sampling by $x_n = t((n - 0.5)d)$, $n \in \{1, ..., N\}$, where $t(\cdot)$ represents the inverse function of the arc length function of the parabola, d is the interval, and N specifies the feature point count. At each discrete point x_n, the orthogonal plane perpendicular to the tangent vector of x_n is computed as $x + (\beta_1 + 2\beta_2 x_n)y - x_n - (\beta_1 + 2\beta_2 x_n)\xi(x_n) = 0$. Feature points are defined as centroids of the intersection areas between these planes and the maxillary/mandibular tooth volumes. These centroids are encoded in 3D label maps with label 1 for maxillary feature points and label 2 for mandibular feature points and processed with $5 \times 5 \times 5$ morphological dilation to create network training targets. This automated pipeline ensures anatomical accuracy while eliminating manual annotation inconsistencies.

2.3 Modified EM Algorithm with Gradient Descent

EM algorithm is an iterative statistical estimation method, particularly effective for parameter optimization in latent variables [8]. Its robustness in handling latent variables makes it particularly suitable for 3D curve fitting challenges. The parameter estimation for Eq. (2.2) employs a modified Expectation-Maximization (EM) framework that integrates gradient descent optimization [3] to address latent variable challenges in 3D curve fitting. This hybrid approach combines the statistical rigor of EM with numerical optimization capabilities.

The initialization step begins with ordered feature point coordinates $\{\boldsymbol{P}_1, \ldots, \boldsymbol{P}_N\} = \{(x_1, y_1, z_1), \ldots, (x_N, y_N, z_N)\}$ sorted by ascending x-values. Each feature point associates with a latent parameter u_i for $i \in \{1, \ldots, N\}$, initialized through centripetal parameterization [4]: $u_i = u_{i-1} + \frac{\|\boldsymbol{P}_i - \boldsymbol{P}_{i-1}\|_2^{1/2}}{\sum_{j=2}^{N} \|\boldsymbol{P}_j - \boldsymbol{P}_{j-1}\|_2^{1/2}}$, with $u_1 = 0$. The error function quantifies cumulative deviation by $E = \sum_{i=1}^{N} \|\boldsymbol{P}_i - \boldsymbol{C}(u_i)\|_2^2$. In the maximization step, the partial derivative $\frac{\partial E}{\partial \theta_x} = 0$ gives the update for $\theta_x = (\theta_1, \theta_2, \theta_3, \theta_4)$, with analogous updates for $\theta_y = (\theta_5, \theta_6, \theta_7, \theta_8)$ and $\theta_z = (\theta_9, \theta_{10}, \theta_{11})$. In the Expectation step, the latent variables $u_1, \ldots, u_N$ are optimized via gradient descent with learning rate η: $u_i^{(k+1)} = u_i^{(k)} - \eta \frac{\partial E}{\partial u_i}$, $i = 1, \ldots, N$ where superscript k denotes iteration index. $\frac{\partial E}{\partial u_1}, \ldots, \frac{\partial E}{\partial u_N}$ are computed through chain rule differentiation of the error function. In the iteration step, iteration alternates between coefficient updates and latent variable optimization until convergence or fixed iteration numbers. This dual optimization strategy combines the global convergence properties of EM with local refinement through gradient descent, thus balancing efficiency and accuracy.

2.4 Curvilinear Volume Parameterization

Given a fitted dental arch curve $\boldsymbol{C}_{fit}(u)$, we define tubular coordinates as $\{(x, y, z) | (x, y, z) = \boldsymbol{C}_{fit}(u) + \alpha \boldsymbol{B}(u) + \gamma \boldsymbol{N}(u), u \in [0, 1], \alpha \in [-40, 40], \gamma \in [t_1, t_2]\}$, where $\boldsymbol{T}(u) = \frac{\boldsymbol{C}'_{fit}(u)}{|\boldsymbol{C}'_{fit}(u)|}$, $\boldsymbol{N}(u) = \frac{\boldsymbol{T}'(u)}{|\boldsymbol{T}'(u)|}$, and $\boldsymbol{B}(u) = \boldsymbol{T} \times \boldsymbol{N}$ are the unit tangent, normal, and binormal vectors, $[t_1, t_2] = [-40, 56]$ for the maxillary teeth and $[-56, 40]$ for the mandibular teeth. Let the length of $\boldsymbol{C}_{fit}(u)$ with $u \in [0, 1]$ be L. This tubular coordinates unwinds the vicinity of the dental arch curve $\boldsymbol{C}_{fit}(u)$ into a rectilinear 3D volume $V \in \mathcal{R}^{L \times 80 \times 96}$ through discretely sampling R_v at $\Delta u = 1/L$, $\Delta \alpha = \Delta \gamma = 1$ using bicubic interpolation and $(u, \alpha, \gamma) \leftarrow (x, y, z)$ via diffeomorphic mapping. This unwinding process is reversible naturally.

3 Experiments and Discussions

3.1 Materials

This study utilizes a hybrid dataset of 110 3D CBCT images with corresponding voxel-level tooth segmentation ground truth volumes, comprising 98 cases from [6,7] and 12 cases from [15]. The dataset [6,7] contains 4531 CBCT volumes, of which 148 are publicly available. Among these 148 volumes, 50 are small field-of-view (FOV) CBCT images lacking complete maxillary and mandibular structures, while the remaining 98 large FOV CBCT volumes constitute our utilized subset. The dataset [15] comprises 12 CBCT volumes, all of which were employed in this study. The hybrid dataset encompasses 15 distinct acquisition protocols with spatial resolutions ranging from $0.25 \times 0.25 \times 0.27$ mm^3 to $0.4{\times}0.4{\times}0.4$ mm^3 and field-of-view dimensions spanning $12.1{\times}12.1{\times}8.51$ cm^3 to $16{\times}16{\times}13.1$ cm^3. To address the absence of manual tooth numbering, we implemented the FDI World Dental Federation notation system [10] as illustrated in Fig. 1 through manual labeling, creating a classification strategy comprising 33 distinct anatomical categories: 32 permanent tooth identifiers (combining 4 jaw quadrants and 8 tooth types) plus background.

3.2 Experimental Setup

Experiments were performed on a GIGABYTE G292-Z42 workstation featuring an Intel Xeon Platinum 8352V processor, NVIDIA RTX 4090 GPU, NVIDIA L20 GPU, and 64GB DDR4 memory, operating under Ubuntu 22.04 LTS. From the complete dataset of 110 CBCT scans with voxel-level annotations, we employed stratified sampling to construct training (88 cases) and testing (22 cases) cohorts while preserving anatomical diversity and scanner manufacturer balance. The training set comprised 79 scans from [6,7] and 9 cases from [15], while the test set included 19 scans from [6,7] and 3 from [15]. This partitioning strategy ensured representative coverage of both conventional and challenging dental arch morphologies across different imaging protocols.

3.3 Feature Point Detection Performance

Since the detected feature points reside within the CBCT volumetric space and are represented as small cubic regions, feature point detection accuracy was quantified through the Dice Similarity Coefficient (DSC) [25], defined as $DSC = \frac{2|P \cap G|}{|P|+|G|}$, where P and G denote predicted and ground truth feature point regions. The range of DSC is [0,1], with a larger value indicating better prediction accuracy. As shown in Fig. 2(a), our feature point network achieves mean DSC scores of $85.39 \pm 3.81\%$ (maxillary feature points, Class 1) and $83.9 \pm 0.036\%$ (mandibular feature points, Class 2), demonstrating its localization accuracy. Notably, case 5 (DSC$=$ 74.43% for Class 1) and case 9 (DSC$=$ 72.39% for Class 2) presented unique challenges: case 5 exhibited metal artifacts in the maxillary region with partial dentition loss, while case 9 contained two impacted mandibular wisdom teeth with associated positional anomalies.

Visual analysis of these challenging cases as shown in Figs. 2(b)-(c) revealed three main characteristics: True positive regions (blue regions) consistently captured essential dental arch trajectory features despite anatomical complexities; false negative regions (red regions) predominantly occurred in interproximal regions where feature point ambiguity naturally exists; and false positive regions (green regions) localized to regions excluded from natural dental arch trajectory, specifically metal artifacts in case 5 and impacted mandibular wisdom teeth in case 9. This strategic error distribution patterns in Figs. 2(b)-(c) indicate the feature point network learned to prioritize anatomically meaningful feature points.

3.4 Dental Arch Curve Fitting Analysis

The convergence characteristics of our modified EM algorithm are demonstrated through progressive curve fitting outcomes across multiple iterations as shown in Fig. 2(d). Employing 1,000 gradient descent steps with a conservative learning rate $\eta = 1 \times 10^{-6}$ per EM iteration, the method achieves acceptable accuracy within just one iteration cycle. While increased iterations (10–50) further refine the fit, diminishing returns become evident, as evidenced by near-identical 10- and 50-iteration fitting function curves in Fig. 2(d). This rapid convergence stems from the algorithm's hybrid optimization strategy that synergizes partial derivative parameter solutions with gradient descent-based latent variable updates. Computational efficiency analysis reveals linear time scaling relative to iteration count, with single-iteration processing requiring 0.394 ± 0.047 seconds for maxilla and 0.367 ± 0.052 seconds for mandible seconds and 10 iterations requiring 3.664 ± 0.414 seconds for maxilla and 3.643 ± 0.549 seconds for mandible. The network's ability to maintain feature points' anatomical plausibility, even in suboptimal detection scenarios, confirms its robustness for the subsequent dental arch curve fitting procedure.

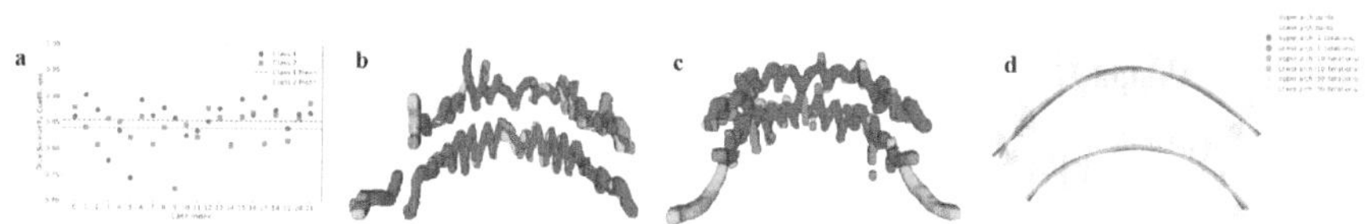

Fig. 2. Evaluations of dental arch curve detection. a. Accuracy of feature point detection. b. Feature point detection results of Case 5. c. Feature point detection results of case 9. d. A case for dental arch curve fitting with 1, 10, and 50 EM iteration cycles.

3.5 Feasibility Analysis of Dental Arch Curve Fitting Function

When defining the fitting function in Eq. (1), we assume that this fitting function can fit a 3D dental arch curve that primarily lies around a plane. This hypothesis of dental arch morphology was validated through geometric analysis of 220 fitted curves (110 in maxilla, 110 in mandible) from their corresponding ground truth feature points. For each fitted curve, we computed the optimal approximation plane by minimizing the orthogonal distance. All orthogonal distances are larger than 0, with mean orthogonal deviation of 0.053 ± 0.056 mm. This confirms the feasibility of our parametric curve fitting function in capturing the near-planar 3D dental arch curve.

3.6 Curvilinear Volume Parameterization for Tooth Segmentation

We propose curvilinear volume parameterization to establish 3D dental arch detection as a plug-and-play tool for tooth segmentation. To validate this tool's efficacy, we compared four popular segmentation architectures: nnU-Net 2D [12], nnU-Net 3D [13], SegResNet [21], and MedNext [23]. For each architecture, training and testing were performed separately on both: (1) the original 3D CBCT volumes, and (2) their transformed cuboid volumes generated through curvilinear volume parameterization. Comparative analysis extends to recent tooth segmentation methods [6,14,18,20,24,26] with their reported performance metrics and 3D CBCT images used. Quantitative results are presented in Table 1. Let TP, TN, FP, FN represent true positives, true negatives, false positives, and false negatives, three metrics [25] quantify segmentation accuracy including $Dice = \frac{2TP}{2TP+FP+FN}$, $Precision = \frac{TP}{TP+FP}$, and $Recall = \frac{TP}{TP+FN}$. Experimental results show that the dental arch curve successfully guides tooth segmentation, achieving segmentation metrics equivalent to state-of-the-art methods.

Table 1. Comparison with existing methodologies in individual tooth segmentation

Methodology	Dental arch guide	3D CBCT images used	Metrics (%)		
			Precision	Dice	Recall
nnUNet 2D [12]	No	110	74.05	72.15	71.34
	Yes		93.83	93.57	93.30
nnUNet 3D [13]	No	110	74.07	72.37	72.77
	Yes		93.72	93.91	94.09
SegResNet [21]	No	110	74.47	73.34	74.25
	Yes		93.66	93.88	94.10
MedNext [23]	No	110	74.10	72.66	73.34
	Yes		94.33	94.33	94.32
Cui et al. [6]	-	20	-	91.98	-
Jang et al. [14]	-	97	95.97	94.79	93.71
Li et al. [18]	-	350	92.13	91.13	91.23
Tan et al. [26]	-	314	-	95.78	-
Shaheen et al. [24]	-	186	-	90	-
Liu et al. [20]	-	451	-	94.3	-

4 Conclusion

This study first proposes 3D dental arch curve detection from volumetric CBCT image and demonstrates that precise 3D dental arch curve detection serves as a plug-and-play tool for automated tooth segmentation. Experimental results show our 3D dental arch curve detection is accurate and robust. The dental arch curve guided tooth segmentation benchmarking methodologies are much more accurate than the corresponding benchmarking methodologies without dental arch curve guide.

Acknowledgments. This work was supported in part by the Guangdong Higher Education Key Platform and Research Project under Grant 2020ZDZX3039, in part by the Guangdong Provincial Key Laboratory of Interdisciplinary Research and Application for Data Science under Grant 2022B1212010006.

References

1. Alom, M.Z., Yakopcic, C., Hasan, M., Taha, T.M., Asari, V.K.: Recurrent residual u-net for medical image segmentation. J. Med. Imaging **6**(1), 014006–014006 (2019)
2. Alpaydin, E.: Machine learning. MIT press (2021)
3. Andrychowicz, M., et al.: Learning to learn by gradient descent by gradient descent. In: Advances in Neural Information Processing Systems, vol. 29 (2016)
4. Balta, C., Öztürk, S., Kuncan, M., Kandilli, I.: Dynamic centripetal parameterization method for b-spline curve interpolation. IEEE Access **8**, 589–598 (2019)
5. Braun, S., Hnat, W.P., Fender, D.E., Legan, H.L.: The form of the human dental arch. Angle Orthod. **68**(1), 29–36 (1998)
6. Cui, W., et al.: Ctooth: a fully annotated 3d dataset and benchmark for tooth volume segmentation on cone beam computed tomography images. In: International Conference on Intelligent Robotics and Applications, pp. 191–200. Springer (2022)
7. Cui, Z., et al.: A fully automatic AI system for tooth and alveolar bone segmentation from cone-beam CT images. Nat. Commun. **13**(1), 2096 (2022)
8. Do, C.B., Batzoglou, S.: What is the expectation maximization algorithm? Nat. Biotechnol. **26**(8), 897–899 (2008)
9. Duan, Y., et al.: Optimizing semi-supervised medical image segmentation with imbalanced filtering and nnu-net enhancement. Visual Comput. 1–13 (2025)
10. Federation, F.W.D.: The 2018 FDI policy statements. Int. Dent. J. **69**(1), 3 (2020)
11. Hagan, P.S., West, G.: Interpolation methods for curve construction. Appl. Math. Finance **13**(2), 89–129 (2006)
12. Isensee, F., Jaeger, P.F., Kohl, S.A., Petersen, J., Maier-Hein, K.H.: nnu-net: a self-configuring method for deep learning-based biomedical image segmentation. Nat. Methods **18**(2), 203–211 (2021)
13. Isensee, F., et al.: nnu-net revisited: a call for rigorous validation in 3D medical image segmentation. In: International Conference on Medical Image Computing and Computer-Assisted Intervention, pp. 488–498. Springer (2024)
14. Jang, T.J., Kim, K.C., Cho, H.C., Seo, J.K.: A fully automated method for 3D individual tooth identification and segmentation in dental CBCT. IEEE Trans. Pattern Anal. Mach. Intell. **44**(10), 6562–6568 (2021)
15. Jiang, B., Zhang, S., Shi, M., Liu, H.L., Shi, H.: Alternate level set evolutions with controlled switch for tooth segmentation. IEEE Access **10**, 76563–76572 (2022)
16. Kwon, T., Choi, D.i., Hwang, J., Lee, T., Lee, I., Cho, S.: Panoramic dental tomosynthesis imaging by use of CBCT projection data. Sci. Reports **13**(1), 8817 (2023)

17. Lee, S.J., Lee, S., Lim, J., Park, H.J., Wheeler, T.T.: Method to classify dental arch forms. Am. J. Orthod. Dentofac. Orthop. **140**(1), 87–96 (2011)
18. Li, P., Liu, Y., Cui, Z., Yang, F., Zhao, Y., Lian, C., Gao, C.: Semantic graph attention with explicit anatomical association modeling for tooth segmentation from CBCT images. IEEE Trans. Med. Imaging **41**(11), 3116–3127 (2022)
19. Lin, G., et al.: Transfarchnet: predicting dental arch curves based on facial point clouds in personalized panoramic x-ray imaging. Expert Syst. Appl. 126577 (2025)
20. Liu, Y., et al.: Fully automatic ai segmentation of oral surgery-related tissues based on cone beam computed tomography images. Int. J. Oral Sci. **16**(1), 34 (2024)
21. Myronenko, A.: 3D MRI brain tumor segmentation using autoencoder regularization. In: International MICCAI Brainlesion Workshop, pp. 311–320. Springer (2018)
22. Qiu, L., Ye, C., Chen, P., Liu, Y., Han, X., Cui, S.: Darch: Dental arch prior-assisted 3D tooth instance segmentation with weak annotations. In: Proceedings of the IEEE/CVF Conference on Computer Vision and Pattern Recognition, pp. 20752–20761 (2022)
23. Roy, S., et al.: Mednext: transformer-driven scaling of convnets for medical image segmentation. In: International Conference on Medical Image Computing and Computer-Assisted Intervention, pp. 405–415. Springer (2023)
24. Shaheen, E., et al.: A novel deep learning system for multi-class tooth segmentation and classification on cone beam computed tomography. a validation study. J. Dentistry **115**, 103865 (2021)
25. Taha, A.A., Hanbury, A.: Metrics for evaluating 3d medical image segmentation: analysis, selection, and tool. BMC Med. Imaging **15**, 1–28 (2015)
26. Tan, M., Cui, Z., Zhong, T., Fang, Y., Zhang, Y., Shen, D.: A progressive framework for tooth and substructure segmentation from cone-beam ct images. Comput. Biol. Med. **169**, 107839 (2024)
27. Theodoridis, S., Koutroumbas, C.: Pattern recognition: Elsevier inc (2009)
28. Treichel, T., Gessat, M., Prietzel, T., Burgert, O.: Dicom for implantations–overview and application. J. Digit. Imaging **25**, 352–358 (2012)
29. Yun, Z., Yang, S., Huang, E., Zhao, L., Yang, W., Feng, Q.: Automatic reconstruction method for high-contrast panoramic image from dental cone-beam CT data. Comput. Methods Programs Biomed. **175**, 205–214 (2019)
30. Zhong, X., Zhang, Z.: 3d dental biometrics: automatic pose-invariant dental arch extraction and matching. In: 2020 25th International Conference on Pattern Recognition (ICPR), pp. 6524–6530. IEEE (2021)

Robust Dental Arch Curve Optimization Using a Standard Arch Form for Panoramic Reconstruction

Songze Zhang[1,2], Benxiang Jiang[1,2], Jingyi Lyu[1,2], and Hongjian Shi[1,2](✉)

[1] Guangdong Provincial Key Laboratory of Interdisciplinary Research and Application for Data Science, Beijing Normal–Hong Kong Baptist University, Zhuhai 519087, China
shihj@bnbu.edu.cn
[2] Hong Kong Baptist University, Hong Kong 999077, China

Abstract. This study presents a robust dental arch curve optimization method for panoramic image reconstruction from CBCT images. The proposed approach integrates prior maxillofacial anatomical knowledge through a statistical standard arch form and introduces an assessment function to guide the fitting of anatomically accurate and convex dental arch curves. Experimental validation in clinically diverse CBCT datasets demonstrates the effectiveness of the method in challenging scenarios, including orthodontic appliances, rigid internal fixation, mixed dentition, complete edentulism, and impacted teeth. The results confirm that the proposed method enables high-quality panoramic image reconstruction suitable for various dental imaging applications.

Keywords: Dental arch · Panoramic imaging · Polynomial curve fitting · CBCT

1 Introduction

Cone-beam computed tomography (CBCT) provides high-resolution imaging of intraoral and maxillofacial structures and has become increasingly prevalent in dental clinical practice [1]. In contrast, panoramic radiography has been widely used for decades, offering a convenient overview of the entire maxillofacial region in a single image [2]. These two modalities are often used in combination for diagnosis and treatment planning. Reconstructing panoramic images from CBCT volumes enables extraction of both 3D and 2D information from a single scan, thereby reducing patient radiation exposure [3].

Since panoramic reconstruction involves projecting the 3D CBCT volume onto a plane defined by the dental arch curve, the accuracy of dental arch curve detection is critical to the quality of the reconstructed panoramic image. A common strategy involves generating an axial maximum intensity projection (MIP)

F. Bolelli et al. (Eds.): ODIN 2025, LNCS 16473, pp. 13–22, 2026.
https://doi.org/10.1007/978-3-032-20711-1_2

of the tooth crown slices, segmenting the teeth and jawbone, refining the segmentation mask, and fitting the dental arch curve using splines or polynomial interpolation over sampled points [4–6]. While these methods are straightforward and computationally efficient, they typically ignore the geometric convexity of the dental arch and fail to incorporate prior anatomical knowledge of maxillofacial structures. Moreover, existing approaches are rarely validated on clinically complex cases such as orthodontic appliances, rigid internal fixation, mixed dentition, complete edentulism, or impacted teeth.

In this study, we propose a dental arch curve optimization method based on a statistical standard arch form [7], which integrates prior knowledge of typical maxillofacial anatomy. An assessment function is introduced to guide the optimization process, ensuring that the resulting curve is both anatomically accurate and geometrically convex. The proposed method enables robust and high-quality panoramic image reconstruction across a wide range of clinically challenging CBCT datasets.

2 Method

2.1 Overview

This section describes our dental arch optimization method based on a standard form for robust panoramic image reconstruction from CBCT images. The process begins by identifying the axial range that includes the tooth crowns. Based on this range, MIP images of the crowns and mandible are generated. A standard dental arch curve is then fitted to the jawbone structures visible in these MIP images. Subsequently, the curve is further optimized using the standard form as a prior, and the resulting dental arch is employed for panoramic image reconstruction. This method detects accurate dental arch curves across diverse CBCT datasets.

2.2 Axial MIP Image Generation

Generating the axial MIP image from a carefully selected stack of axial slices significantly improves the accuracy of dental arch curve detection. The selected range should primarily include the tooth crowns. If the MIP image is generated from all axial slices, it introduces redundant bone structures surrounding the dental arch, which impairs curve detection, as illustrated in Fig. 1(a). Inspired by the axial MIP generation method in [4], we propose an axial MIP image generation method for dental arch curve optimization.

Oral CBCT images mainly consist of three tissue types: air, soft tissue, and bone. We apply K-means clustering with $k = 3$ on the coronal MIP image (Fig. 2(a) and (d)) to segment these regions. Since tooth crowns exhibit higher intensity than other bony structures, we select the intensity value at the bone cluster center as the threshold for crown segmentation. This yields the tooth crown masks shown in Fig. 2(b) and (e). To identify the axial range containing crowns, we count the number of crown pixels in each row to construct a histogram

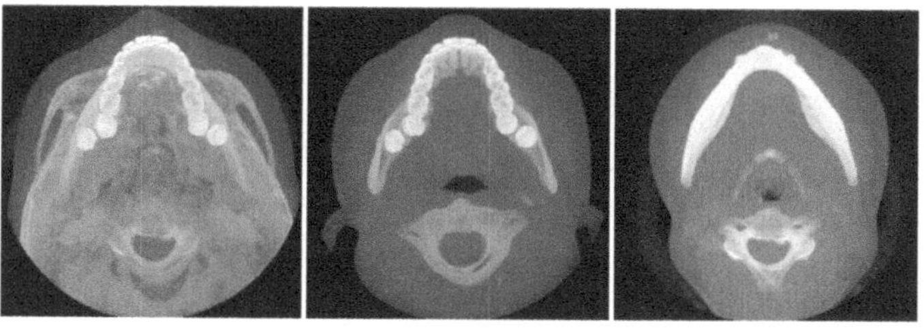

Fig. 1. From left to right: (a) the axial MIP image of all slices; (b) the axial MIP image of tooth crowns; (c) the axial MIP image of mandible below the tooth crowns.

(blue bars in Fig. 2(c) and (f)). A Gaussian Mixture Model (GMM) is then used to fit the histogram. To determine the optimal number of GMM components, we test models with 1 to $K_{max} = 5$ components and evaluate each using the Bayesian Information Criterion (BIC):

$$\text{BIC} = p \ln N - 2 \ln L, \tag{1}$$

where p is the number of model parameters, N is the number of data points, and L is the model likelihood. Although, the BIC penalizes complexity via the $p \ln N$ term, we observed that the models with $K_{\max}$ components often yield the lowest BIC, suggesting under-penalization. Therefore, we introduce a modified BIC, BIC_{mod}, to more strongly penalize complex models:

$$\text{BIC}_{mod} = \alpha p \ln N - 2 \ln L, \tag{2}$$

where $\alpha > 1$ could increase the penalty for additional parameters, helping to avoid overfitting and $\alpha = 20$ in the experiments. The GMM with the lowest BIC_{mod} is selected as the fitted histogram model, as the red curves depicted in Fig. 2(c) and (f).

Let μ_h, α_h and p_h denote the mean, standard deviation, and peak value of the dominant component. If no other component within $[\mu_h - 3\sigma_h, \mu_h + 3\sigma_h]$ exceeds $0.8\,p_h$, then this range defines the axial slices range of tooth crown: $[R_s, R_e] = [\mu_h - 3\sigma_h, \mu_h + 3\sigma_h]$, shown by green lines in Fig. 2(b). Otherwise, if two prominent components are detected, as in Fig. 2(f), we denote their statistics as (μ_{up}, σ_{up}) and $(\mu_{low}, \sigma_{low})$. The tooth crown-containing slice range is defined as: $[R_s, R_e] = [\mu_{up} - 3\sigma_{up}, \mu_{low} + 3\sigma_{low}]$ as the green lines in Fig. 2(e). Based on the determined slice range, two axial MIP images are generated: one from $[R_s, R_e]$, representing the tooth crowns, and the other from $[R_e + 1, end]$, representing the mandible below the crowns, as shown in Fig. 1(b) and (c), respectively. Here, *end* denotes the index of the bottom axial slice. These two MIP images are used for standard dental arch curve fitting as follows.

2.3 Standard Dental Arch Curve Fitting

The dental arch represents the anatomical layout of the dentition and jaw. Based on population statistics, Welander et al. [7] configured a standard dental arch

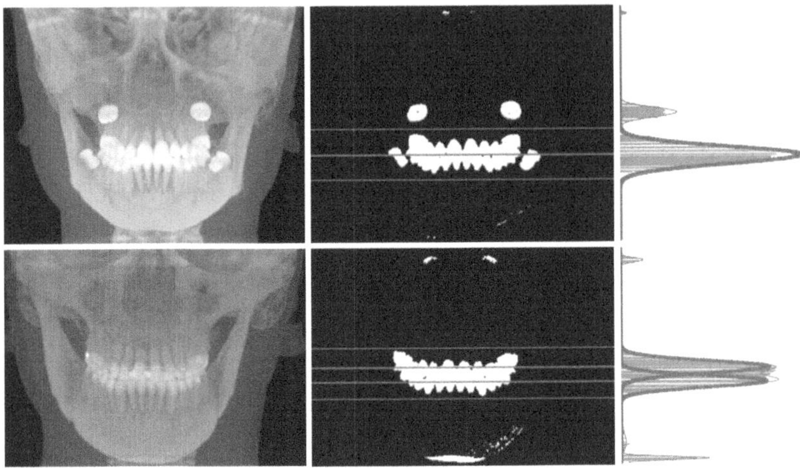

Fig. 2. From top to the bottom, left to right: (a) the coronal MIP image; (b) corresponding crown mask, red line shows the center of the dominant GMM component in (c), green lines indicate axial slice range containing crowns; (c) histogram of crown pixels (blue bars), red curve is GMM fit, green curve is the dominant component; (d)-(f) are analogous results for another dataset with two prominent GMM components. (Color figure online)

form composing a dentition curve y_D and a mandible curve y_M, defined as:

$$y_D = d_2x^2 + d_4x^4, \tag{3}$$

$$y_M = m_0 + m_2x^2 + m_4x^4 + m_6x^6, \tag{4}$$

with coefficients $d_2 = -0.014097$ and $d_4 = -7.3814 \times 10^{-5}$, $m_0 = -5.4341$, $m_2 = -0.040436$, $m_4 = 1.0507 \times 10^{-5}$, $m_6 = -2.7483 \times 10^{-9}$, units are millimeter (mm).

These curves characterize the standard morphology of the dentition and mandible and must be spatially aligned to individual CBCT datasets. Alignment is performed using two axial MIP images: one representing the tooth crowns (Fig. 1(b)) and the other representing the mandible region below the crowns (Fig. 1(c)). Jawbone structures are segmented from these images as follows:

1. The axial MIP images are first denoised using a Gaussian filter.
2. K-means clustering with $k = 3$ is applied to classify pixels into bone, soft tissue, and air; the bone cluster is retained.
3. The largest connected component is extracted and smoothed via morphological operations to generate jawbone masks (Fig. 3(a) and (b)).

To locate the highest points on the jawbone, we analyze the central 10 mm column of each axial MIP image. The upmost jaw bones points from top to bottom and from bottom to top in the central 10 mm are identified. These may

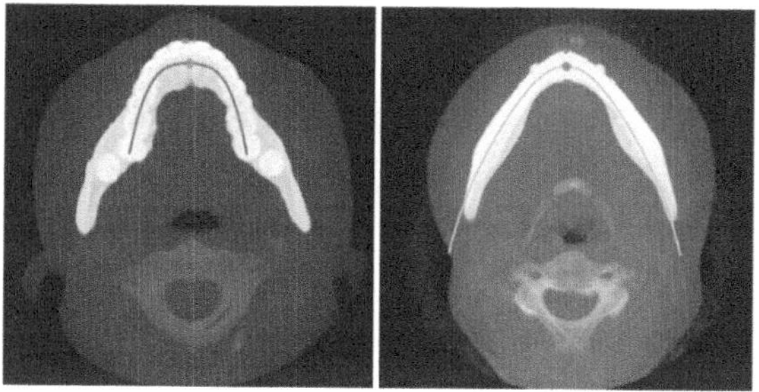

Fig. 3. Superimposing images (white masks represent the segmented jawbones) from left to right: (a) jawbone mask from Fig. 1(b); (b) jawbone mask from Fig. 1(c).

include multiple local maxima on each side, shown as green points in Fig. 3(a) and (b). The mean coordinates of upmost points in top and bottom sides are computed, and the average of these means defines the vertex of each standard curve (shown as red points). Using these vertex points, the standard dentition and mandible curves are spatially shifted and overlaid as the purple and orange curves in Fig. 3.

The shifted curves serve as the initial representations of the individual's dentition and mandible geometry. To obtain a unified initial standard dental arch curve, these two curves are fused using a smooth blending function. A window function $W(x)$ is defined as:

$$W(x) = [\frac{x-a}{b-a}]^4, x \in [a,b], a < b. \tag{5}$$

Let $P_L = (x_{PL}, y_{PL})$ and $P_R = (x_{PR}, y_{PR})$ denote the leftmost and rightmost intersections between the dentition and mandible curves. Let $V_M = (x_{VM}, y_{VM})$ be the vertex of the mandible curve, and $R_D = 42\,mm$ be the half horizontal span of the dentition curve. The piecewise initial standard dental arch curve $C_S(x)$ is then defined as:

$$C_S(x) = \begin{cases} C_M(x), & x < x_{VM} - R_D \\ W(x)C_D(x) + [1 - W(x)]C_M(x), & x_{VM} - R_D \leq x \leq x_{PL} \\ C_D(x), & x_{PL} < x < x_{PR} \\ W(-x)C_D(x) + [1 - W(-x)]C_M(x), & x_{PR} \leq x \leq x_{VM} + R_D \\ C_M(x), & x > x_{VM} + R_D \end{cases} \tag{6}$$

where $C_D(x)$ and $C_M(x)$ are the shifted dentition and mandible curves, as the purple and orange curve shown in Fig. 4(a). The initialized standard dental arch curve is optimized to fit the individual dataset in following step.

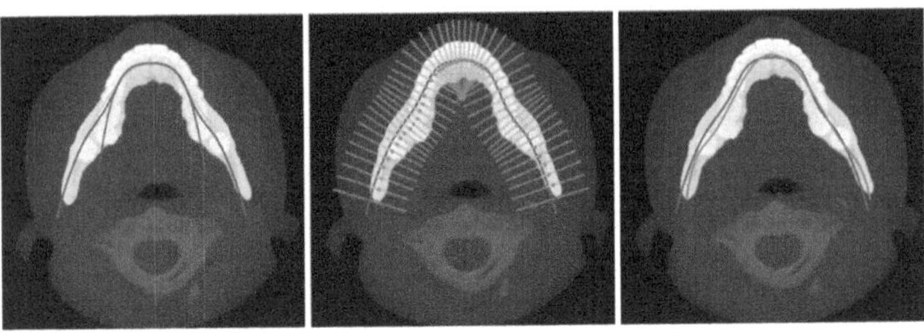

Fig. 4. Jawbone masked axial MIP image of tooth crowns from left to right: (a) the blue curve is the initial standard dental arch; purple and orange curves are the shifted dentition and mandible curves; (b) green lines represent perpendiculars to the blue curve, their intersections with jawbone masks (orange segments) define central points (red); (c) red curve shows the optimized dental arch. (Color figure online)

2.4 Dental Arch Curve Optimization

The initial standard dental arch curve serves as a prior template and must be adapted to the individual's jawbone morphology. To achieve this, we extract central points of the jawbone from the axial MIP image of the tooth crown slices. Perpendicular lines are drawn at each point along the initial standard dental arch curve (green lines in Fig. 4(b)). Each perpendicular intersects the segmented jawbone mask, producing intersection segments (orange lines in Fig. 4(b)). The center of each segment is computed by averaging the coordinates of its endpoints, forming a set of central points (red dots in Fig. 4(b)). While Fig. 4(b) shows sampled lines for visualization, in practice, perpendiculars are generated at every point along the initial curve to obtain a dense set of central points.

These points are then used to fit a new dental arch curve using polynomial regression. However, the optimal polynomial degree varies across datasets and must balance accuracy, simplicity, and geometric stability. To address this, we adopt the following criteria:

1. Minimize the average distance between the fitted curve and the central points.
2. Use the lowest polynomial degree that satisfies criterion 1 to reduce overfitting.
3. Ensure the fitted curve is as convex as possible for anatomical plausibility.

To integrate these criteria, we define an assessment function that combines mean squared error (MSE), polynomial degree penalty, and convexity regularization:

$$\mathcal{L}(f_D) = \sum_{i=1}^{n} (y_i - f_D(x_i))^2 + \beta D + \gamma (1 - r_{\text{convex}}), \tag{7}$$

where (x_i, y_i) are the coordinates of the i-th central points, n is the number of the central points, $f_D(x) = \sum_{j=0}^{D} a_j x^j$ is the D-degree polynomial model, r_{convex} is the proportion of the curve domain over which the second derivative $f''_D(x) > 0$, and $\beta = 1.5$, $\gamma = 100$ are empirically chosen weighting factors. Polynomial models with degrees ranging from 2 to 20 are fitted to the central points, and the one yielding the lowest value of $\mathcal{L}(f_D)$ is selected as the optimized dental arch curve, shown as the red curve in Fig. 4(c).

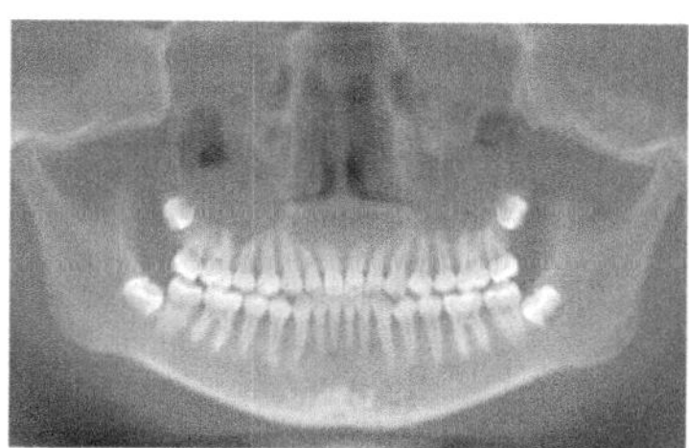
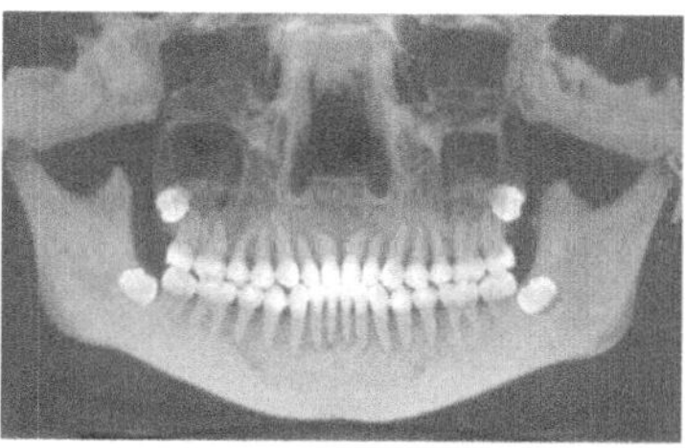

Fig. 5. From left to right: (a) ray-sum panoramic image; (b) MIP panoramic image.

Finally, panoramic images are reconstructed using the optimized dental arch curve with equal-arc-length sampling and a fixed arch thickness of 2 cm. Both ray-sum and MIP rendering techniques are applied to produce the final panoramic projections, as illustrated in Fig. 5.

3 Results

3.1 Datasets

This study utilized a partially open-access CBCT dataset released by Cui et al. [8–10], which comprises 150 CBCT volumes. Among these, 95 CBCT volumes include a complete dentomaxillofacial field of view (FOV). The remaining volumes contain either partial dentition and were therefore excluded from evaluation.

Given that panoramic images depict the full dentomaxillofacial structure, we used the 95 CBCT volumes to evaluate the proposed dental arch curve optimization method. These volumes include a wide range of clinically challenging cases commonly encountered in dentistry. Notably, some cases present multiple co-occurring conditions, including: orthodontic appliances (7 cases), mixed dentition (1 case), rigid internal fixation (9 cases), root canal (40 cases), crown restoration (49 cases), implants (36 cases), partial edentulism (74 cases), complete edentulism (2 cases) and impacted teeth (13 cases).

3.2 Experiment Results

In this study, panoramic images were reconstructed for all 95 CBCT volumes to validate the robustness of our proposed dental arch curve optimization method. The polynomial degree used for curve fitting was selected based on the assessment function defined in Eq. 7. Table 1 summarizes the distribution of the selected polynomial degrees.

Approximately 90% of the fitted dental arch curves were modeled using either 6th- or 8th-degree polynomials. This aligns with the design of the initial standard dental arch curve, which is formed by blending a 4th-degree dentition curve and a 6th-degree mandible curve, making a 6th- or 8th-degree polynomial generally sufficient for most cases. Additionally, most selected degrees were even, which may be attributed to their geometric suitability for producing convex-shaped curves.

Table 1. Statistical analysis of polynomial fitting degrees

Degree	6	8	9	12	14	Total
Number	26	58	2	6	3	95
Rate	27.37%	61.05%	2.10%	6.32%	3.16%	100%

The proposed method demonstrated well performance across various complex clinical scenarios. It effectively identified individualized dental arch curves and enabled high-quality panoramic image reconstruction. While Fig. 5 displays a case involving impacted teeth, Fig. 6 showcases four additional representative examples. In each case, the first column shows jawbone-masked axial MIP images of the crown slice, where the blue and red curves denote the initial standard and optimized dental arch curves, respectively. The second column presents the corresponding ray-sum panoramic images. These four cases cover a broad range of clinical challenges:

1. Orthodontic appliances and rigid internal fixation (1st row);
2. Mixed dentition with impacted teeth (2nd row);
3. Rigid internal fixation, dental implants, and partial edentulism (3rd row);
4. Complete edentulism with root canal treatment and crown restorations (4th row).

Despite the anatomical complexity in these examples, the reconstructed panoramic images retain high anatomical fidelity. These results suggest that the proposed method generalizes well to diverse and challenging clinical conditions, demonstrating notable robustness and adaptability.

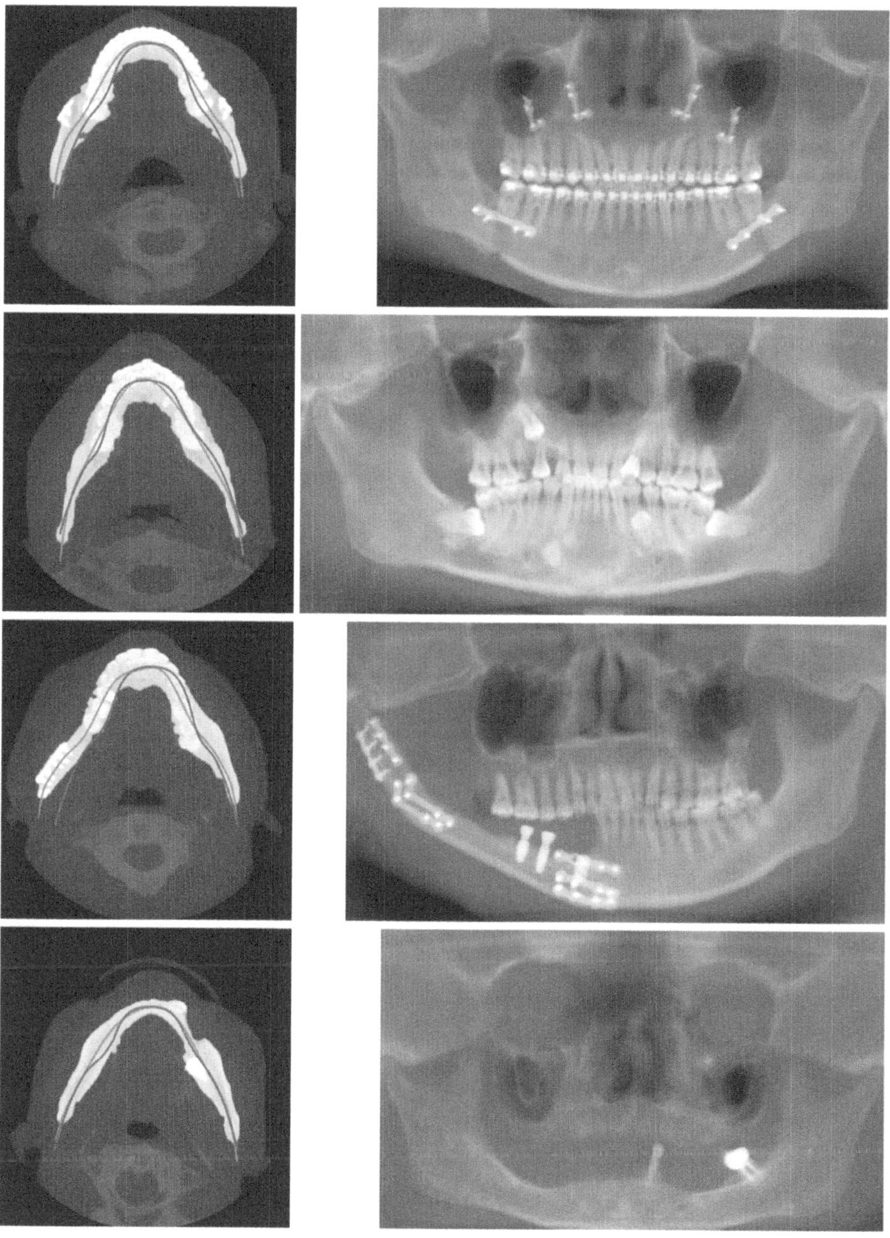

Fig. 6. The optimized dental arch curves (the first column) and the corresponding ray-sum panoramic images of four complex cases (the second column). *Note that the panoramic images have varying widths because the lengths of the detected dental arch curves differ.*

4 Conclusions

This paper presents a dental arch curve optimization method that incorporates prior maxillofacial anatomical knowledge through a standard arch form. An assessment function is designed to guide the fitting process, ensuring anatomically accurate and convex dental arch curves. The proposed method exhibits strong robustness and accuracy across a wide range of clinically challenging CBCT cases and enables high-quality panoramic image reconstruction. These results highlight the method's potential for reliable application in dental imaging and treatment planning.

Acknowledgments. This work was supported in part by the Guangdong Higher Education Key Platform and Research Project under Grant 2020ZDZX3039, in part by the Guangdong Provincial Key Laboratory of Interdisciplinary Research and Application for Data Science under Grant 2022B1212010006.

References

1. Scarfe, W.C., Farman, A.G.: What is cone-beam CT and how does it work? Dent. Clin. North Am. **52**, 707–730 (2008)
2. Ameli, N., Miri Moghaddam, M., Lai, H., Pacheco-Pereira, C.: Automated quality evaluation of dental panoramic radiographs using deep learning. Imaging Science in Dentistry **55**, (2025)
3. Zhang, S., Jiang, B., Shi, H.: Dental Arch Curve Optimization from Standard Dental Arch Curves. In: 2nd International Conference on Pattern Recognition, Machine Vision and Intelligent Algorithms (PRMVIA), pp. 98–102 (2024)
4. Yun, Z., Yang, S., Huang, E., Zhao, L., Yang, W., Feng, Q.: Automatic reconstruction method for high-contrast panoramic image from dental cone-beam CT data. Comput. Methods Programs Biomed. **175**, 205–214 (2019)
5. Oliveira, L., et al.: Dental arch definition in computed tomographs using two semi-automatic methods. Med. Biol. Eng. Comput. **60**, 3499–3508 (2022)
6. Zhang, J., Jiang, Y., Gao, F., Zhao, S., Yang, F., Song, L.: A fast automatic reconstruction method for panoramic images based on cone beam computed tomography. Electronics **11**(15), 2404 (2022)
7. Welander, U., Nummikoski, P., Tronje, G., McDavid, W.D., Legrell, P.E., Langlais, R.P.: Standard forms of dentition and mandible for applications in rotational panoramic radiography. Dentomaxillofacial Radiol. **18**, 60–67 (1989)
8. Cui, Z., et al.: A fully automatic AI system for tooth and alveolar bone segmentation from cone-beam CT images. Nat. Commun. **13**, 2096 (2022)
9. Cui, Z., Li, C., Wang, W.: ToothNet: automatic tooth instance segmentation and identification from cone beam CT images. In: IEEE/CVF Conference on Computer Vision and Pattern Recognition (CVPR), pp. 6361–6370 (2019)
10. Cui, Z., et al.: Hierarchical morphology-guided tooth instance segmentation from CBCT images. In: Information Processing in Medical Imaging (IPMI), pp. 150–162. Springer International Publishing (2021)

Self-configuring 3D Segmentation of Pediatric Dentition

Enzo Tulissi[1,2], Alban Gaydamour[1,2], Juan C. Prieto[3], Claudia Mattos[4], Renata R. Rosa[4], Sara Tinawi[1], Dylan J. Keener[1], Aron Aliaga Del Castillo[1], Eduardo Caleme[6], Brent Larson[7], Antonio C. de Oliveira Ruellas[8], Luis E. Arriola-Guillén[9], Jonas Bianchi[10], Heesoo Oh[10], Marcela Lima Gurgel[11], Erika Benavides[1], Fabiana Soki[1], Yalil A. Rodríguez-Cárdenas[12], Gustavo A. Ruíz-Mora[12], Bruno M. R. Braga[5], Ana B. Teodoro[13], Selene Barone[14], Martin Styner[3], Roberto Bespalez-Neto[15], and Lucia H. Cevidanes[1](✉)

[1] University of Michigan, Ann Arbor, MI, USA
luciacev@umich.edu
[2] CPE Lyon, Villeurbanne, France
[3] University of North Carolina, Chapel Hill, NC, USA
[4] Universidade Federal Fluminense, Rio de Janeiro, Brazil
[5] Hospital for Rehabilitation of Craniofacial Anomalies, University of São Paulo, São Paulo, Brazil
[6] Universidade Positivo, Curitiba, Paraná, Brazil
[7] University of Minnesota, Minneapolis, MN, USA
[8] Federal University of Rio de Janeiro, Rio de Janeiro, Brazil
[9] Universidad Científica del Sur, Lima, Peru
[10] University of the Pacific, San Francisco, CA, USA
[11] Federal University of Ceara, Fortaleza, Brazil
[12] Universidad Nacional de Colombia, Bogotá, Colombia
[13] Federal University of Goiás, Goiânia, Brazil
[14] Magna Graecia University, Catanzaro, Italy
[15] University Anhanguera/Uniderp, Campo Grande, MS, Brazil

Abstract. Robust 3D segmentation of primary and permanent teeth in cone-beam CT (CBCT) is critical for pediatric and orthodontic care. We propose a fully automatic deep-learning pipeline built on the self-configuring nnU-Net v2 framework, tailored for high-fidelity dental shape modeling. Our approach learns fine-scale tooth geometries directly from volumetric data, eliminating manual tuning. On a pediatric CBCT cohort (369 training, 93 validation, 55 test scans), our model attains a mean Dice score of 0.87 across 55 dental and supporting anatomical structures. Key components include adaptive preprocessing (isotropic resampling, automatic craniofacial cropping, intensity normalization), on-the-fly 3D augmentations, and lightweight postprocessing to remove spurious segment. The resulting segmentations are consistent and clinically actionable, supporting advanced 3D morphometric analysis and digital treatment planning. By extending state-of-the-art volumetric segmentation to mixed dentition CBCT data, our work facilitates

F. Bolelli et al. (Eds.): ODIN 2025, LNCS 16473, pp. 23–32, 2026.
https://doi.org/10.1007/978-3-032-20711-1_3

integration of AI-driven geometric learning into routine pediatric dentistry workflows.

Keywords: 3D segmentation · pediatric dentistry · Cone-beam CT (CBCT) · deep learning · nnU-Net · dental morphometry

1 Introduction

Understanding and analyzing the 3D shape of anatomical structures is a cornerstone of medical image computing. In dentistry, tooth morphology including crown and root geometries directly impacts diagnosis, treatment planning, and monitoring. Recent advances in artificial intelligence, particularly convolutional neural networks (CNNs) have significantly improved the segmentation of anatomical structures in medical images. They now learn shape representations from voxel data, overcoming the limitations of thresholding or region growing caused by partial volume effects and anatomical variability [1,2]. Accurate, automatic segmentation of individual teeth in cone-beam CT (CBCT) is especially critical for pediatric mixed dentition, which involves coexisting primary and erupting permanent teeth, unerupted buds, resorbing roots, and impacted teeth all of which introduce significant shape variability. While previous methods have shown strong results for permanent teeth [1], few have addressed the challenge of comprehensive shape segmentation across all dentition types in pediatric CBCTs. This paper explores a fully automatic segmentation approach using the self-configuring nnU-Net v2 framework [3,4]. Unlike traditional pipelines that require manual network tuning or rule-based preprocessing, nnUNet v2 adapts its architecture and training plan to the geometry of the input data. This makes it particularly well-suited for tasks involving complex, irregular, and densely packed structures such as mixed dentition. Our study represents the first application of nnUNet v2 to the joint segmentation of both primary and permanent teeth, including all 52 dental and 3 skeletal supporting structures, treated

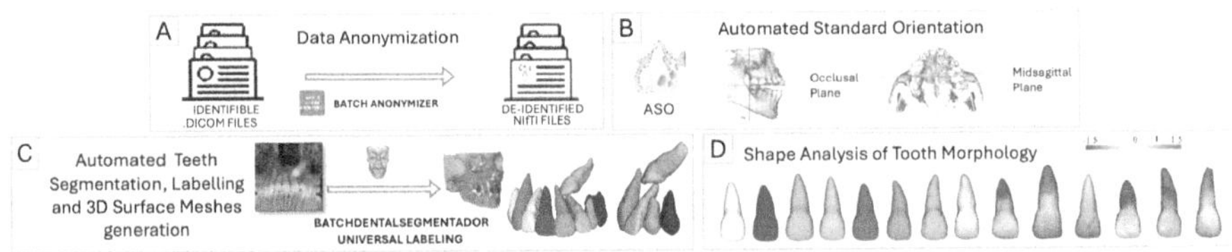

Fig. 1. End-to-end automated dental analysis, deployed as modules of 3D Slicer software [5] (A) *Batch Anonymizer* converts identifiable DICOM image stacks into de-identified NIfTI volumes. **(B)** *Automated Standard Orientation* (ASO) aligns each volume to the occlusal and midsagittal planes, ensuring consistent orientation across patients. **(C)** The *BatchDentalSegmentador* module performs fully automatic tooth segmentation. **(D)** Individual tooth meshes undergo statistical shape analysis to quantify morphological variability.

as independent classes in a high-resolution 3D domain. Our contributions are twofold: (1) to design and evaluate a self-configuring deep learning pipeline tailored to pediatric dental anatomy in CBCT; and (2) to demonstrate how this approach enables high-fidelity geometric modeling of the entire dentition, facilitating downstream applications such as orthodontic planning, eruption tracking, and surgical guidance.

2 Methods

2.1 Segmentation Method: Overview and Novelty w.r.t. nnUNet v2

We build on nnU-Net v2 for 3D dental segmentation, with two focused departures from the vanilla framework. First, we perform mixed-dentition *single-head* labeling across **55 classes**: in a single forward pass the network predicts all primary and permanent teeth (52 dental labels) together with the mandible, maxilla, and mandibular canal. Prior nnU-Net applications typically address permanent teeth only or a substantially smaller label set.

Second, to preserve laterality, we explicitly disable left–right flips in both data augmentation and test-time augmentation. This deviation from nnU-Net's default flip policy mitigates contralateral swaps in mixed dentition and stabilizes side-specific tooth labels across upper and lower arches.

2.2 Dataset and Annotation Strategy

To enable robust shape modeling of the mixed dentition (Fig. 1), we curated a retrospective dataset of 517 pediatric CBCT scans exhibiting both primary and permanent teeth [6]. Each volume encompasses complete maxillary and mandibular arches and captures a broad spectrum of tooth development stages, including unerupted buds, resorbing roots, and impactions, each presenting unique geometric challenges. On average, each scan includes 6–8 primary teeth and over 28 permanent teeth in varying states of eruption. Initial segmentations were generated using the DentalSegmentator module in 3D Slicer [7] and refined manually in ITK-SNAP [8] to assign anatomically precise voxel-wise labels for each discernible tooth. This resulted in a dense multi-class segmentation with 55 total unique anatomical structures, each representing 52 distinct dental shapes, the upper jaw/cranium, lower jaw and the mandibular canal. To make class balance explicit across the 55 classes, Fig. 2 reports, for each label, how many of the 517 scans contain that structure (presence $>$ 0 voxels). Permanent teeth and supporting structures are nearly universal (e.g., upper-right first premolar: 517/517; most premolars/molars $\geq$92%), whereas age-dependent classes vary widely: third molars appear in $\sim$56–62% of scans (UR 61.7%, UL 59.0%, LL 57.1%, LR 56.7%), and primary incisors are scarce (2.7–13.3%), with primary canines/molars ranging 34–51%.

Importantly, our labeling captures detailed morphologies, including curved roots, crown morphology, and interproximal spacing, thereby supporting downstream geometric analysis. Unerupted or malformed structures were included

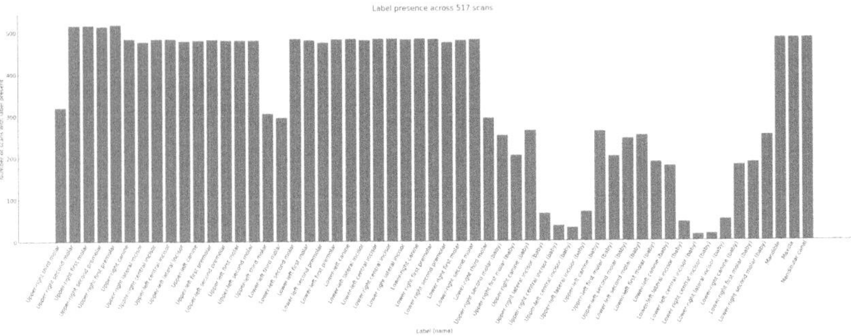

Fig. 2. Per-label prevalence across the cohort (n = 517).

when identifiable, ensuring anatomical completeness. The dataset was split into 369 scans for training, 93 for validation, and 55 for testing. This diverse set provides a strong basis for generalizable 3D learning across a spectrum of pediatric dental geometries.

2.3 Self-configuring Segmentation Pipeline

We implemented the nnU-Net v2 pipeline [3,4], which offers a fully automated segmentation framework that configures all aspects of preprocessing, network architecture, and training strategy based on data-driven heuristics (Fig. 2) [9]. This design is especially suited for medical shape analysis tasks, where anatomical variability and image heterogeneity demand robust adaptation (Fig. 3).

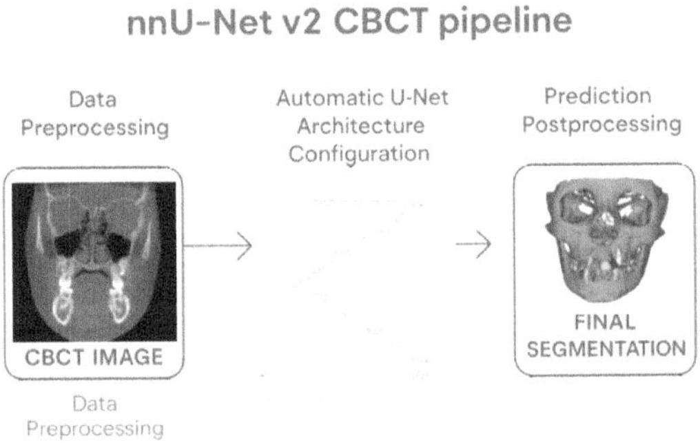

nnU-Net v2 CBCT pipeline

Data Preprocessing

Automatic U-Net Architecture Configuration

Prediction Postprocessing

CBCT IMAGE

FINAL SEGMENTATION

Data Preprocessing

Fig. 3. Illustration of the nnU-Net v2 segmentation pipeline. Left: coronal slice from the original pediatric CBCT volume. Right: voxel-wise prediction showing all 55 teeth individually.

Preprocessing: To prepare the CBCT volumes for geometric learning Fig. 4, nnU-Net performs: (1) Resolution normalization. All scans are resampled to a consistent isotropic spacing, preserving geometric proportions and enabling scale-invariant feature learning. (2) Spatial cropping. The field-of-view is restricted to the craniofacial region via automatic bounding box detection, focusing the learning process on relevant anatomical context. (3) CT-based intensity normalization. Voxel intensities are clipped and z-normalized to homogenize grayscale representations of bone and soft tissue, preserving contrast critical for shape boundaries. (4) On-the-fly 3D augmentation. During training, randomized transformations such as elastic deformations, rotations, and intensity shifts are applied to simulate anatomical variation and imaging noise without distorting the underlying geometry. These steps produce standardized yet anatomically diverse inputs that allow the network to learn generalizable shape features

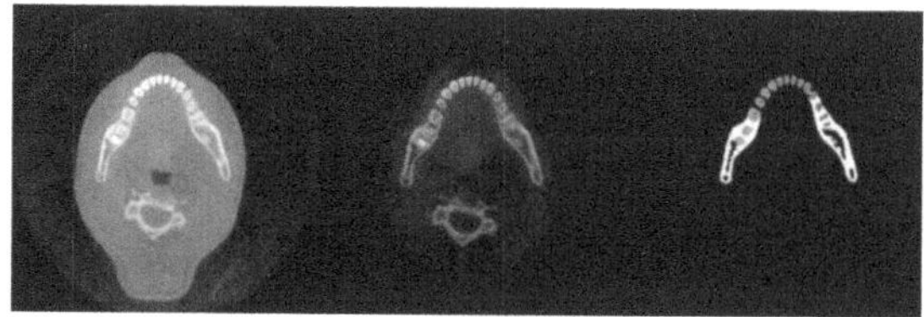

Fig. 4. nnU-Net v2 preprocessing. (Left) Original axial pediatric CBCT. (Center) After automatic cropping and intensity normalization. (Right) Segmentation of 55 anatomical structure (52 dental and 3 skeletal), plus background (label 0), in the preprocessed space.

Architecture Configuration: nnU-Net v2 automatically selected a full-resolution 3D U-Net with six resolution levels (about 30 M parameters), omitting low-resolution cascades since our volumes fit in GPU memory. Training patches measured $112 \times 128 \times 128$ voxels, covering several teeth while respecting memory limits Fig. 5. The encoder applies successive strides to downsample, and a symmetric decoder with skip-connections reconstructs spatial detail. The network concludes with a $1 \times 1 \times 1$ convolution followed by softmax activation and a voxel-wise argmax over 56 classes. This full-resolution setup proved both accurate and efficient, without needing 2D or multi-resolution variants.

Automated Training Schedule: We trained using the default nnU-Net v2 optimization, which automatically configures hyperparameters, learning rate scheduling, and optimizer selection. A combined soft Dice and cross-entropy loss handled the severe class imbalance across 56 labels. Each iteration sampled two random $112 \times 128 \times 128$ patches, with on-the-fly augmentations (rotations, elastic deformations, zooms, noise) to improve generalization. We trained for 150 epochs (3000 iterations per epoch) per fold using 5-fold cross-validation and ensembled the softmax outputs, to produce consistent, anatomically robust segmentations.

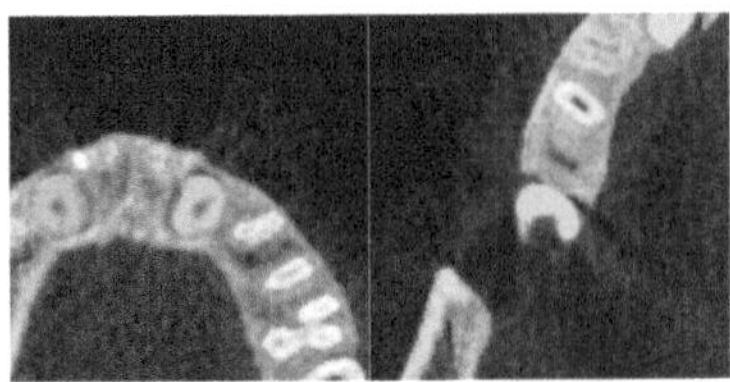

Fig. 5. 112×128^2 voxel training patches: (A) deciduous incisors and permanent buds; (B) deciduous molars with an erupting first permanent molar. Colored overlays show tooth labels on the CBCT. (Color figure online)

Postprocessing: After inference, connected components are extracted per class and small isolated false positives are removed, retaining the largest anatomically plausible shape per label. This preserves the integrity of each tooth's morphology and ensures separation of closely spaced structures. This light-weight post-processing step helps preserve geometric consistency without requiring external priors or templates. Post-segmentation, surface meshes are generated and made available for shape analysis. We enforced shape smoothness via Laplacian regularization.

3 Results

3.1 Quantitative Segmentation Performance

We tested our nnU-Net v2 on 55 pediatric CBCT scans, reporting Dice (DSC) and Intersection-over-Union (IoU) across all 55 labels. As Fig. 6 and Table 1 show, permanent teeth average DSC about 0.90, while smaller primary teeth average about 0.85. All annotated structures were recovered (no missing labels), matching prior CBCT segmentation benchmarks [11].

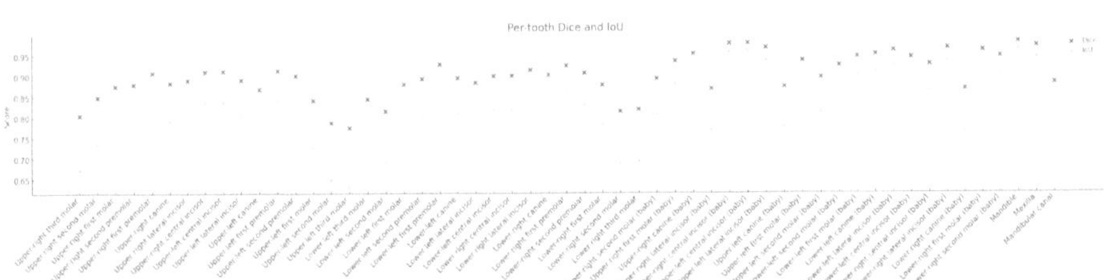

Fig. 6. Per-class accuracy on the test set. Blue circles = Dice, orange triangles = IoU, for the 55 labels ordered from the upper right third molar. Most permanent teeth score Dice ≥ 0.90, primary teeth around 0.90. Lower values appear only for the rare third molars. (Color figure online)

To further characterize the segmentation performance at the voxel level, we computed per-class confusion matrices grouped by dentition type. Figure 7 shows the normalized confusion matrices separately for permanent and deciduous teeth,

Table 1. Results demonstrate the model's capacity to robustly segment both primary and permanent teeth across all regions of the dentition. Lower Dice and higher variability are observed for third molars and primary incisors, reflecting anatomical variation and limited sample representation.

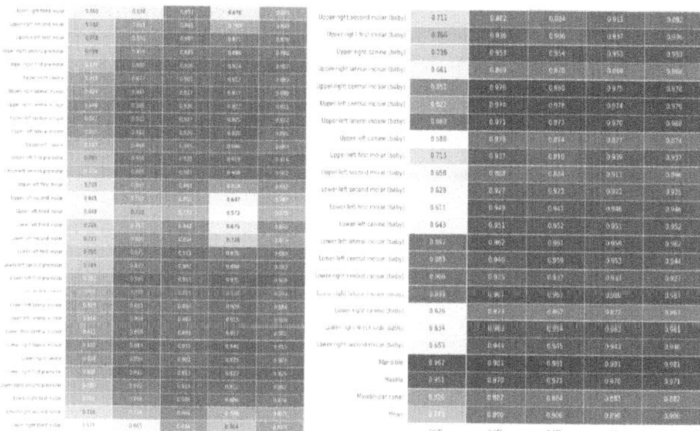

divided into upper and lower arches. The matrices highlight that misclassifications, when present, are mostly limited to adjacent teeth or homologous structures, especially among primary teeth with similar shapes.

3.2 Qualitative Visual Assessment

Figure 8 shows a representative test-set CBCT with the nnU-Net v2 segmentation overlaid. The automatic masks align closely with true tooth boundaries, isolating each tooth in a distinct color and accurately separating adjacent structures even unerupted buds and resorbing roots. No major label swaps were observed.

Figure 9 presents, from left to right, the ground truth, our model's output and the output of DentalSegmentator (nnU-Net v2). Semi-transparent bone surfaces reveal the tooth labels. Compared with *DentalSegmentator*, our method more faithfully reproduces the reality especially at inter-tooth contacts resulting in clearer individualization of teeth and fewer merge errors.

Clinically, our open-source method [10], deployed in the 3D Slicer platform delivers a patient specific digital twin within minutes: each tooth becomes a separate 3D object for measurement or virtual extraction. Segmentation takes 2 min on GPU (NVIDIA RTX A6000) or <7 min on CPU, cutting manual effort by > 90% and enabling chair-side deployment [11].

4 Discussion

Our results confirm that nnU-Net v2 accurately segments primary and permanent teeth in pediatric CBCT, achieving a mean Dice of 0.87, performance that approaches expert level [11]. We discuss clinical implications, compare with prior dental-segmentation work, and outline limitations and future directions.

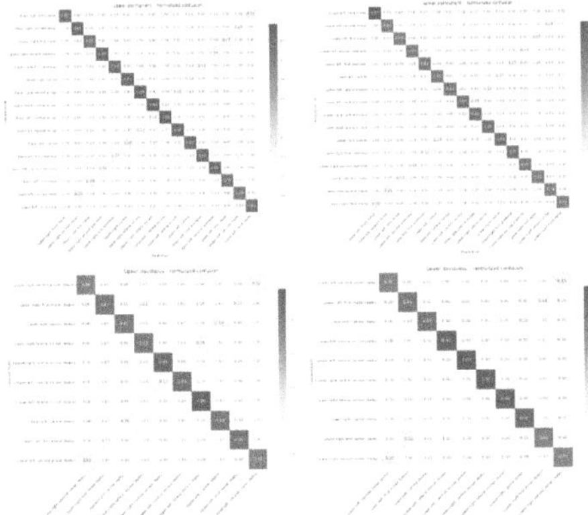

Fig. 7. Normalized confusion matrices for upper/lower permanent and upper/lower primary teeth. Notably, errors are rare and usually limited to neighboring classes or to the same tooth on the opposite side (i.e., right–left confusion), especially among primary incisors and molars.

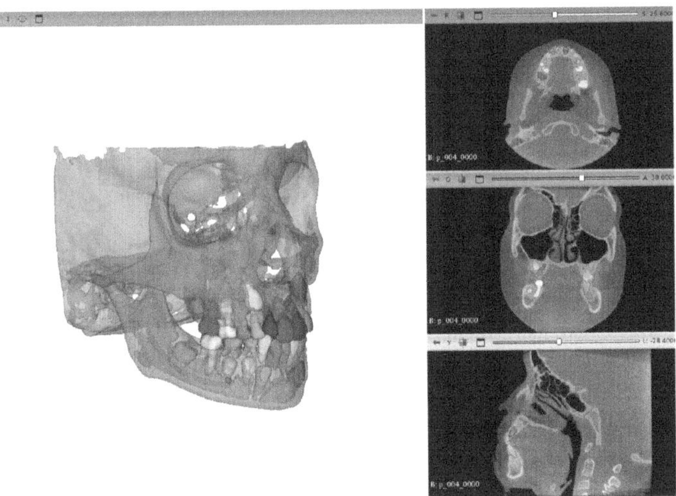

Fig. 8. Qualitative example of the automatic segmentation. **Left:** 3-D surface rendering of the maxilla, mandible and teeth generated from the predicted labels. **Right:** axial, coronal and sagittal CBCT slices with the same labels over-laid in semi-transparency.

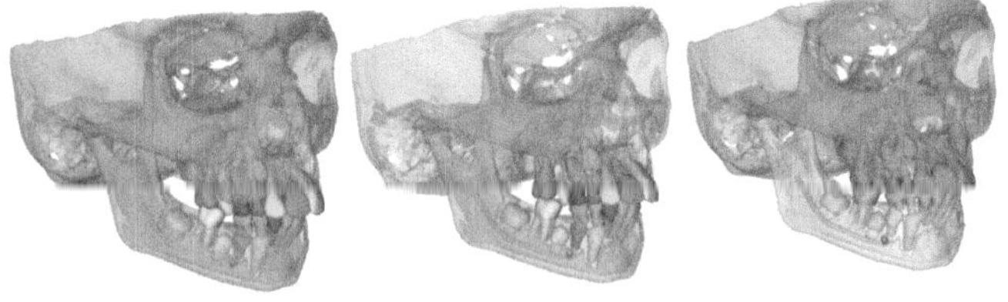

Fig. 9. Ground Truth vs. Ours vs. DentalSegmentator.

Precise 3D tooth segmentation enables advanced geometric analyses in pediatric dentistry. Mixed dentition presents variable anatomy unerupted buds, erupting premolars, resorbing roots while 2D imaging fails to capture these shapes and manual segmentation is slow and inconsistent. We reconstruct the entire dentition volumetrically, each tooth as a separate 3D object. These models support applications like extraction simulation, eruption-path prediction, surgical guidance, and 3D orthodontic planning. Our pipeline is fast, reliable, and maximizes clinical CBCT value. While we emphasize enhancing the utility of already prescribed scans, we also stress the importance of judicious CBCT use in pediatric populations [12].

We demonstrate how nnU-Net v2, a self-configuring framework, extends DentalSegmentator for pediatric tooth shape modeling [1,13], segmenting 55 classes in pediatric CBCT while preserving inter-class 3D geometry. A single nnU-Net generalizes across tooth types and stages without custom tuning, leveraging shape priors during augmentation and outputting semantic labels directly, avoiding heuristic post-processing. Unlike watershed or atlas methods [14], our model infers tooth morphology directly while maintaining anatomical coherence.

Where classical methods fail near weak separation or artifacts, our network remains robust through targeted data augmentation. Although Metal artifacts continue to limit segmentation accuracy [15], training with bracketed scans may help [16]. Reported per-tooth Dice ranges (0.75–0.93) [15] place our mean of 0.87 in the mid-range: better than early CNNs but below top permanent tooth only pipelines, yet we uniquely handle mixed dentition in one pass. We disabled left–right flips to avoid laterality errors (e.g., mis-labelling contralateral teeth) and achieved 56-class segmentation in a single forward pass streamlining over previous binary or hierarchical approaches while preserving anatomical fidelity.

Limitations include underrepresented anatomical outliers (e.g., syndromic cases) and unmodeled cross-scanner variability. Future work will aim to: (i) expand training to include rare anatomies, (ii) incorporate shape-aware loss functions, (iii) fuse with intraoral scans, (iv) integrate geometric learning tools [17].

5 Conclusion

We have presented a fully automatic segmentation pipeline that leverages the self- configuring nnU-Net v2 framework to model the complete mixed dentition in pediatric CBCT volumes. Our approach accurately segments all 55 anatomical structures, including both primary and permanent teeth, while preserving the geometric fidelity of the voxel level. The method achieves a mean Dice score of 0.87 and delivers anatomically coherent segmentations suitable for clinical and computational applications. By capturing the full spatial extent and inter-class relationships of dental structures, our pipeline enables the generation of patient-specific digital twins in which each tooth is represented as a manipulable 3D object. These models support shape-based clinical tasks such as eruption assessment, surgical planning, and orthodontic treatment design. Critically, the workflow runs in near real-time, enabling seamless integration into diagnostic pipelines without manual post processing.

Acknowledgments. This work was funded by NIH, grant number R01-DE024450.

Disclosure of Interests. The authors have no competing interests to declare that are relevant to the content of this article.

References

1. Lahoud, P., EzEldeen, M., Beznik, T., et al.: Artificial intelligence for fast and accurate 3-dimensional tooth segmentation on cone-beam computed tomography. J. Endod. **47**(5), 827–835 (2021)
2. Tarce, M., Zhou, Y., Antonelli, A., Becker, K.: The application of artificial intelligence for tooth segmentation in CBCT images: a systematic review. Appl. Sci. **14**(14), 6298 (2024)
3. Isensee, F., Jäger, P.F., Kohl, S.A.A., Petersen, J., Maier-Hein, K.H.: nnU-Net: a self-configuring method for deep learning-based biomedical image segmentation. Nat. Methods **18**(2), 203–211 (2021)
4. Isensee, F., Kirchhoff, Y., Kraemer, L., Rokuss, M., Ulrich, C., Maier-Hein, K.H.: Scaling nnU-Net for CBCT Segmentation. arXiv:2411.17213 [cs.CV] (2024)
5. Slicer Automated Dental Tools github. https://github.com/DCBIA-OrthoLab/SlicerAutomatedDentalTools. Accessed 22 July 2025
6. Cui, W., Wang, Y., Zhang, Q., et al.: CTooth: a fully annotated 3d dataset and benchmark for tooth volume segmentation on cone beam computed tomography images. arXiv:2206.08778 [cs.CV] (2022)
7. 3D Slicer page. https://www.slicer.org/. Accessed 22 July 2025
8. ITK-SNAP page. https://www.itksnap.orgto. Accessed 22 July 2025
9. Beser, B., Reis, T., Berber, M.N., et al.: YOLO-V5 based deep learning approach for tooth detection and segmentation on pediatric panoramic radiographs in mixed dentition. BMC Med. Imaging **24**, 172 (2024)
10. BATCHDENTALSEG Module. https://github.com/DCBIA-OrthoLab/SlicerAutomatedDentalTools/tree/main/BATCHDENTALSEG. Accessed 07 Aug 2025
11. Elsonbaty, S., Elgarba, B.M., Fontenele, R.C., Swaity, A., Jacobs, R.: Novel AI-based tool for primary tooth segmentation on CBCT using convolutional neural networks: a validation study. Int. J. Pediatr. Dent. **35**(1), 31–40 (2025)
12. Oenning, A.C., Jacobs, R., Pauwels, R., Stratis, A., Hedesiu, M., Salmon, B.: Cone-beam CT in paediatric dentistry: DIMITRA project position statement. Pediatr. Radiol. **48**(3), 308–316 (2018)
13. Shaheen, E., Leite, A., Alqahtani, K.A., et al.: A novel deep learning system for multi-class tooth segmentation and classification on cone beam computed tomography: a validation study. J. Dent. **115**, 103865 (2021)
14. Galibourg, A., Dumoncel, J., Telmon, N., Calvet, A., Michetti, J., Maret, D.: Assessment of automatic segmentation of teeth using a watershed-based method. Dentomaxillofacial Radiol. **47**(3), 20170220 (2018)
15. Polizzi, A., Quinzi, V., Ronsivalle, V., et al.: Tooth automatic segmentation from CBCT images: a systematic review. Clin. Oral Invest. **27**(6), 3363–3378 (2023)
16. Alqahtani, K.A., Jacobs, R., Smolders, A., et al.: Deep convolutional neural network-based automated segmentation and classification of teeth with orthodontic brackets on cone-beam computed tomographic images: a validation study. Eur. J. Orthod. **45**(2), 169–174 (2023)
17. Zhang, Y., Liu, Z., Feng, Y., Xu, R.: 3D-U-SAM network for few-shot tooth segmentation in CBCT images. arXiv:2309.11015 [cs.CV] (2023)

From Prediction to Prompt: Leveraging nnU-Net Outputs to Guide SAM for Active Learning in 3D Dental Segmentation

Nicolas Martin[1,2(✉)], Jean-Pierre Chevallet[2], and Philippe Mulhem[2]

[1] PEEKTORIA, Grenoble, France
nicolas.martin@peektoria.com

[2] Univ. Grenoble Alpes, CNRS, Grenoble INP (Institute of Engineering Univ. Grenoble Alpes), LIG, Grenoble, France
{jean-pierre.chevallet,philippe.mulhem}@univ-grenoble-alpes.fr

Abstract. To enhance annotation efficiency in 3D dental Cone Beam Computed Tomography (CBCT) image segmentation, this paper explores an active learning (AL) approach that leverages nnU-Net predictions to generate prompts for a specialized 3D Segment Anything Model (SAM). The objective is to minimize the annotation burden without relying on prompts during the inference phase. First, our experiments showed that AL offers similar segmentation performance with less than 20% of the original annotations. Second, random selection offers similar results than more complex sampling method with less more computing demand. Third, the predictions of nnU-Net on unannotated images provided effective prompts for the SAM model specialized in 3D medical images (i.e., SAM-Med3D). Combining these two approaches reduced the required amount of manual annotation by up to 50%. This paper paves the way for more easily obtaining new annotated datasets in the dental domain while simultaneously training a segmentation model, by leveraging SAM-like models.

Keywords: Active Learning · nnU-Net · Segment Anything · Segmentation · 3D dental CBCT

1 Introduction

Organ segmentation is a highly active research area within computer vision for medical imaging. In the dental domain, the widespread adoption of imaging technologies like Cone Beam Computed Tomography (CBCT) and panoramic X-rays in clinical settings has underscored the critical need for automated solutions to effectively leverage this information. Precisely segmenting anatomical structures (e.g., teeth) is often an essential step for robust computer-aided detection systems [19]. Despite dental issues affecting a significant global population, dedicated computer vision tools for dentistry remain less developed, largely due to

F. Bolelli et al. (Eds.): ODIN 2025, LNCS 16473, pp. 33–44, 2026.
https://doi.org/10.1007/978-3-032-20711-1_4

a scarcity of annotated datasets outside the scope of recent MICCAI challenges (e.g., ToothFairy [2], 3DTeethSeg [1]). As highlighted by these challenges, accurately segmenting dental organs, particularly in 3D images, presents a major difficultly, and currently often relies on adaptations of the nnU-Net model [10] specialized for dental datasets (e.g., [11,31]).

On the other hand, inspired by the success of large language models (LLMs), which are pre-trained using self-supervised learning (SSL) on very large datasets and fine-tuned to follow instructions (prompt-based models) [24], the Segment Anything Model (SAM) [15] has been proposed. The initial SAM model [15] have been trained on approximately one billion image-mask pairs. This attention-based model is designed to be applied to any image, aiming to address nearly any segmentation task. Despite this initial assertion, these models are unable to correctly segment specific image types, such as medical images [9], necessitating fine-tuning (e.g., MedSAM [21,22], SAM-Med3D [30]). Furthermore, such SAM-like models heavily rely on "prompts" (e.g., bounding boxes, points), which serve as strong indicators for defining the image region to be segmented [15]. In practice, in daily clinical routine, the introduction of SAM is barely impossible, as it requires a precise bounding box or multiple points to perform accurate segmentation [16]. Consequently, it remains essential to train segmentation models on annotated data. This paper investigates the integration of Active Learning (AL) with SAM-like models to reduce the expert annotation burden in 3D dental segmentation tasks.

2 Related Work

Prior studies on active learning (AL) have shown that not all data points are equally informative [25]. Their annotations can significantly influence both the training process and the final performance of the model [28]. Selecting the most informative images should be more beneficial to model performance than random selection of images [32]. This assumption has led to the development of numerous AL methods designed to select the most informative samples for annotation [25,28].

In the dental domain, obtaining images for diagnostic or archival purposes has become standard practice, leading to the availability of large datasets [33]. However, these datasets are rarely annotated [5]. Thus, selecting the most informative images using AL methods presents a valuable opportunity to significantly alleviate the annotation workload for experts, thereby promoting the creation of more efficient medical tools based on deep learning algorithms: see [3] for a review of AL for medical images. In 3D dental domain, Huang et al. [8] and Jung et al. [14] showed that AL can improve the segmentation performance.

In the context of 2D medical images, Li et al. [18] explored the combination of nnU-Net and a generic SAM model. SAM predictions are directly integrated into the nnU-Net architecture as an external module to enhance segmentation performance. Stock el al. [29] investigated the integration of nnU-Net with SAM for 3D images. However, due to computational constraints, their approach is applied in a 2D slice-by-slice manner. On the other hand, interactive annotation relying on SAM-like models have been proposed: Isensee et al. [12] trained nnU-Net model on 120+ 3D datasets to produce segmentation masks using prompts.

In this paper, we explore the integration of active learning with promptable segmentation models (e.g., SAM-like models). To the best of our knowledge, no prior study has investigated the combination of nnU-Net and SAM for 3D dental image segmentation within an active learning framework.

3 Method

This paper investigates two key aspects: (1) the impact of various AL sampling strategies on 3D image segmentation performance and (2) the performance of SAM like models (i.e., SAM-Med3D [30]) when integrated with nnU-Net-derived prompts during AL training.

3.1 Datasets

The dataset ToothFairy2 [2] have been used in the following experiments. It is composed of 480 Cone Beam Computed Tomography (CBCT) with 42 classes. To reduce computational complexity and focus our analysis, the original anatomical classes were re-categorized into the following 6 broader classes for segmentation:

- Background
- Jawbones: Lower and Upper
- Inferior Alveolar Canal (IAC): Left and Right
- Sinus: Left and Right
- Pharynx
- Teeth (32 classes originally)

Due to their sparse representation in the dataset, the Bridge, Crown, Implant, and NA classes were excluded from segmentation and assigned to the background.

3.2 Metrics

The segmentation performance was evaluated using the Dice Similarity Coefficient (DSC in %). For a given image i and a specific target class C, let Sg_i^C represent the set of pixels assigned to class C in the ground truth segmentation, and Sa_i^C denote the corresponding set of pixels predicted by the automatic segmentation model. The *Dice* score for class C on image i quantifies the overlap between these two segmentations and is defined by Eq. (1):

$$Dice(Sg_i^C, Sa_i^C) = \frac{2|Sg_i^C \cap Sa_i^C|}{|Sg_i^C| + |Sa_i^C|} \tag{1}$$

DSC ranges from 0 to 1, where 1 indicates perfect agreement between the predicted and ground truth segmentations for that specific class. The overall performance is typically reported as the mean of these per-image, per-class Dice scores averaged across all relevant classes and images in the dataset.

To evaluate the effectiveness of SAM-Med3D [30] in facilitating annotation, we calculated the Symmetric Difference (SD). This metric quantifies the total volume of discrepancy between two segmentations, representing the exact voxels an expert would need to adjust (either add or remove) to align a prediction with the ground truth. It is defined as the sum of false positives (FP) and false negatives (FN), as shown in Eq. (2):

$$SD(A, B) = FP + FN \tag{2}$$

This metric is normalized (Normalized Symmetric Difference – NSD) per class by the union of predicted and the ground truth for the corresponding voxels. That ensures a fair comparison between classes with large regions (e.g., jawbones) and those with small regions (e.g., IAC). NSD ranges from 0 to 100, where 0 indicates perfect masks not requiring any modification.

To account for differences in organ size across classes (e.g., large regions such as Jawbones versus small regions such as the Sinus), SD was normalized by the union of predicted and ground-truth voxels, resulting in the Normalized Symmetric Difference (NSD). NSD ranges from 0 to 100, where 0 indicates perfectly overlapping masks that require no modification.

3.3 Active Learning Sampling Methods

Two AL sampling methods have been evaluated: Naive sampling (random selection) and Least confidence sampling. The random sampling consists into randomly select N images at each AL round. The least confidence [17] approach involves selecting the images for which the model is the least confident. The least confidence score for a single pixel is defined in Eq. (3):

$$Uncertainty_{LeastConfidence}(\hat{y}) = |1 - \hat{y}| \tag{3}$$

where $\hat{y}$ is the predicted value for pixel y of an input image. The uncertainty score for an entire image is obtained by averaging the individual pixel uncertainty scores across all considered classes.

3.4 Workflow

During the AL process (see Fig. 1), round 0 corresponds to the cold-start and consists of the following: (1) N images are randomly selected for annotation, (2) a data fingerprint is generated and used to prepare the dataset for nnU-Net, and (3) the model is trained.

The following steps are performed in each subsequent AL round.

1. the informativeness of each unlabeled image is computed using previously trained model,
2. the most informative images are selected,

3. these images are annotated and incorporated into the set of images labeled in previous AL rounds,
4. the images are prepared for nnU-Net. Following the approach of [7], a fixed data fingerprint (generated in round 0) is reused across iterations to accelerate data preparation,
5. a new model is fine-tuned, and
6. the model is evaluated, with the best checkpoint always used to make predictions at each AL round.

This AL process is repeated until the annotation budget is exhausted.

Concerning the SAM predictions, the following steps are performed (see Fig. 2):

1. Predictions are generated using the nnU-Net model.
2. Prompts (i.e., simulated clicks on relevant areas corresponding to classes) are generated based on these predictions.
3. The images and prompts are fed into SAM-Med3D to produce 3D segmentations.

3.5 Network Architecture

The segmentation is performed using the nnU-Net model [10]. It builds upon the successful U-Net architecture [26] and offers a self-configuring approach that minimizes the need for manual parameter tuning. nnU-Net has consistently demonstrated high performance across various medical datasets [10] and becomes the default model for medical image segmentation [13,27]. Concerning prompt-based models for segmentation, the SAM-Med3D model [30] has been used. This model has been specialized for 3D medical images and adapted to handle click-based prompts.

3.6 Hyper-Parameters

Concerning nnU-Net [10], the default parameters were used, with three exceptions. To reduce computational demands and mitigate overfitting, since AL involves significantly fewer annotated examples than standard training, the number of iterations per epoch was limited to 100. Additionally, the number of epochs per AL round was limited to 50. Lastly, only the 3D low-resolution configuration of nnU-Net was used.

Concerning the AL part, prospective comparison of AL methods (i.e., actually asking an expert to annotate the selected images) is problematic, since image selection influences subsequent selections and, consequently, the results. To enable a fair comparison, the AL process was simulated using the fully annotated dataset. The following parameters was used:

- Number of AL rounds: 10
- Number of images selected at each AL round: 5

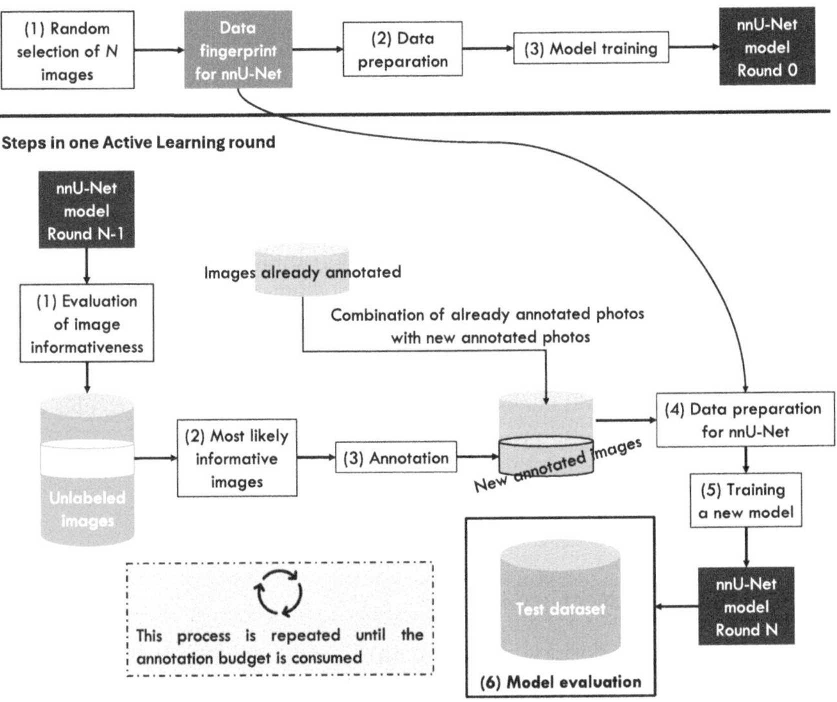

Fig. 1. Active Learning (AL) workflow. Round 0: A predefined number of images are randomly selected to generate the nnU-Net data fingerprint and train the initial model. Steps in a single AL round: (1) evaluate the informativeness of each image in the unlabeled pool using the current model, (2) select the most informative images, (3) annotate the selected images, (4) prepare the images for nnU-Net using the existing data fingerprint, (5) fine-tune the model with both previously and newly annotated images, and (6) evaluate the updated model. Steps 1–6 in are repeated until the annotation budget is exhausted.

- Cold start (round 0): 5% of annotated data (20 images) have been randomly selected images and used to initialize model training
- At each AL round, in accordance with the survey of Budd et al. [3], the model was finetuned using all available annotated data (previously + newly annotated images), from prior best checkpoint at the previous round.

For the evaluation, 15% of the dataset (72 images) was randomly sampled to form the test dataset. For a fair comparison, a nnU-Net model was also trained on the fully annotated dataset for the same number of iterations (50,000) as used in the 10 AL iterations (called "Internal Test" in Table 1).

Concerning the SAM-Med3D model [30], the default parameters were used.

Experiments were performed on a system with an NVIDIA A6000 GPU (48 GB VRAM), Intel Xeon Silver 4208 CPU (16 cores), and 128 GB RAM.

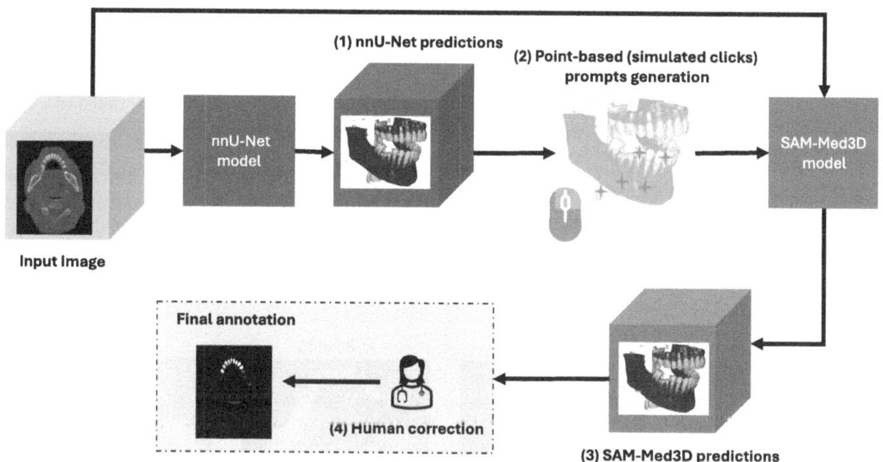

Fig. 2. Overview of 3D-assisted annotation using nnU-Net and a SAM-like model. The process consists of four steps: (1) generating pixel-wise predictions with nnU-Net, (2) creating point-based prompts (simulated clicks) from these predictions, (3) producing pixel-wise predictions with SAM-Med3D using these prompts, and (4) performing human corrections on the generated masks to obtain the final annotation.

The code used for the experiments is publicly available at https://github.com/martinicmrim/sam_nnunet.

4 Results

4.1 Active Learning Sampling Methods on Segmentation Performance

The comparison between Active Learning (AL) sampling methods is depicted in Table 1. The performance of the AL sampling methods was evaluated using the model weights from the final AL round (i.e., round 10). We also report the performance obtained using the fully annotated dataset ("Internal Test"), as well as the performance of random sampling AL with the 3D full-resolution configuration of nnU-Net.

The AL methods demonstrated performance comparable to training on the full dataset, utilizing less than 20% of the original training data, with the exception of "Sinus" segmentation. Similar segmentation performance is observed between the random selection method and least confidence selection, although training time is 5 time longer.

Figure 3 depicts the qualitative evaluation of segmentation across AL rounds.

4.2 Evaluation of SAM-Med3D Masks with Prompts Derived from nnU-Net Predictions

To evaluate the potential of SAM-Med3D [30] in facilitating the annotation of 3D dental images, we simulated an additional Active Learning (AL) iteration. The

Table 1. Mean Dice Score (in %) at the last AL round (round 10) and training time on grouped ToothFairy2 classes according to Active Learning sampling method

Method	Average DSC	Jawbones DSC	IAC DSC	Sinus DSC	Pharynx DSC	Teeth DSC	Training time Hours	Data used %
Full dataset (FD) [2]	70.92	90.31	71.34	64.81	95.66	73.17	NA	100
Random Samp. AL	74.33	98.5	88.38	0	96.73	88.38	5	18
Least Conf. Samp. AL	73.7	98	86.02	0	96.82	87.67	27	18
Internal Test FD	74.33	98.15	88.38	0.0	96.74	88.37	5	100
Random Samp. AL - Full resolution	72.62	97.89	85.42	0.0	95.16	84.60	7	100

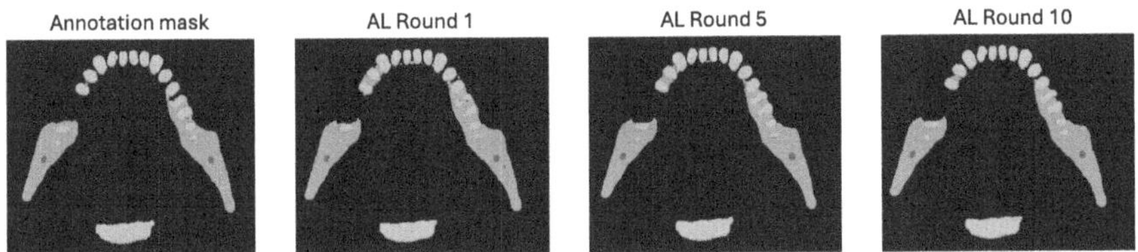

Fig. 3. Qualitative visualization of predictions for image 58 (ToothFairy dataset) at AL rounds 1, 5, and 10, compared with the annotation mask (axial slice S: 43.8 mm, 3D Slicer).

objective was to assess, if SAM-Med3D were deployed at the step 3 of the AL process, how much annotation effort could be reduced through the combination of nnU-Net and SAM-Med3D. Specifically, the quality of the masks generated by SAM-Med3D from prompts derived from nnU-Net predictions was evaluated. The procedure was as follows, based on the last AL iteration (with random sampling method):

1. Randomly select 5 images,
2. Generate 3D predictions using the most recently trained nnU-Net model,
3. Generate point-based prompts (i.e., simulated clicks) for each predicted class,
4. Use SAM-Med3D with the prompts and input images to produce 3D annotation masks,
5. Evaluate the quality of the generated 3D annotation masks.

The influence of the number of prompts per class (i.e., 1, 5, and 10 clicks per class) on the quality of the masks was also evaluated. The quality of the generated masks was quantitatively assessed using the Normalized Symmetric Difference (NSD), with Table 2 reporting the percentage of voxels requiring expert annotation or correction based on the combination of nnU-Net and SAM-Med3D.

5 Discussion

Concerning AL, estimating informativeness at each AL round is computationally expensive. In this paper, we focus exclusively on the least confidence method to

Table 2. Evaluation of SAM-Med3D performance (Normalized Symmetric Difference, in %) with varying numbers of prompts per class.

Number of Prompts	Average	Jawbones	IAC	Sinus	Pharynx	Teeth
1 click	62.61	88.92	37.94	98.60	98.97	0
5 clicks	50.75	76.59	37.58	98.12	97.38	0
10 clicks	51.52	69.34	35.38	97.56	97.30	0

compare to random selection. While other strategies, such as entropy or Monte Carlo (MC) dropout, may improve the performance, they come with significantly higher computational costs. For example, MC dropout requires multiple forward passes per image, substantially increasing the overall runtime. The choice of cold-start images may also influence the outcomes, as noted in [20]. Moreover, consistent with findings in other medical domains (e.g., [6, 23]), random selection has shown performance comparable to more complex selection strategies such as least confidence.

The preliminary results on the annotation using Med-SAM3D show that with 5 simulated point-based prompt (i.e., simulated clicks) from nnU-net prediction allows to reduce the number of pixels to annotate or verify to up to 50%. Other SAM models exploiting other type of prompt (e.g., [21]) could be explored to improve this pre-annotation.

Moreover, contrary to 2D image segmentation, where training U-Net-like models can be very fast and require fewer iterations, 3D image training demands significantly more computational time. Adding the use of SAM generate also a lot of time between each AL round. An asynchronous iteration need to be considered to limit the waiting for the experts during the annotation. Moreover, even if random is very hard to beat to selection the images to annotate, other sampling methods could be considered in the future. The trade-off between gain in term of quality in selection and the computing power required as well as computing time to select the images seems to be an essential criteria to develop new methods.

It is important to note that the selected test dataset may not be entirely representative of the underlying distribution of the full dataset. Furthermore, the chosen class grouping strategy appears to have significantly impacted segmentation performance. On one hand, this grouping led to increased performance for classes with a large pixel representation in the images (e.g., Teeth), as the aggregation of pixels likely facilitated model training. On the other hand, it severely degraded performance for the "Sinus" class, which became largely undetected. This degradation could be attributed to the increased class imbalance introduced by the grouping, which disproportionately affects minority or less complex classes such as "Sinus".

This paper presents a preliminary work on the combination of traditional segmentation models (nnU-net [10]) and prompt-based segmentation models (SAM-Med3D [30]) to facilitate data annotation and model training in the 3D dental domain. In future studies, other dental datasets (e.g., 3DTeethSeg [1]) will be considered. Moreover, nnU-Net is a complex model due to its automated configuration capabilities, which accelerate model setup. Other models, such as TransUNet (e.g., [4]), could also be considered in future work, especially to evaluate other AL sampling methods.

Acknowledgments. This work has been supported by MIAI@Grenoble Alpes (ANR-19-P3IA-0003). This work benefited from state aid managed by the National Research Agency under France 2030 bearing the reference ANR-23-IACL-0006.

Disclosure of Interests. Philippe Mulhem and Jean-Pierre Chevallet have no competing interests to declare that are relevant to the content of this article. Nicolas Martin owns stock in PEEKTORIA.

References

1. Ben-Hamadou, A., et al.: 3DTeethSeg'22: 3D teeth scan segmentation and labeling challenge (2023). https://doi.org/10.48550/arXiv.2305.18277. arXiv:2305.18277 [cs]
2. Bolelli, F., et al.: Segmenting maxillofacial structures in cbct volumes. In: Proceedings of the Computer Vision and Pattern Recognition Conference (CVPR), pp. 5238–5248 (2025)
3. Budd, S., Robinson, E.C., Kainz, B.: A survey on active learning and human-in-the-loop deep learning for medical image analysis. Med. Image Anal. **71**, 102062 (2021). https://doi.org/10.1016/j.media.2021.102062
4. Chen, J., et al.: TransUNet: rethinking the U-Net architecture design for medical image segmentation through the lens of transformers. Med. Image Anal. **97**, 103280 (2024). https://doi.org/10.1016/j.media.2024.103280
5. Dao, L., Ly, N.Q.: A comprehensive study on medical image segmentation using deep neural networks. Int. J. Adv. Comput. Sci. Appl. **14**(3) (2023). https://doi.org/10.14569/IJACSA.2023.0140319
6. Ekner, A.B., et al.: Active learning with nnUNet for coronary artery lumen segmentation using a centerline prior. In: Petersen, J., Dahl, V.A. (eds.) Image Analysis, pp. 227–239. Springer, Cham (2025). https://doi.org/10.1007/978-3-031-95918-9_16
7. Föllmer, B., Schulze, K., Wald, C., Stober, S., Samek, W., Dewey, M.: Active learning with the nnUNet and sample selection with uncertainty-aware submodular mutual information measure. In: Proceedings of The 7nd International Conference on Medical Imaging with Deep Learning, pp. 480–503. PMLR (2024). https://proceedings.mlr.press/v250/follmer24a.html. iSSN: 2640-3498
8. Huang, J., et al.: Uncertainty-based active learning by bayesian U-net for multi-label cone-beam CT segmentation. J. Endodont. **50**(2), 220–228 (2024). https://doi.org/10.1016/j.joen.2023.11.002
9. Huang, Y., et al.: Segment anything model for medical images? Med. Image Anal. **92**, 103061 (2024). https://doi.org/10.1016/j.media.2023.103061
10. Isensee, F., Jaeger, P.F., Kohl, S.A.A., Petersen, J., Maier-Hein, K.H.: nnU-Net: a self-configuring method for deep learning-based biomedical image segmentation. Nat. Methods **18**(2), 203–211 (2021). https://doi.org/10.1038/s41592-020-01008-z

11. Isensee, F., Kirchhoff, Y., Kraemer, L., Rokuss, M., Ulrich, C., Maier-Hein, K.H.: Scaling nnU-Net for CBCT Segmentation (2024). https://doi.org/10.48550/arXiv.2411.17213. arXiv:2411.17213 [cs]
12. Isensee, F., et al.: nnInteractive: redefining 3D Promptable Segmentation (2025). https://doi.org/10.48550/arXiv.2503.08373. arXiv:2503.08373 [cs]
13. Isensee, F., et al.: nnU-net revisited: a call for rigorous validation in 3D medical image segmentation. In: Linguraru, M.G., et al. (eds.) Medical Image Computing and Computer Assisted Intervention MICCAI 2024, pp. 488–498. Springer, Cham (2024). https://doi.org/10.1007/978-3-031-72114-4_47
14. Jung, S.K., Lim, H.K., Lee, S., Cho, Y., Song, I.S.: Deep active learning for automatic segmentation of maxillary sinus lesions using a convolutional neural network. Diagnostics **11**(4), 688 (2021). https://doi.org/10.3390/diagnostics11040688
15. Kirillov, A., et al.: Segment anything. In: 2023 IEEE/CVF International Conference on Computer Vision (ICCV), pp. 3992–4003 (2023). https://doi.org/10.1109/ICCV51070.2023.00371
16. Li, B., Yuan, Y., Tan, W.: Optimization of MedSAM model based on bounding box adaptive perturbation algorithm (2025). https://doi.org/10.48550/arXiv.2503.19700. arXiv:2503.19700 [cs]
17. Li, X., et al.: HAL-IA: a hybrid active learning framework using interactive annotation for medical image segmentation. Med. Image Anal. **88**, 102862 (2023). https://doi.org/10.1016/j.media.2023.102862
18. Li, Y., Jing, B., Li, Z., Wang, J., Zhang, Y.: Plug-and-play segment anything model improves nnUNet performance. Med. Phys. **52**(2), 899–912 (2025). https://doi.org/10.1002/mp.17481
19. Litjens, G., et al.: A survey on deep learning in medical image analysis. Med. Image Anal. **42**, 60–88 (2017). https://doi.org/10.1016/j.media.2017.07.005. arXiv:1702.05747
20. Liu, H., et al.: COLosSAL: a benchmark for cold-start active learning for 3D medical image segmentation (2023). https://doi.org/10.48550/arXiv.2307.12004. arXiv:2307.12004 [cs]
21. Ma, J., He, Y., Li, F., Han, L., You, C., Wang, B.: Segment anything in medical images. Nat. Commun. **15**(1), 1–9 (2024). https://doi.org/10.1038/s41467-024-44824-z
22. Ma, J., et al.: MedSAM2: segment anything in 3D medical images and videos (2025). https://doi.org/10.48550/arXiv.2504.03600. arXiv:2504.03600 [eess]
23. Martin, N., Chevallet, J.P., Mulhem, P., Qu not, G.: Combining image and region uncertainty-based active learning for melanoma segmentation. In: 2024 International Conference on Content-Based Multimedia Indexing (CBMI), pp. 1–7. IEEE, Reykjavik (2024). https://doi.org/10.1109/CBMI62980.2024.10859208
24. Ouyang, L., et al.: Training language models to follow instructions with human feedback (2022). https://doi.org/10.48550/arXiv.2203.02155. arXiv:2203.02155 [cs]
25. Ren, P., et al.: A survey of deep active learning. ACM Comput. Surv. **54**(9), 180:1–180:40 (2021). https://doi.org/10.1145/3472291
26. Ronneberger, O., Fischer, P., Brox, T.: U-net: convolutional networks for biomedical image segmentation (2015). arXiv:1505.04597 [cs]
27. Russell, E., Boyd, A., Finlay, D., Trindade, L.: Machine learning-based anatomical segmentation: a systematic review of methodologies and applications. Open J. Clin. Med. Images **4**(1), 1187 (2024)
28. Settles, B.: Active Learning Literature Survey. Computer Sciences Technical Report 1648, University of Wisconsin Madison (2009). http://axon.cs.byu.edu/~martinez/classes/778/Papers/settles.activelearning.pdf

29. Stock, R., Kirchhoff, Y., Rokuss, M.R., Ravindran, A., Maier-Hein, K.: Segment anything in medical images with nnUNet. In: Ma, J., Zhou, Y., Wang, B. (eds.) Medical Image Segmentation Foundation Models. CVPR 2024 Challenge: Segment Anything in Medical Images on Laptop, pp. 167–179. Springer, Cham (2025). https://doi.org/10.1007/978-3-031-81854-7_11
30. Wang, H., et al.: SAM-Med3D: towards general-purpose segmentation models for volumetric medical images (2024). https://doi.org/10.48550/arXiv.2310.15161. arXiv:2310.15161 [cs]
31. Wang, Y., et al.: STS MICCAI 2023 challenge: grand challenge on 2D and 3D semi-supervised tooth segmentation (2024). https://doi.org/10.48550/arXiv.2407.13246. arXiv:2407.13246 [cs]
32. Yoo, D., Kweon, I.S.: Learning loss for active learning. In: 2019 IEEE/CVF Conference on Computer Vision and Pattern Recognition (CVPR), pp. 93–102. IEEE, Long Beach (2019). https://doi.org/10.1109/CVPR.2019.00018
33. Zeng, X., Wen, L., Xu, Y., Ji, C.: Generating diagnostic report for medical image by high-middle-level visual information incorporation on double deep learning models. Comput. Methods Programs Biomed. **197**, 105700 (2020)

Bits2Bites: Intra-oral Scans Occlusal Classification

Lorenzo Borghi[1], Luca Lumetti[1], Francesca Cremonini[2], Federico Rizzo[2], Costantino Grana[1], Luca Lombardo[2], and Federico Bolelli[1(✉)]

[1] University of Modena and Reggio Emilia, Modena, Italy
{lorenzo.borghi,luca.lumetti,costantino.grana,federico.bolelli}@unimore.it
[2] University of Ferrara, Ferrara, Italy
{francesca.cremonini,federico.rizzo,luca.lombardo}@unife.it

Abstract. We introduce *Bits2Bites*, the first publicly available dataset for occlusal classification from intra-oral scans, comprising 200 paired upper and lower dental arches annotated across multiple clinically relevant dimensions (sagittal, vertical, transverse, and midline relationships). Leveraging this resource, we propose a multi-task learning benchmark that jointly predicts five occlusal traits from raw 3D point clouds using state-of-the-art point-based neural architectures. Our approach includes extensive ablation studies assessing the benefits of multi-task learning against single-task baselines, as well as the impact of automatically-predicted anatomical landmarks as input features. Results demonstrate the feasibility of directly inferring comprehensive occlusion information from unstructured 3D data, achieving promising performance across all tasks. Our entire dataset, code, and pretrained models are publicly released to foster further research in automated orthodontic diagnosis.

Keywords: Intra-oral Scans · Dental Occlusion · 3D Point Cloud

1 Introduction

Deep learning has become a key enabler in dental healthcare, supporting the automation and enhancement of diagnostic workflows. The growing availability of public 3D imaging datasets related to dental healthcare has significantly contributed to the research community (Fig. 1). For instance, in recent years, different datasets introduced labeled CBCT scans with dozens of anatomical structures, fostering research in segmenting complex regions such as the inferior alveolar canal, teeth, jaws, and dental implants [2–5,7,8,17]. In the domain of intra-oral 3D scanning (IOS), large-scale datasets like 3DTeethSeg [1] offer full-tooth segmentation annotations

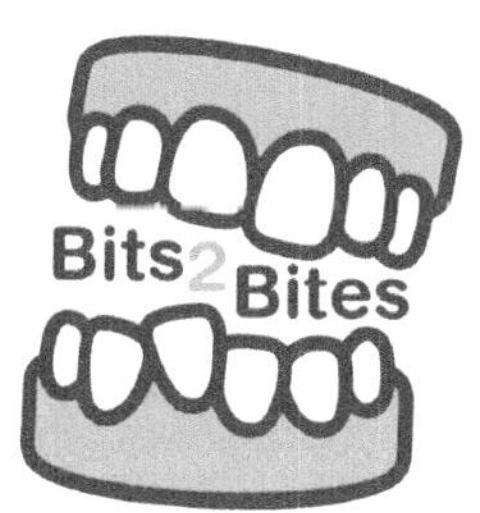

Fig. 1. *Bits2Bites* logo.

L. Borghi and L. Lumetti—Authors are allowed to list their name first on their CVs.

F. Bolelli et al. (Eds.): ODIN 2025, LNCS 16473, pp. 45–54, 2026.
https://doi.org/10.1007/978-3-032-20711-1_5

across hundreds of scans, while the TeethLand dataset, released by the same authors, provides detailed landmark annotations for each tooth. These resources have catalyzed the development of a wide range of methods—from voxel-based and surface-based segmentation networks to point-based landmark detection approaches [10,13,14,16,19].

Despite these advances, several clinically relevant tasks remain underexplored in the context of 3D IOS analysis, largely due to the lack of publicly available annotations. One such task is *occlusal classification*, which involves determining the relationship between the upper and lower dentition when the mouth is closed. Accurate occlusion assessment is fundamental for orthodontic diagnosis and treatment planning, as it directly informs the strategy for interventions such as braces or clear aligners and serves as a baseline for evaluating treatment success. While prior work has investigated malocclusion detection from 2D snapshots of 3D models [11], these modalities lack the rich 3D surface information captured in IOS scans. Consequently, they omit crucial depth and structural cues that are essential for a fine-grained and comprehensive occlusion analysis.

To the best of our knowledge, no existing 3D deep learning method directly operates on paired upper and lower IOS meshes to predict occlusion classes. Addressing this gap, our work introduces new resources and benchmarks to facilitate progress in this direction.

Contribution. In summary, the contributions of this work are outlined below:

- We present *Bits2Bites*, the first publicly available dataset of 200 paired intra-oral scans with multi-dimensional clinical labels for occlusion classification, including sagittal, vertical, transverse, and midline relationships;[1]
- A robust multi-task and single-task learning benchmark is introduced for this task, evaluating two state-of-the-art point cloud backbones and demonstrating the effectiveness of jointly learning multiple occlusal traits;
- Detailed ablation studies are carried out to analyze the impact of using automatically-predicted anatomical landmarks as input features and to validate our multi-task learning strategy against single-task baselines;
- We release our entire codebase and pretrained models to ensure reproducibility and foster further research in the community.[2]

2 Dataset

The dataset comprises 200 pairs of registered intra-oral scans in STL format, with separate high-resolution meshes for the upper and lower dental arches. All scans are spatially aligned to preserve the true occlusal relationship between the jaws and are transformed to a shared reference RAS (Right-Anterior-Superior) frame, a standardized coordinate system where axes are oriented toward the patient's right, anterior, and superior directions. Scan bases were removed to retain only

[1] https://ditto.ing.unimore.it/bits2bites

[2] https://github.com/AImageLab-zip/Bits2Bites

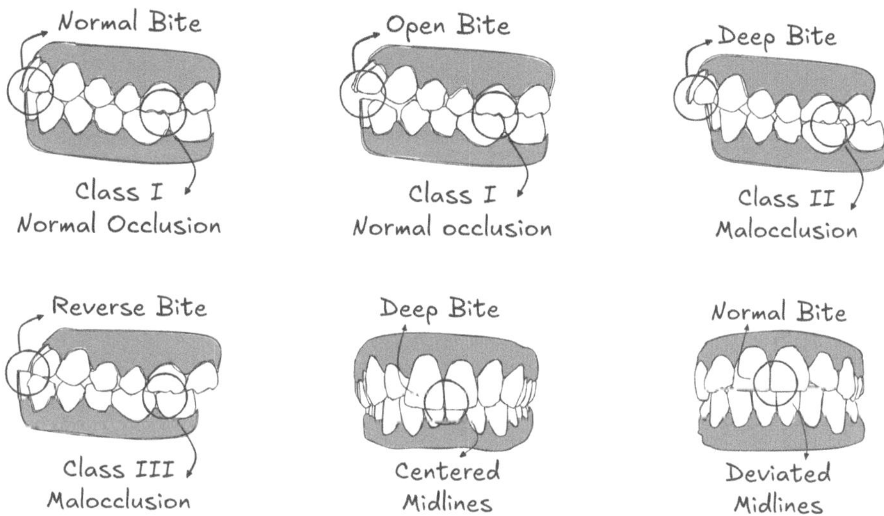

Fig. 2. Example of different occlusal classes present in our dataset.

the gingival and dental structures. Meshes average $92,201 \pm 28,140$ vertices and $182,444 \pm 55,862$ faces, with bounding-box dimensions of approximately 65.9 ± 4.12 mm (width), 53.84 ± 4.5 mm (depth), and 17.9 ± 1.9 mm (height). The mean mesh surface area is $\sim 3,780 \pm 409\,\text{mm}^2$.

Scans were acquired using two different intra-oral scanners, Carestream and 3Shape TRIOS, to capture variability in acquisition technologies. The scans included were selected randomly without any filtering criteria to reflect the natural diversity and distribution observed in clinical practice.

Annotations were performed by a single orthodontic specialist with five years of experience in the field. Each scan pair includes detailed, clinically relevant occlusion labels across multiple dimensions. Sagittal classifications are provided separately for the left and right sides, following a subset of Angle's standard classification [9] (i.e., *Class I*, *Class II edge-to-edge*, *Class II full*, *Class III*). Vertical anterior–posterior relationships are labeled as *Normal*, *Deep Bite*, *Reverse Bite*, or *Open Bite*. Transverse relationships are identified as *Normal*, *Cross Bite*, or *Scissor Bite*, using reference teeth. Finally, midline alignment is annotated as *Centered* or *Deviated*. Fig. 2 provides illustrations of these different characteristics. This multi-label annotation scheme enables clinically meaningful classification across sagittal, vertical, and transverse planes. The class distribution inside the proposed dataset is reported in Fig. 4.

Ethical Approval. Approval of all ethical and experimental procedures and protocols, as well as the release of data, was granted by the Comitato Etico di Ateneo di Ferrara under Approval No. 262/2025/Oss/UniFe.

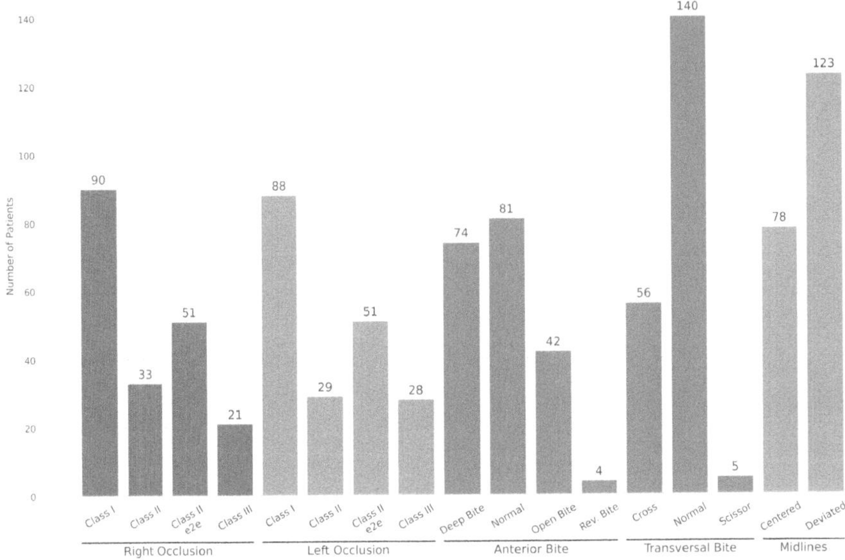

Fig. 4. Distribution of dataset classes. Distinct colors indicate different tasks.

3 Method

To address the challenge of multi-dimensional occlusion classification from intraoral scans, we developed a multi-task, point-based classification pipeline built on the open-source *Pointcept* framework [6]. Our approach jointly predicts five occlusal attributes from a single 3D point cloud representing the combined upper and lower dental arches.

Input Representation. Each sample consists of a registered pair of upper and lower intra-oral scans in STL format. Meshes are combined into a single 3D structure and converted into point clouds, where each point is represented by its *xyz* coordinates. This representation is optionally enriched with one-hot encoded per-tooth landmark features (Fig. 3) to capture anatomical context better. These landmarks are not manually annotated, but automatically predicted using the publicly available[3] state-of-the-art method from the 3DTeethLand challenge [15].

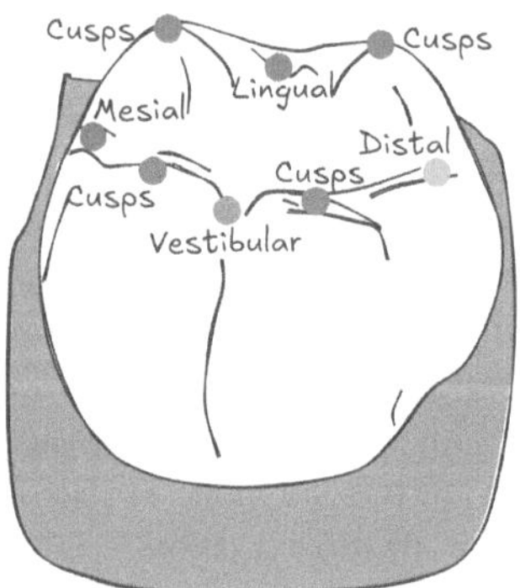

Fig. 3. Landmarks employed as additional input features.

[3] https://github.com/nnistelrooij/3dteethland, *final_test_phase* commit.

The dataset was split into five folds of 40 scans each to support a robust 5-fold cross-validation schema.

Preprocessing and Augmentation. To improve generalization, our training procedure leverages a carefully designed data augmentation pipeline. Each scan is normalized to a unit sphere, randomly scaled in all directions ($[0.95, 1.05]$), shifted (± 0.02 mm), rotated ($\pm 18^\circ$ on z-axis), and subjected to random dropout (50% of points with 50% probability). Finally, it is processed with grid sampling (voxel size 0.01 mm) and converted to a tensor. Validation and testing only apply normalization and grid sampling.

Task Formulation. We frame occlusion analysis as a multi-task classification problem with a single common backbone and five independent output heads, each corresponding to: (*i*) right sagittal classification (3 classes), (*ii*) left sagittal classification (3 classes), (*iii*) anterior vertical bite type (4 classes), (*iv*) transverse bite type (3 classes), and (*v*) midline alignment (2 classes). Each head performs categorical classification using ground-truth annotations.

Model Architecture. We evaluated two state-of-the-art point cloud backbones, PointTransformerV3 [18] and SPUNet [12], both already integrated within the Pointcept framework [6]. Our benchmark formulates occlusion analysis as a multi-task classification problem, where a single shared feature extractor is followed by five independent task-specific classification heads. Each head is implemented as a two-layer multilayer perceptron (MLP) with a final softmax activation. To assess the effectiveness of this approach, Sec. 4 also conducts an ablation study comparing the multi-task learning (MTL) setup with a single-task learning (STL) strategy that trains a separate dedicated model per task.

Training Configuration. Training was performed for 200 epochs with a batch size of 8. The PointTransformerV3 models used the AdamW optimizer (learning rate 1×10^{-4}, weight decay 0.01) with a cosine annealing scheduler, while SPUNet models employed the SGD optimizer (learning rate 1×10^{-3}, weight decay 0.01) with a multistep schedule. Mixed-precision training and gradient clipping set to 1.0 were used to stabilize learning for both backbones and in all the training performed. The total loss is computed as the unweighted mean of the five task-specific losses. Each of these task-specific losses is a cross-entropy function with pre-computed class weights to address label imbalance. The exact weights are available in the source code inside the configuration files.

Evaluation Protocol. We adopted a 5-fold cross-validation scheme. In each fold, 160 scans were used for training and 40 for testing. No dedicated validation split was used. Final results are reported as the mean and standard deviation of per-task classification scores across the five folds.

Table 1. Ablation study on input features. All classification metrics are macro-averaged across the five occlusal tasks and reported as mean ± std (%) over the 5 cross-validation folds. Inference time is the average time in seconds to process a single scan.

Input Features	Model	Accuracy	Precision	Recall	F1-Score	Time (s)
Mesh	PointTr.V3	0.69 ± 0.03	0.62 ± 0.02	0.61 ± 0.04	0.60 ± 0.03	0.11
Landmarks		0.70 ± 0.04	0.62 ± 0.04	0.63 ± 0.05	0.61 ± 0.04	0.04
Mesh + Landmarks		**0.71 ± 0.03**	**0.64 ± 0.03**	**0.64 ± 0.02**	**0.63 ± 0.03**	0.11
Mesh	SPUNet	0.64 ± 0.01	0.56 ± 0.03	0.58 ± 0.03	0.56 ± 0.04	0.05
Landmarks		0.60 ± 0.02	0.56 ± 0.06	0.56 ± 0.06	0.58 ± 0.05	**0.02**
Mesh + Landmarks		0.65 ± 0.01	0.59 ± 0.05	0.61 ± 0.04	0.58 ± 0.05	0.05

4 Experiments

Experimental Setup and Metrics. We conducted our experiments following a 5-fold cross-validation protocol. For each fold, models were trained on four partitions and evaluated on the remaining held-out split, ensuring that every sample is used for testing exactly once. We evaluated two different backbones, PointTransformerV3 and SPUNet, to provide a robust benchmark for future research. Both backbones were trained using identical data processing and augmentation strategies to ensure a fair and direct comparison.

Given the significant class imbalance inherent in clinical dental datasets, we selected the macro-averaged *F1-score* as our primary evaluation metric. This metric provides a balanced measure of a model's performance by calculating the F1-score for each class independently and then averaging them. In our context, such an approach ensures a more informative evaluation w.r.t. using the overall accuracy. For a more comprehensive analysis, particularly in our ablation studies, we also report accuracy, precision, recall, and model inference time.

On the Impact of Input Features. To determine the optimal input representation, we first conducted an ablation study on the input features. We compared the performance of models trained using three different input configurations: (*i*) the raw 3D mesh only, (*ii*) automatically-predicted landmark coordinates only, and (*iii*) a combination of both mesh and landmark features.

The results, summarized in Table 1, show that combining mesh and landmark features yields the best overall performance for both backbones, with PointTransformerV3 achieving the highest F1-score of 0.63 ± 0.03. Interestingly, using only landmark coordinates as input provides results that are only marginally lower than using the full mesh. This is a noteworthy finding, as the landmark-only models are exceptionally efficient; for instance, training takes approximately 15 minutes, compared to over 2 hours for models that process the entire mesh. Despite the efficiency of the landmark-only approach, to maximize performance, we chose configuration (*iii*) for all subsequent experiments.

Table 2. Ablation study on Multi-Task Learning (MTL) vs. Single-Task Learning (STL). All classification metrics are macro-averaged across the five occlusal tasks and reported as mean ± std (%) over the 5 cross-validation folds. Inference time is the average time in seconds to process a single scan.

Model	Learning Strategy	Accuracy	Precision	Recall	F1-Score	Time (s)
PointTr.V3	Single-Task (STL)	0.72 ± 0.13	0.66 ± 0.14	0.65 ± 0.14	0.64 ± 0.13	1.10
	Multi-Task (MTL)	0.71 ± 0.03	0.64 ± 0.03	0.64 ± 0.02	0.63 ± 0.03	0.11
SPUNet	Single-Task (STL)	0.67 ± 0.14	0.61 ± 0.13	0.61 ± 0.14	0.60 ± 0.13	0.50
	Multi-Task (MTL)	0.65 ± 0.01	0.59 ± 0.05	0.61 ± 0.04	0.58 ± 0.05	0.05

Table 3. Per-task F1-score (%) across occlusal classification tasks. Results are macro-averaged over 5-fold cross-validation and reported as mean ± std (%).

Model	Strategy	Right Occl.	Left Occl.	Anter. Bite	Tran. Bite	Midline	Avg.
PointTr.V3	STL	0.71 ± 0.05	0.67 ± 0.07	0.77 ± 0.14	0.59 ± 0.10	0.49 ± 0.06	0.64 ± 0.13
	MTL	0.69 ± 0.05	0.68 ± 0.04	0.74 ± 0.14	0.57 ± 0.12	0.46 ± 0.05	0.63 ± 0.03
SPUNet	STL	0.60 ± 0.02	0.57 ± 0.02	0.78 ± 0.13	0.58 ± 0.14	0.48 ± 0.04	0.62 ± 0.14
	MTL	0.54 ± 0.07	0.59 ± 0.04	0.68 ± 0.15	0.61 ± 0.15	0.51 ± 0.08	0.60 ± 0.13

Multi-task vs. Single-task Learning. Having established the optimal input features, we then evaluated the difference in performance between multi-task learning (MTL), i.e., a single backbone with a head for each different task, versus a single-task learning (STL) approach, i.e., a dedicated network (backbone + head) for each task. For this comparison, we trained five separate single-task models (one for each of our classification tasks) and evaluated their performance against that of our single, unified multi-task model.

As shown in Table 2, the STL approach, where each task is handled by a specialized model, achieves superior performance in terms of F1-score. However, this gain comes at a significant cost in computational resources and complexity. The STL strategy requires training and maintaining five distinct models per backbone, resulting in an increase in total training time and inference overhead compared to the unified MTL model. Table 3 provides a more granular, per-task breakdown of the F1-scores, confirming the strong performance of the STL models across the individual tasks.

These results present a clear trade-off: the MTL framework offers an efficient and scalable solution well-suited for clinical application where speed may be critical, while the STL approach can provide higher accuracy if computational cost is not a primary constraint. Across all experiments, the PointTransformerV3 backbone consistently outperformed SPUNet, establishing it as the more robust architecture for this problem domain.

Qualitative and Error Analysis. To better illustrate model performance beyond quantitative metrics, Fig. 5 shows example predictions from our test set, highlighting both successful classifications and common failure modes. These

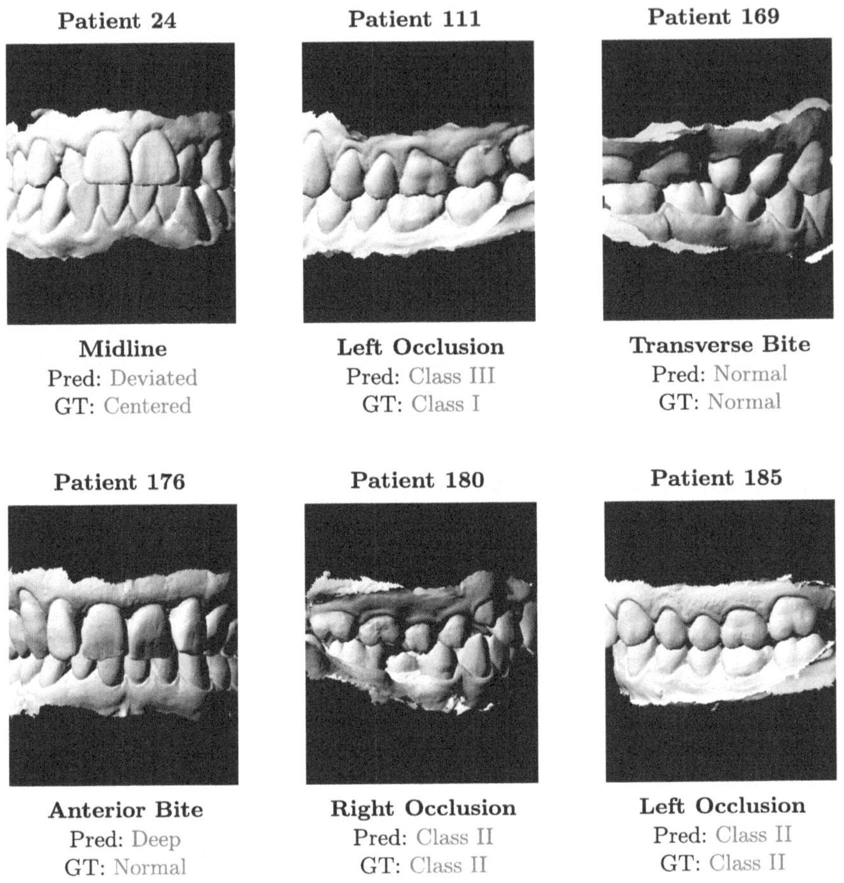

Patient 24

Midline
Pred: Deviated
GT: Centered

Patient 111

Left Occlusion
Pred: Class III
GT: Class I

Patient 169

Transverse Bite
Pred: Normal
GT: Normal

Patient 176

Anterior Bite
Pred: Deep
GT: Normal

Patient 180

Right Occlusion
Pred: Class II
GT: Class II

Patient 185

Left Occlusion
Pred: Class II
GT: Class II

Fig. 5. Qualitative analysis of PointTransformerV3 model predictions on various occlusal classification tasks. The figure showcases both correct classifications , where the model's prediction matches the ground truth, and failures , where the model misclassifies one task in the scan. Each example compares the model's prediction (Pred) with the expert-annotated ground truth (GT) for a specific patient from the test set.

visualizations provide insight into the models' ability to interpret complex inter-arch relationships and offer a qualitative understanding of their predictive behavior in challenging clinical cases.

5 Conclusion

In this paper, we introduced *Bits2Bites*, a novel benchmark for occlusal classification from intra-oral scans. We provided the first public dataset of 200 paired IOS scans with detailed, multi-dimensional clinical annotations. Our evaluation of state-of-the-art point cloud backbones within a multi-task learning framework demonstrates the feasibility of directly predicting multiple occlusal attributes from raw 3D point clouds. The results of our experiments lay the groundwork for developing automated tools that can assist orthodontists in diagnosis and treatment planning.

Future work will proceed in three main directions. First, we plan to expand the dataset to include a larger and more diverse cohort of patients, capturing a wider range of rare malocclusions. Second, we will validate the clinical annotations by involving multiple experts to establish inter-rater reliability, further strengthening the quality of the ground truth. Finally, once the dataset is enriched, support for the previously merged Class II edge-to-edge and Class II full sagittal classifications, as well as for tooth-level identification in crossbite and scissor bite cases, will be reinstated and fully integrated.

References

1. Ben-Hamadou, A., et al.: 3DTeethSeg'22: 3D teeth scan segmentation and labeling challenge. arXiv preprint arXiv:2305.18277 (2023)
2. Bolelli, F., et al.: Segmenting the inferior alveolar canal in CBCTs volumes: the ToothFairy challenge. IEEE Trans. Med. Imag. **44**(4), 1890–1906 (2024)
3. Bolelli, F., et al.: Segmenting maxillofacial structures in CBCT volumes. In: IEEE/CVF Conference on Computer Vision and Pattern Recognition (2025)
4. Cipriano, M., Allegretti, S., Bolelli, F., Di Bartolomeo, M., Pollastri, F., Pellacani, A., Minafra, P., Anesi, A., Grana, C.: Deep Segmentation of the Mandibular Canal: a New 3D Annotated Dataset of CBCT Volumes. IEEE Access (2022)
5. Cipriano, M., Allegretti, S., Bolelli, F., Pollastri, F., Grana, C.: Improving Segmentation of the Inferior Alveolar Nerve through Deep Label Propagation. In: IEEE/CVF Conference on Computer Vision and Pattern Recognition (2022)
6. Contributors, P.: Pointcept: a codebase for point cloud perception research. https://github.com/Pointcept/Pointcept (2023)
7. Cui, Z., et al.: a fully automatic AI system for tooth and alveolar bone segmentation from cone-beam CT images. Nature Commun. **13**(1) (2022)
8. Di Bartolomeo, M., et al.: Inferior alveolar canal automatic detection with deep learning CNNs on CBCTs: development of a novel model and release of open-source dataset and algorithm. Appl. Sci. **13**(5) (2023)
9. Graber, L.W., Vanarsdall, R.L., Vig, K.W., Huang, G.J.: Orthodontics: Current Principles and Techniques (1994)
10. Isensee, F., Kirchhoff, Y., Kraemer, L., Rokuss, M., Ulrich, C., Maier-Hein, K.H.: Scaling nnU-net for CBCT segmentation. In: Supervised and Semi-supervised Multi-structure Segmentation and Landmark Detection in Dental Data (2025)
11. Juneja, M., Saini, S.K., Kaur, H., Jindal, P.: Application of convolutional neural networks for dentistry occlusion classification. Wireless Personal Commun. **136**(3) (2024)
12. Liu, X., Liu, X., Liu, Y.S., Han, Z.: SPU-Net: self-supervised point cloud upsampling by coarse-to-fine reconstruction with self-projection optimization. IEEE Trans. Image Process. **31** (2022)
13. Lumetti, L., Pipoli, V., Bolelli, F., Ficarra, E., Grana, C.: Enhancing patch-based learning for the segmentation of the mandibular canal. IEEE Access **12** (2024)

14. Ma, Q., et al.: Video foundation model for medical 3D segmentation. In: Supervised and Semi-supervised Multi-structure Segmentation and Landmark Detection in Dental Data (2025)
15. van Nistelrooij, N., Vinayahalingam, S.: ToothInstanceNet: comprehensive information from intra-oral scans by integration of large-context and high-resolution predictions. In: Supervised and Semi-supervised Multi-structure Segmentation and Landmark Detection in Dental Data (2025)
16. Rekik, A., Ben-Hamadou, A., Smaoui, O., Bouzguenda, F., Pujades, S., Boyer, E.: TSegLab: multi-stage 3D dental scan segmentation and labeling. Comput. Biol. Med. **185** (2025)
17. Wang, C., et al.: MMDental-a multimodal dataset of tooth CBCT images with expert medical records. Sci. Data **12**(1) (2025)
18. Wu, X., et al.: Point Transformer V3: simpler, faster, stronger. In: IEEE/CVF Conference on Computer Vision and Pattern Recognition (2024)
19. Zou, B., et al.: Teeth-SEG: an efficient instance segmentation framework for orthodontic treatment based on anthropic prior knowledge. In: IEEE/CVF Conference on Computer Vision and Pattern Recognition (2024)

Extended Partial Angle Based Motion Compensation for Dental CBCT

Cristina Sarti, Mikhail Mikerov, and Claudio Landi(✉)

See Through S.r.l, via Bolgara 2, 24060 Brusaporto BG, Italy
{cristina.sarti,claudio.landi}@seethrough.one

Abstract. Motion artifacts can degrade image quality in dental cone-beam CT and complicate diagnosis. In some cases, an exam retake is necessary, resulting in additional radiation exposure for the patient, without any guarantee of improved image quality. Therefore, motion compensation methods play a crucial role. Many methods are time-consuming since they require several reconstructions. We propose a very efficient method that requires only two partial-angle reconstructions. It assumes that the patient remains still during the acquisition, except for a short interval. In this situation, two motion-free partial-angle reconstructions, one before and one after patient motion, can be reconstructed. Motion compensation is achieved by registering forward projections of the two volumes. To enhance the robustness of the registration step, we simulate an extended angular range covered by the two partial volumes using a conditioned U-Net trained on a target-specific dataset. Qualitative analysis shows that we can significantly reduce the appearance of motion artifacts even in the case of challenging motion patterns.

Keywords: Dental CBCT · Motion compensation · Partial-angle reconstruction · Angular range extension

1 Introduction

Dental cone-beam CT (CBCT) is a fully 3D imaging modality that provides accurate volumetric images of the oral cavity. Its applications include implant planning, detection of caries and periodontal diseases, orthodontic treatment, and exodontics [9]. A typical dental CBCT device consists of a C-arm with mounted x-ray source and detector on the opposite sides, which can rotate in the horizontal plane around the patient's head. The patient can either stand or sit, although the standing position is more common. During the scan, the patient's chin is resting on a chin rest, the head is stabilized using head fixation, and the patient's arms hold a handle to minimize body movement. Additionally, the patient may be asked to bite on a bite block that is attached to the chin rest for more stability. The absence of motion is crucial for good image quality since image reconstruction algorithms rely on a well defined geometry at each acquisition step.

F. Bolelli et al. (Eds.): ODIN 2025, LNCS 16473, pp. 55–63, 2026.
https://doi.org/10.1007/978-3-032-20711-1_6

Despite fixation, the patient can still move during scans with a typical duration between 5 and 40 s. The images affected by motion artifacts are often characterized by blurry edges, undefined contours or doubled appearance of structures [7]. Due to the ALARA[1] principle, image retakes should be avoided to reduce radiation dose even at the cost of image quality. Therefore, it becomes important to be able to reduce the appearance of motion artifacts in the image domain using non-optimal projection data.

Several solutions have been proposed in recent years to perform motion correction in dental CBCT. One class of such solutions relies on additional motion tracking hardware installed on the C-arm that enables the estimation of the motion direction and amplitude to modify the projection data [11]. These solutions are rarely used in clinical practice, since they increase device costs and complicate installation, calibration, and maintenance.

Another class of solutions relies on extracting the necessary motion parameters from the acquired projection data and imperfect reconstructions. Sun *et al.* proposed an iterative joint motion estimation and image update method [12]. Maur *et al.* estimates the motion parameters by detecting, reconstructing and forward projecting the contours of anatomical features [6]. Autofocus approaches aiming to improve some metric in the image domain, e.g., image sharpness in the bone region, have also been applied to this problem [10].

Previously, we presented an approach for motion compensation based on the registration of two volumes reconstructed using only limited angular ranges [8].We assumed that the patient remained still in an initial position, then briefly moved and remained still in a second position. We reconstructed two partial volumes corresponding to the two motion-free segments of the full scan and we added the projections affected by motion to one of the two volumes. In general, very little common information is present in both volumes since they are reconstructed using non-overlapping projection data. However, if two volumes do share common edges, it is possible to register their forward-projected data to estimate more reliably the motion parameters needed for correction. By excluding the projections affected by motion from both reconstructions can also have a positive impact on the final motion parameter estimation, especially if the motion duration exceeds one second.

In this work, we extend and optimize our previous method. We exclude the motion-affected projections from each partial reconstruction and incorporate a conditioned U-Net to modify partial-angle reconstructions to cover a larger angular range, thus increasing the amount of common features when the volumes are forward projected.

2 Materials and Methods

In this section, we provide details about all the steps of our motion compensation method. These steps include generation of two partial-angle reconstructions,

[1] As Low As Reasonably Achievable.

optimization of the motion compensation parameters with 2D-3D registration and training and application of a conditioned U-Net for volume modification in the image domain.

2.1 Geometric Calibration

During installation, a CBCT device is usually calibrated with an offline calibration process. A geometric calibration using specially designed phantoms is performed to calculate so-called *projection matrices* corresponding to each detector position i of a total of N positions assumed by the C-arm during the X-ray scan. They contain the parameters describing the projection geometry of the 3D patient head onto the 2D detector. Each matrix $P_i \in \mathbb{R}^{3\times4}$ can be written as a product of two matrices:

$$P_i = K \cdot G_i, \quad i = 0, \ldots, N. \tag{1}$$

The matrix $G_i = [R_i|t_i] \in \mathbb{R}^{4\times4}$ contains the extrinsic parameters, i.e., the parameters describing the relative translation and rotation of the X-ray source with respect to the patient's position. The matrix $K \in \mathbb{R}^{3\times4}$ contains the intrinsic parameters of the projections such as the source-detector-distance, the detector origin and the pixel size [4].

Patient motion during acquisition can partially or entirely invalidate the parameters estimated during calibration. The goal of motion compensation is to restore a correct geometry and to output an artifact-free reconstruction. To reach this goal, our method calculates a transformation matrix $G_i{}' = [R_i{}'|t_i{}'] \in \mathbb{R}^{4\times4}$ for each device position i such that

$$P_i{}' = K \cdot G_i \cdot G_i{}', \quad i = 0, \ldots, N. \tag{2}$$

The matrix $G_i{}'$ contains the rotation and translation parameters that best compensate for patient motion.

2.2 Partial-Angle Reconstruction

Similarly to our perviously proposed method [8], we perform motion compensation by partial-angle volume registration. With *partial-angle reconstruction* we describe a reconstruction that only includes a small subset of the full set of projections collected during a scan. Figure 1 compares a complete reconstruction and a partial-angle reconstruction covering 60 degrees. Both volumes are reconstructed using the Feldkamp-Devis-Kress (FDK) algorithm [3]. The partial-angle reconstruction shows artifacts due to the fact that only the information contained in a small subset of the projections is reconstructed.

In our approach, we assume that the patient remains still during the first portion of the scan, then moves and remains still in a new position during the final part of the scan. In our previous method, we registered the two partial-angle volumes assuming that the portion of the scan affected by motion was

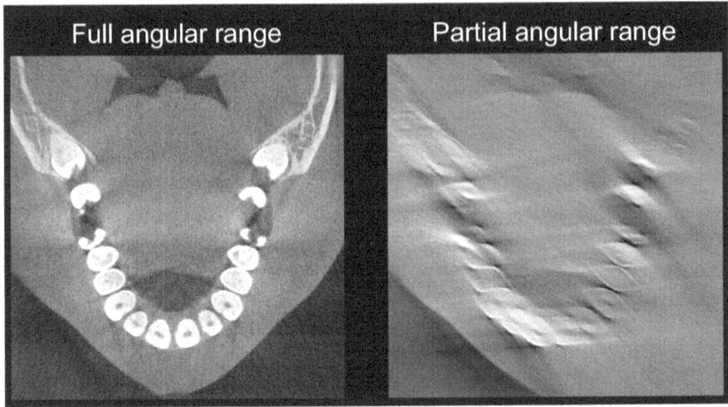

Fig. 1. Complete reconstruction and partial-angle reconstruction (60°).

small compared to the one or the other partial reconstruction. So, we included the projections affected by motion in one or in the other reconstruction. The method turned out to be very robust for abrupt motion covering 0.5 s but reliability decreased for motion exceeding 1 s.

To be able to compensate for longer motion, we propose a new strategy and modify some of the steps to generate the reference partial-angle reconstructions and to perform registration: (1) The projections affected by motion are no longer included in one of the partial reconstructions. This means that two partial-angle reconstructions are obtained using only motion-free projection data acquired before and after patient motion. The angular gap between the two partial reconstruction corresponds to the motion extent. (2) In order to extend the angular range covered by each partial volume, we apply a suitably trained U-Net. We simulate the addition of projections within the angular gap to each of the two original partial volumes. This leads to a higher number of common structures and stabilizes the subsequent 2D-3D registration step.

2.3 Conditioned U-Net

U-Nets are widely used for image-to-image translations in medical imaging. We apply a U-Net architecture to transform partial-angle reconstructions obtained from data acquired over a limited angular range $\Delta\theta$, so that they approximate reconstructions covering a slightly extended range $\Delta\theta + \Delta\phi$. In general, the appearance of the partial volumes will vary depending on whether the additional angular range $\Delta\phi$ is added before the first or after the last angle in the initial reconstruction. We control the output of the network by defining the side to which the additional angular range should be added.

Architecture. For this task, we added a control mechanism in form of simple Feature-wise Linear Modulation (simple FiLM) layers to the encoder block of a standard 3D U-Net working on 3D patches [2]. The simple FiLM layer is an additional fully connected layer in each double convolution block that receives an indicator of extension direction as either 0 or 1 and outputs two scalars, the multiplicative factor γ and the offset β. They are used to modify the output of the block. The network's architecture is displayed in Fig. 2.

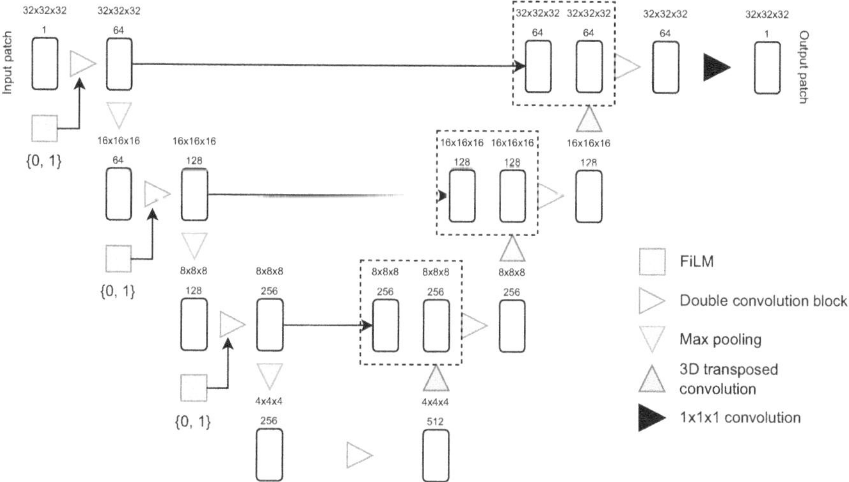

Fig. 2. Architecture of a 3D U-Net with simple FiLM modulation layers. Black arrows represent skip connections; dashed rectangles represent data concatenation. Patch size and number of channels are displayed above each patch.

Dataset Preparation. Dental cone-beam CT data is characterized by high variability. For example, some patients may have implants, crowns, or other metal inserts which can lead to significant image artifacts even without motion. Moreover, missing teeth are a common pathology. The operator can influence the image, too, by instructing the patient to bite on a bite block, thereby introducing an additional visible structure into the scan. Finally, another source of variability is the time point at which the patient moves and the motion extent. We constructed our dataset to account for as much variability as possible.

We started by selecting seven highly variable patients. Then, we randomly sampled the starting projection number of a partial-angle reconstruction from a uniform distribution of possible projection numbers. If the projection number was too close to an already added projection number in the dataset, it was not included. Finally, for each angle, we randomly assigned one of the seven patients. Figure 3 displays the distribution of the input volumes corresponding to the selected patients and projection numbers in the dataset. The same reconstruction is included twice in the dataset if it can be extended in both directions. Otherwise, it appears in the dataset only once.

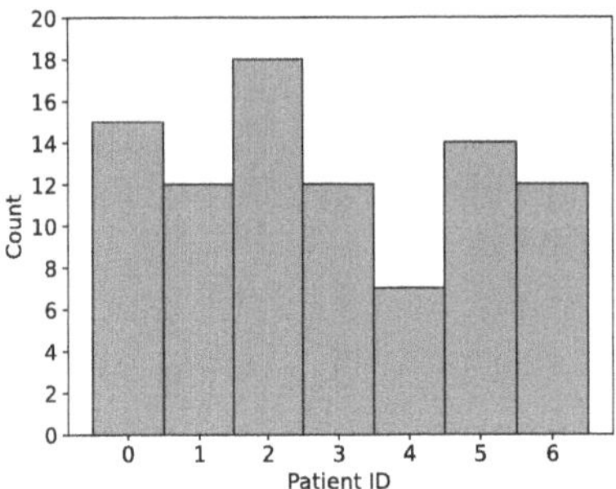

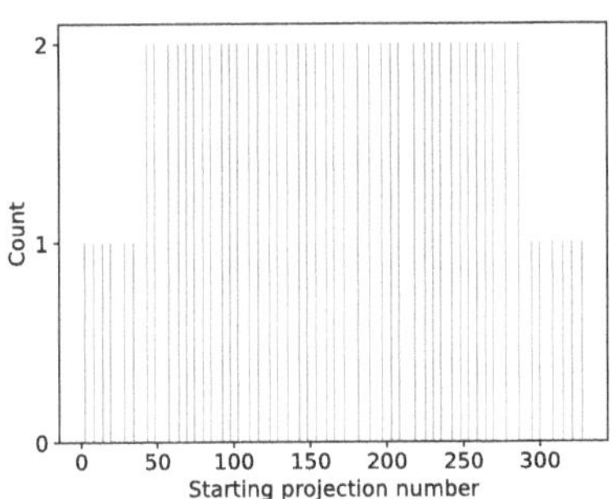

Fig. 3. Left: number of input images in the dataset per patient. Right: number of input images in the dataset per starting projection number in the partial-angle reconstruction.

Training. The conditioned U-Net was trained using PyTorch's automatic mixed precision package with early stopping regularization for 13 epochs on $32 \times 32 \times 32$ patches with stride 16 in all three directions. The patches were extracted from $316 \times 316 \times 344$ volumes with 320 mm voxel size. The training dataset contained reconstructions from the first six patients. The learning rate of the Adam optimizer was set to 0.0001. No learning scheduler was used. We used MSE loss as a cost function for this task. The data of the seventh patient were used for validation.

2.4 Partial-Angle Reconstruction Registration

After modification using the U-Net, the two partial-angle volumes share common structures corresponding to the data within the angular gap. The volumes are normalized and binarized by applying an experimentally estimated threshold. This operation enables the extraction of hard tissue structures like bones and teeth and the removal of soft tissues and possible artifacts that could affect the subsequent registration process. The binarized volumes are forward projected at M sampling positions within the gap. For each position j, we have pair of projections (r_j, r'_j) defined as

$$r_j = P_j \cdot V_I, \quad r_j{}' = P_j \cdot G_j{}' \cdot V_{II}, \quad j = 1, \ldots, M. \tag{3}$$

The volumes V_I and V_{II} are the partial volumes. The matrix P_j is the projection matrix that corresponds to the acquisition position j. The compensation matrix $G_j{}'$ is defined in Eq. (2).

The process of retrieving the parameters of $G_j{}'$ is formulated as a minimization problem. Since small translations can be well approximated by small rotations [5] we limit our estimation to the rotation parameters (rX, rY, rZ). As explained in [8] we start the minimization process by extracting hard tissue edges on the forward-projected images. We apply a gradient operator $\boldsymbol{\nabla} = (\nabla_x, \nabla_y)$ and generate corresponding gradient images $(\boldsymbol{\nabla} r_j, \boldsymbol{\nabla} r_j{}')$. We define the cost function $\Phi(\nabla r_j, \nabla r_j')$ as explained in [8] and for each sampling position j we retrieve the entries of the matrix $G_j{}'$ repeating the 2D-3D registration step until the function Φ reaches a minimum.

The final matrix used to align V_I and V_{II} is the average of the matrices estimated for each position $j = 1, \ldots, M$. To correct the motion-affected projections within the angular gap and to ensure a smooth transition between the first and the second part of the final volume, we linearly interpolate the values from 0 to (rX, rY, rZ) across the angular gap.

3 Data

We tested our method with real patient data acquired using the CBCT device Seethrough Max (See Through s.r.l, Brusaporto, Italy). The acquisitions lasted 14 s and covered an angle slightly larger than 180 degrees. The size of the reconstructed field of view is 10×11 centimeters. Since the collected data did not present motion artifacts, we simulated different motion patterns (nodding, tilting, axial rotation, translation) and durations modifying the projection matrices at some angular points. We used the strategy described in [1]. We particularly focused on movements of about 1.5–2.0 s duration for which our previously implemented method did not perform reliably. Furthermore, we focused on movements that occurred either at the very beginning or the very end of the acquisition, as these are especially challenging to compensate for. In the next section, we present exemplary results for three cases: (1) nodding or axial rotation with translation (1.5 s); (2) combined nodding, tilting, axial rotation, and translation (1.5 s); (3) nodding only (2 s). A comparison with our previous method [8] is also provided.

4 Results

On the left, Fig. 4 shows the results of our motion compensation method for Case 1. Strong motion as a combination of a single rotation (nodding, axial rotation) and a translation was simulated. In both cases artifacts are almost fully corrected or strongly attenuated even in the case that the patient has metal inserts. The same can be observed for more complicated types of motion resulting from a combination of rotations (nodding, tilting, axial rotation) and a translation (Case 2). Also in this case, artifacts could be almost completely corrected or significantly attenuated, as shown in Fig 4 on the right. Finally, we compared our current approach with our previous method. Figure 5 shows that the current method also performs very well in the case of a longer nodding motion of about 2 s (Case 3).

5 Discussion and Conclusion

In this paper, we present a robust optimized method to compensate for motion in dental CBCT images. The current method preserves the advantages of the

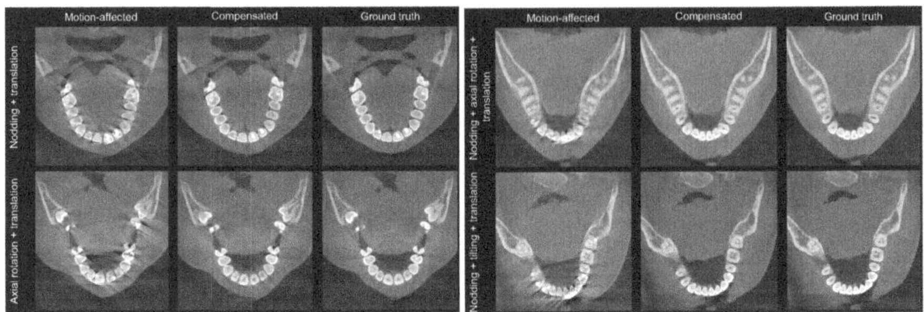

Fig. 4. Left: Case 1. Right: Case 2.

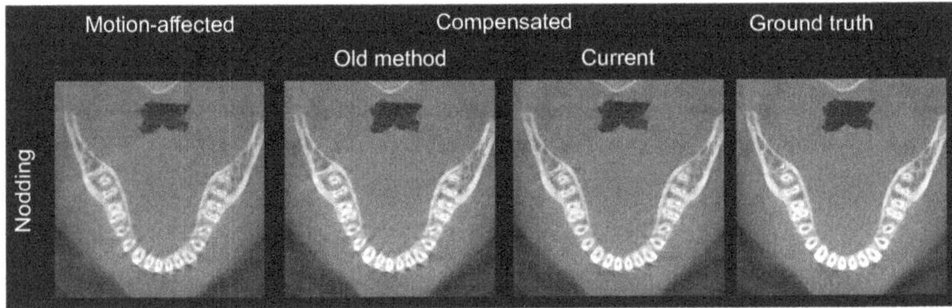

Fig. 5. Case 3.

previous method [8]. It is robust and fast, since only forward-projected data are registered and only two partial-angle volumes are reconstructed. Very few projections, taken at predefined sampling angles within the angular gap, are necessary for the 2D-3D registration process to recover the motion compensation parameters. The novelty of the current approach relies on a combination of our previous strategy with a deep learning approach. With a suitably trained conditioned U-Net, we could modify each partial-angle volume to cover a larger angular range. In this way, we were able to compensate for longer and more complex motion patterns

Our current results are very promising and suggest the possibility of using the optimized method to compensate for motions longer than two seconds. It is also conceivable to apply the method to compensate for artifacts due to multiple motion patterns. Multiple partial-angle volumes could be reconstructed and iteratively aligned using the motion compensation approach. Once motion artifacts are sufficiently compensated, the diagnostic quality of the final fully reconstructed volume may be restored. Finally, additional experiments are necessary involving various patient pathologies and various types of motion to determine whether some data types and artifacts are more challenging to compensate for than others.

Acknowledgments. The authors thank Lorenzo Arici, Andrea Delmiglio, Luca Fracassetti, and Ivan Tomba for their valuable contributions to the implementation of the reconstruction library.

Disclosure of Interests. C. Sarti, M. Mikerov, and C. Landi are employed by See Through s.r.l.

References

1. Asraf Ali, A.S.R., Fusiello, A., Landi, C., Sarti, C., Siswadi, A.A.P.: Motion artifacts detection in short-scan dental cbct reconstructions. arXiv preprint arXiv:2304.10154 (2023)
2. Brocal, G.M., Peeters, G.: Conditioned-u-net: introducing a control mechanism in the u-net for multiple source separations (2019). https://doi.org/10.5281/ZENODO.3527766. https://zenodo.org/record/3527766
3. Feldkamp, L.A., Davis, L.C., Kress, J.W.: Practical cone-beam algorithm. Josa A **1**(6), 612–619 (1984)
4. Hartley, R., Zisserman, A.: Multiple View Geometry in Computer Vision. Cambridge University Press, Cambridge (2004). https://books.google.fr/books?id=e30hAwAAQBAJ
5. Hernandez, J., Eldib, M., Hegazy, M., Cho, M., Cho, M., Lee, S.: A head-motion estimation algorithm for motion artifact correction in dental ct imaging. Phys. Med. Biol. **63** (2018). https://doi.org/10.1088/1361-6560/aab17e
6. Maur, S., Stsepankou, D., Hesser, J.: CBCT auto-calibration by contour registration. In: Schmidt, T.G., Chen, G.H., Bosmans, H. (eds.) Medical Imaging 2019: Physics of Medical Imaging, vol. 10948, p. 109481N. International Society for Optics and Photonics, SPIE (2019). https://doi.org/10.1117/12.2512181
7. Moratin, J., et al.: Head motion during cone-beam computed tomography: analysis of frequency and influence on image quality. Imaging Sci. Dent. **50**(3), 227–236 (2020). https://doi.org/10.5624/isd.2020.50.3.227
8. Sarti, C., Mikerov, M., Landi, C.: Single motion compensation by fast partial volume registration in dental cbct. In: Proceedings of the 18th International Meeting on Fully Three-Dimensional Image Reconstruction in Radiology and Nuclear Medicine (2025)
9. Schulze, R., Drage, N.: Cone-beam computed tomography and its applications in dental and maxillofacial radiology. Clin. Radiol. **75**(9), 647–657 (2020). https://doi.org/10.1016/j.crad.2020.04.006
10. Sisniega, A., Stayman, J.W., Yorkston, J., Siewerdsen, J., Zbijewski, W.: Motion compensation in extremity cone-beam ct using a penalized image sharpness criterion. Phys. Med. Biol. **62**(9), 3712 (2017)
11. Spin-Neto, R., Matzen, L.H., Schropp, L.W., Sørensen, T.S., Wenzel, A.: An ex vivo study of automated motion artefact correction and the impact on cone beam ct image quality and interpretability. Dentomaxillofacial Radiol. **47**(5), 20180013 (2018). https://doi.org/10.1259/dmfr.20180013
12. Sun, T., Jacobs, R., Pauwels, R., Tijskens, E., Fulton, R., Nuyts, J.: A motion correction approach for oral and maxillofacial cone-beam ct imaging. Phys. Med. Biol. **66**(12), 125008 (2021). https://doi.org/10.1088/1361-6560/abfa38

Landmarks Are Alike Yet Distinct: Harnessing Similarity and Individuality for One-Shot Medical Landmark Detection

Xu He[1,2], Zhen Huang[3,4], Qingsong Yao[5], Xiaoqian Zhou[1,2], and S. Kevin Zhou[1,2](✉)

[1] School of Biomedical Engineering, Division of Life Sciences and Medicine, University of Science and Technology of China, Hefei 230026, Anhui, People's Republic of China
skevinzhou@ustc.edu.cn

[2] Suzhou Institute for Advanced Research, University of Science and Technology of China, Suzhou 215123, Jiangsu, People's Republic of China

[3] School of Computer Science and Technology, University of Science and Technology of China, Hefei 230026, Anhui, People's Republic of China

[4] School of Information Science and Technology, Eastern Institute of Technology (EIT), Ningbo 315200, Zhejiang, People's Republic of China

[5] Stanford University, Palo Alto, CA 94305, USA

Abstract. Landmark detection plays a crucial role in medical imaging applications such as disease diagnosis, bone age estimation, and therapy planning. However, training models for detecting multiple landmarks simultaneously often encounters the "seesaw phenomenon", where improvements in detecting certain landmarks lead to declines in detecting others. Yet, training a separate model for each landmark increases memory usage and computational overhead. To address these challenges, we propose a novel approach based on the belief that "landmarks are distinct" by training models with pseudo-labels and template data updated continuously during the training process, where each model is dedicated to detecting a single landmark to achieve high accuracy. Furthermore, grounded on the belief that "landmarks are also alike", we introduce an adapter-based fusion model, combining shared weights with landmark-specific weights, to efficiently share model parameters while allowing flexible adaptation to individual landmarks. This approach not only significantly reduces memory and computational resource requirements but also effectively mitigates the seesaw phenomenon in multi-landmark training. Experimental results on publicly available medical image datasets demonstrate that the single-landmark models significantly outperform traditional multi-point joint training models in detecting individual landmarks. Although our adapter-based fusion model shows slightly lower performance compared to the combined results of all single-landmark models, it still surpasses the current state-of-the-art methods while achieving a notable improvement in resource efficiency.

X. He and Z. Huang—Contribute equally to this work.

F. Bolelli et al. (Eds.): ODIN 2025, LNCS 16473, pp. 64–75, 2026.
https://doi.org/10.1007/978-3-032-20711-1_7

Keywords: Medical landmark detection · One-shot learning

1 Introduction

Accurate medical landmark detection (MLD) has widespread applications in clinical settings, such as disease diagnosis [6,20,26], bone age estimation [4], and therapy planning [1,23]. It also supports various downstream tasks, such as segmentation [14,17], image reconstruction [11], and image registration [5]. With the rapid development of deep learning [9,16], many neural network-based models have been proposed for MLD. For instance, [21] employs a prototypical network for MLD by comparing image features with landmark prototypes, while [28] incorporates dynamic sparse attention into a hybrid Transformer-CNN architecture. However, despite the superior performance of these methods, they generally rely on a large amount of labeled data, which poses a significant challenge due to the time-consuming and labor-intensive annotation process. To address this issue, some studies have proposed *one-shot learning* methods, which use a single annotated medical image for landmark detection [13,24,25].

MLD is typically formulated as a multi-label task, where traditional methods often train a single model to detect all landmarks, sharing the same network weights and thus ignoring the individuality of different landmarks. Since different landmarks may have distinct features and local variations, training them in the same network may lead to the so-called "seesaw phenomenon" [19], that is, improving the detection of certain landmarks could degrade the performance of others. In multi-task learning [27], some studies have used hard parameter sharing [2] to facilitate joint learning. [8] introduced the Mixture of Experts (MoE) model, which shares some experts at the bottom layers and combines them through a gating network. [19] proposed Progressive Layered Extraction (PLE) to alleviate the seesaw phenomenon. Inspired by these approaches, we introduce the concept of multi-task learning into landmark detection and propose a novel single-landmark approach (SLA) to harness the *landmark individuality* and improve the accuracy of one-shot landmark detection.

We use the Cascade Comparing to Detect (CC2D) framework [24], a pioneering one-shot MLD method, as the foundation and propose the CC2D-SLA method, which eliminates the interdependencies between different landmarks by training a separate model for each landmark, thereby addressing the seesaw phenomenon at its core. Our experiments demonstrate that CC2D-SLA brings improved MLD accuracy over CC2D. To further enhance the detection accuracy of each landmark, we leverage the idea of augmented template data (ATD) [7], which leads to an improved SLA method called CC2D-SLA-ATD.

However, both CC2D-SLA and CC2D-SLA-ATD require training a separate model for each landmark, which leads to a substantial computational overhead. To address the issue of resource inefficiency and redundancy bought by multiple single-landmark models and further mitigate the seesaw phenomenon, we introduce an adapter to harness the *landmark similarity and individuality*. By combining shared weights with landmark-specific weights, we enable the model

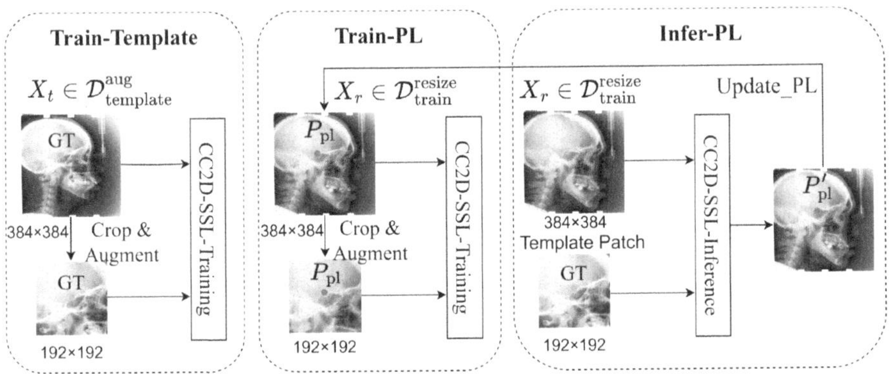

Fig. 1. Training framework of CC2D-SLA-ATD, which consists of three stages at each epoch: Train-Template, Train-PL, and Infer-PL. CC2D-SLA training, on the other hand, is composed of only the Train-PL and Infer-PL stages.

to learn the features of all landmarks through a single end-to-end model. Ultimately, this leads to the proposed CC2D-SLA-ATD-Adapter method, which not only reduces computational and memory overhead but also maintains high precision in landmark detection performance.

We evaluate our models on the ISBI 2015 Challenge dataset [20]. Experimental results show that the single-landmark models significantly outperform traditional multi-point joint training models in landmark detection. Although our adapter-based fusion model (CC2D-SLA-ATD-Adapter) slightly underperforms compared to the best results from combining all single-landmark models, it still outperforms the current state-of-the-art (SOTA), demonstrating the potential of our method for medical imaging applications.

2 Method

Below, we first introduce CC2D-SLA and its improved variant, CC2D-SLA-ATD. We then describe how to integrate the adapter. Finally, we present the architecture of our CC2D-SLA-ATD-Adapter. Figure 1 shows the training framework.

2.1 CC2D-SLA

The training of CC2D-SLA in each epoch consists of two stages: 1) Train-PL, in which the model is trained using pseudo-labels (PLs), and 2) Infer-PL, in which the pseudo-labels are inferred and updated.

Train-PL Stage. Let $\mathcal{D}_{\text{train}}$ be the training dataset. We first resize all images to 384×384, forming the resized set $\mathcal{D}^{\text{resize}}_{\text{train}}$. Initially, each image $X_r \in \mathcal{D}^{\text{resize}}_{\text{train}}$ is assigned a random pseudo-label $P_{pl} = (x_{pl}, y_{pl})$. As training proceeds, these pseudo-labels are updated at the end of each epoch. During the Train-PL stage, for each image X_r, we first crop a patch centered at P_{pl} and then apply data augmentation to obtain X_p. Both X_r and X_p are subsequently used as inputs to the CC2D-SSL framework in its training stage, referred to as CC2D-SSL-Training. Note that CC2D-SSL-Training encompasses the entire training pipeline of CC2D-SSL after receiving the image inputs, and is distinct from our CC2D-SLA approach. Here, we simply replace the typical input of CC2D-SSL-Training with the pair (X_r, X_p) to train on the PL-based patches.

Infer-PL Stage. After one pass through the training set, the model enters the Infer-PL stage to update the pseudo-labels. We denote CC2D-SSL-Inference as the complete inference pipeline of the CC2D-SSL framework. Specifically, for a given landmark ID k, a template patch X_{tp} is cropped from the template image around the ground-truth location of the k-th landmark. Next, every image $X_r \in \mathcal{D}_{\text{train}}^{\text{resize}}$ serves as a query image. We feed (X_{tp}, X_r) into the CC2D-SLA-Inference module to infer the new pseudo-label P'_{pl} for the k-th landmark on X_r. Thus, all pseudo-labels in $\mathcal{D}_{\text{train}}^{\text{resize}}$ are updated at the end of the epoch.

CC2D-SLA-ATD. In CC2D-SLA, training relies on pseudo-labels generated from a single template image. To better utilize the template data, we perform data augmentation on the template, following the procedure in FM-OSD [13]. Specifically, we apply random shifting, rotation, and scaling to produce 500 augmented versions of the template, forming the dataset $\mathcal{D}_{\text{template}}^{\text{aug}}$.

As illustrated in Fig. 1, for each augmented template image $X_t \in \mathcal{D}_{\text{template}}^{\text{aug}}$, we crop a patch centered at its ground-truth location and apply additional data augmentation to obtain X_{tp}. We then feed X_t and X_{tp} into the CC2D-SSL-Training pipeline. We refer to this procedure as the Train-Template stage, which is prepended to CC2D-SLA to get CC2D-SLA-ATD.

2.2 Adapter Integration for Multi-landmark Training

To address the seesaw phenomenon and the resource inefficiency of multiple single-landmark models, we introduce adapter layers into our network. By incorporating adapters, all landmarks can be jointly trained using shared and landmark-specific weights, while ensuring only minor performance degradation.

Pre-adapter Feature Extraction. As shown in the upper-left part of Fig. 2, without adapters, a feature map F_i of shape $H \times W \times C$ is transformed by a convolutional layer $Conv$, yielding $F_{i+1} \in \mathbb{R}^{H \times W \times C'}$: $F_{i+1} = Conv(F_i)$.

Adapter-Incorporated Layers. After integrating adapters, each landmark k has its own dedicated convolution $Conv^{A_k}$ alongside the shared convolution $Conv$. The primary difference lies in the output channel dimension: $Conv^{A_k}$ produces a feature map $F_{i+1}^{A_k} \in \mathbb{R}^{H \times W \times C_A}$, where C_A (e.g., 16) is typically

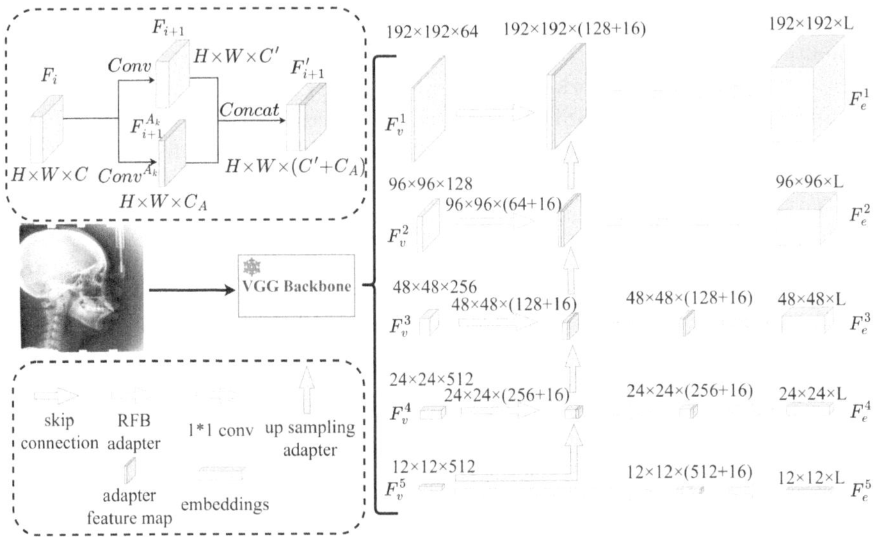

Fig. 2. Network architecture of CC2D-SLA-ATD-Adapter. The upper-left part of the figure shows an illustration of the adapter-based feature map transformation.

much smaller than C'. Formally, $F_{i+1}^{A_k} = Conv^{A_k}(F_i)$. We then concatenate F_{i+1} and $F_{i+1}^{A_k}$ along the channel dimension to obtain

$$F'_{i+1} = \text{Concat}\big(F_{i+1}, F_{i+1}^{A_k}\big) = \text{Concat}\Big(Conv(F_i),\, Conv^{A_k}(F_i)\Big), \tag{1}$$

where $F'_{i+1} \in \mathbb{R}^{H \times W \times (C'+C_A)}$. Equation (1) is simplified as $F'_{i+1} = C^{A_k}(F_i)$. Consequently, the subsequent layer's input channel size is adjusted to $C' + C_A$.

In this scheme, $Conv$ captures shared features across all landmarks, while $Conv^{A_k}$ learns landmark-specific features, activated only during training or inference of landmark k. This design alleviates the seesaw phenomenon, and enables landmark-specific learning without affecting others.

Adapters allow joint training of multiple landmarks, reducing the need for separate models for each, thus improving memory and computational efficiency. This shared-plus-specific design balances accuracy and resource usage, maintaining performance when scaling to multiple landmarks.

2.3 CC2D-SLA-ATD-Adapter

By enhancing CC2D-SLA-ATD with an adapter, we achieve CC2D-SLA-ATD-Adapter, enabling multi-landmark training while mitigating the seesaw phenomenon and improving overall performance.

As illustrated in Fig. 2, for an input image X of size 384×384, we use a pretrained VGG [18] network to extract five layers of feature maps: $F_v = \{F_v^1, F_v^2, \ldots, F_v^5\} = \text{VGG}(X)$. Here, F_v^5 is the deepest layer. We adopt the same

VGG19 model [18] pretrained on ImageNet [3] as in CC2D [24], and keep its weights frozen throughout training. Following [15], each upsampled feature map is concatenated with the corresponding lower-level feature map. Specifically,

$$F_{\text{concat}}^{i} = \text{Concat}\Big(\text{Up}(F_c^{i+1}),\ F_v^{i}\Big), \quad i = 1, 2, 3, 4. \tag{2}$$

Here, F_c is the feature map obtained by applying the adapter-based convolution:

$$F_c^{i} = C^{A_k}\big(F_{\text{concat}}^{i}\big), \quad i = 1, 2, 3, 4, \tag{3}$$

We set $F_c^5 = F_v^5$ to represent the deepest layer (where no upsampling occurs).

In CC2D [24], the third, fourth, and fifth layers employ Receptive Field Block (RFB) modules [10] to enlarge the receptive field. We also integrate adapters into the RFB modules by replacing the $Conv$ and $Conv^{A_k}$ modules with RFB and RFB^{A_k}, then concatenate their outputs. Formally,

$$F_{RFB}^{i} = R^{A_k}\big(F_c^{i}\big) = \text{Concat}\Big(\text{RFB}(F_c^{i}),\ \text{RFB}^{\text{A}_\text{k}}(F_c^{i})\Big), \quad i = 3, 4, 5, \tag{4}$$

where F_{RFB}^{i} is the resulting feature map after applying the RFB with adapters.

Finally, each feature map is passed through a 1×1 convolution to yield a fixed-dimensional embedding F_e^i. In particular,

$$F_e^{i} = \begin{cases} \text{Conv}_{1\times1}\big(F_c^{i}\big), & \text{if } i = 1, 2, \\ \text{Conv}_{1\times1}\big(F_{RFB}^{i}\big), & \text{if } i = 3, 4, 5. \end{cases} \tag{5}$$

3 Experiments

3.1 Settings

Dataset. For this study, we use the widely recognized IEEE ISBI 2015 Challenge dataset [20], which contains 400 radiographs annotated with 19 landmarks by two expert clinicians. The average of their annotations serves as the ground truth. The images are 1935 × 2400 pixels with a 0.1 mm pixel spacing. The dataset is split into 150 training and 250 testing images. One image is selected as the template, and the others are treated as unlabeled data for model training.

Evaluation Metrics. We evaluate the model performance using two common metrics: Mean Radial Error (MRE) and Successful Detection Rate (SDR). MRE calculates the average Euclidean distance between predicted landmarks and ground truth. SDR measures the proportion of landmarks detected within various thresholds (2 mm, 2.5 mm, 3 mm, and 4 mm) from the ground truth. These metrics are widely used in previous studies on landmark detection [13,24,29].

Table 1. Performance comparison of different methods on the Head [20] dataset.

Method	Model Count	MRE(↓) (mm)	SDR(↑)(%)			
			2 mm	2.5 mm	3 mm	4 mm
SAM [22]	1	2.56	54.11	63.66	70.25	80.84
UOD [29]	1	2.43	51.14	62.37	74.40	86.49
CC2D [24]	1	2.04	62.46	71.62	80.00	89.45
FM-OSD(coarse) [13]	1	1.93	63.60	75.43	83.03	91.94
FM-OSD(fine) [13]	2	1.82	67.35	77.92	84.59	91.92
CC2D-SLA(ours)	19	1.82	69.73	76.69	84.04	**92.17**
C-ATD(ours)	19	**1.79**	**72.02**	**78.02**	**84.72**	92.00
C-Adapter(ours)	1	1.96	67.83	75.33	81.89	90.82
C-F2(ours)	3	1.83	70.48	77.35	83.96	91.43

Implementation Details. All experiments are conducted using PyTorch on an NVIDIA RTX 3090 GPU with a learning rate of 0.0001, the Adam optimizer, a batch size of 8, and 300 epochs. In CC2D-SLA-ATD (or C-ATD in short), 19 models are trained, each dedicated to a single landmark. For CC2D-SLA-ATD-Adapter (or C-Adapter in short), we introduce 19 adapters, each with an output channel size of 16. A frozen VGG19 network serves as the feature extractor.

3.2 Performance Comparison

As shown in Table 1, we compare our proposed models with several SOTA methods, including SAM [22], UOD [29], CC2D [24], and the two stages of FM-OSD [13]. We re-trained SAM, UOD, and CC2D on the ISBI 2015 Challenge dataset under the one-shot setting and reported their best results following our experimental protocol. For FM-OSD [13], the fine-stage results are taken from the original paper, while the coarse-stage results are reproduced by us using the official implementation to ensure consistency with our setup. We also implement CC2D-SLA-ATD-Adapter-F2 (or C-F2 in short), which uses our C-Adapter model as the coarse stage of FM-OSD, followed by the fine stage of FM-OSD to perform landmark detection on high-resolution medical images. Note that all models except C-F2 are evaluated on low-resolution images (384×384). We report the MRE and SDR results for these methods on the ISBI 2015 Challenge dataset and compare the number of models used.

It is evident that our C-ATD model achieves the best performance, with a 2 mm SDR of 72.02% and an MRE of 1.79 mm, significantly surpassing previous SOTA methods. This confirms that training individual landmark models effectively enhances detection accuracy, though it requires 19 separate models. To improve efficiency, we introduce adapters, allowing for the fusion of all landmarks into a single model. While this results in a slight performance drop compared to C-ATD, it still performs similarly to FM-OSD's coarse stage. Furthermore, applying FM-OSD's fine stage for high-resolution inference boosts the

Table 2. Performance of different methods on the 19 landmarks. The landmark indices correspond to the positions described in [12]. The MRE is measured in millimeters, and the SDR refers to the 2 mm SDR, with units in percentage.

Landmark	CC2D		FM-OSD		C-ATD		C-F2	
	MRE	SDR(2 mm)	MRE	SDR(2 mm)	MRE	SDR(2 mm)	MRE	SDR(2 mm)
1	1.35	85.2	1.55	84.0	**0.98**	**97.6**	1.26	92.0
2	1.60	74.0	**1.49**	73.2	1.51	**78.0**	1.54	73.6
3	1.58	72.4	1.66	68.4	**1.37**	**84.4**	1.46	78.4
4	1.93	66.4	2.28	55.6	**1.80**	**70.8**	2.00	67.2
5	1.86	62.8	1.72	65.6	**1.54**	**76.0**	1.61	75.2
6	2.50	**50.0**	**2.41**	48.4	2.47	49.2	2.43	48.4
7	1.42	81.6	1.05	88.0	0.96	**94.0**	**0.94**	93.6
8	1.46	78.4	**0.99**	91.6	1.10	**93.2**	1.93	89.6
9	1.08	88.8	**0.83**	94.8	0.84	**96.8**	0.84	95.2
10	4.19	20.4	3.23	33.6	3.59	24.8	**3.17**	**37.6**
11	2.58	42.8	**2.44**	**52.0**	2.85	48.8	2.66	48.8
12	2.60	48.8	1.91	68.0	**1.43**	**86.4**	1.50	80.8
13	1.63	70.0	1.60	68.4	1.56	78.4	**1.52**	**79.2**
14	1.69	71.2	**1.43**	80.0	1.54	79.6	1.47	**80.0**
15	1.73	65.6	**1.69**	**68.8**	2.50	50.0	1.89	59.6
16	3.54	26.4	2.61	47.2	**2.52**	**51.2**	2.56	48.8
17	1.73	67.6	1.55	74.8	**1.24**	**84.0**	1.51	77.6
18	1.77	65.6	**1.67**	**67.6**	2.00	63.2	1.82	66.4
19	2.44	48.8	2.49	49.6	**2.25**	**62.0**	2.75	47.2
Mean	2.04	62.5	1.82	67.4	**1.79**	**72.0**	1.83	70.5

performance of C-Adapter, achieving a 2 mm SDR of 70.48%. This not only exceeds the previous SOTA methods but also sets a new benchmark for MLD performance.

Figure 3 presents the predicted landmark detection results from different methods on the dataset. As shown in the figure, CC2D has the lowest prediction accuracy among the methods displayed, while FM-OSD achieves relatively better accuracy. The prediction accuracy of C-Adapter is comparable to that of FM-OSD. And the C-ATD model shows the best prediction accuracy overall.

As shown in Table 2, we provide the MRE and SDR results for each of the 19 landmarks across different methods. C-ATD achieves the best performance on most landmarks, with significant improvements for landmarks 1, 3, 5, 7, 12, 17, and 19, highlighting the effectiveness of the single-landmark approach. However, its performance is less optimal for landmarks 10, 15, and 18, suggesting that different landmarks have distinct characteristics, and these particular landmarks require absorbing more knowledge in order to achieve higher prediction accuracy. To address this, we introduce adapters, allowing landmarks to learn through shared weights as well as landmark-specific weights. After testing, this adaptation leads to a more balanced performance across all landmarks.

Table 3. The performances of our methods with different channel sizes.

Para.	Value	MRE(↓) (mm)	SDR(↑)(%)			
			2 mm	2.5 mm	3 mm	4 mm
C_A	0	2.30	63.92	72.15	79.68	89.09
	4	1.95	67.64	**75.92**	82.61	**91.07**
	8	1.95	67.07	74.53	81.18	90.48
	16	1.96	67.83	75.33	81.89	90.82
	32	**1.91**	**68.21**	75.64	**82.67**	90.99
CC2D's channels	+16	2.06	62.00	70.38	79.16	88.76
	+16 × 19	**2.02**	**63.68**	**72.32**	**80.38**	**89.68**

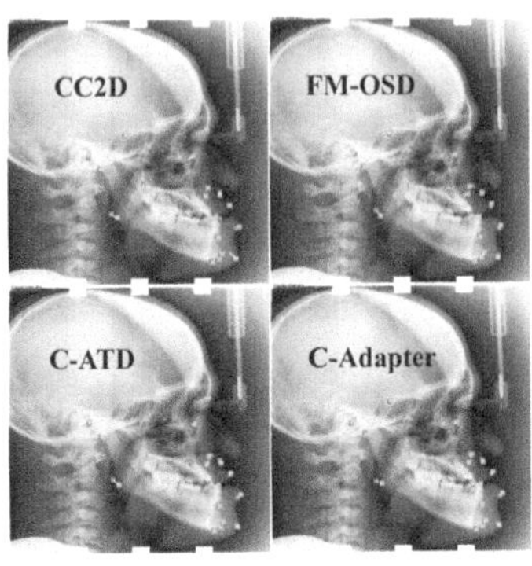

Fig. 3. Visualizations of the prediction results from different methods. The landmarks in red and green represent the predictions and ground truths. (Color figure online)

3.3 Ablation Study

As shown in the upper half of Table 3, we investigate the effect of varying the output channel size, denoted as C_A, for each adapter in the C-Adapter model. We set C_A to 0, 4, 8, 16, and 32. When no adapter is used ($C_A = 0$), the model's performance significantly degrades. However, with adapters, performance remains stable across different C_A values, suggesting that the adapters help the model recognize feature patterns, while shared weights handle main feature extraction.

In the lower half of Table 3, we explore the impact of increasing the number of channels in all convolution layers of the decoder in the original CC2D model, in order to examine how weight scaling affects performance. Specifically, we increased the number of channels by 16 and by 16×19. While increasing weights improves performance slightly, the gain is small, indicating that C-Adapter's performance enhancement is not primarily due to increased model weights.

4 Conclusion

In this paper, we present a progression from exploiting each landmark's individuality—through single-landmark training—to utilizing inter-landmark similarity by incorporating adapters into a unified model. This two-fold approach demonstrates a feasible and effective strategy for improving MLD accuracy. The proposed C-Adapter represents an initial endeavor toward jointly learning multiple landmarks via shared and landmark-specific weights. However, further investigation is needed into more advanced methods of inter-landmark collaboration to simultaneously enhance performance for all landmarks. We believe that continued exploration of this balance between individuality and similarity will yield more robust, efficient, and accurate solutions for one-shot MLD.

Acknowledgment. This work is supported by Natural Science Foundation of China under Grant 62271465 and Suzhou Basic Research Program under Grant SYG202338.

References

1. Bier, B., et al.: X-ray-transform invariant anatomical landmark detection for pelvic trauma surgery. In: Frangi, A., Schnabel, J., Davatzikos, C., Alberola-López, C., Fichtinger, G. (eds.) International Conference on Medical Image Computing and Computer-Assisted Intervention, pp. 55–63. Springer, Cham (2018). https://doi.org/10.1007/978-3-030-00937-3_7
2. Caruana, R.: Multitask learning. Mach. Learn. **28**, 41–75 (1997)
3. Deng, J., Dong, W., Socher, R., Li, L.J., Li, K., Fei-Fei, L.: Imagenet: a large-scale hierarchical image database. In: 2009 IEEE conference on computer vision and pattern recognition, pp. 248–255. IEEE (2009)
4. Gertych, A., Zhang, A., Sayre, J., Pospiech-Kurkowska, S., Huang, H.: Bone age assessment of children using a digital hand atlas. Comput. Med. Imaging Graph. **31**(4–5), 322–331 (2007)
5. Han, D., Gao, Y., Wu, G., Yap, P.T., Shen, D.: Robust anatomical landmark detection for mr brain image registration. In: Golland, P., Hata, N., Barillot, C., Hornegger, J., Howe, R. (eds.) Medical Image Computing and Computer-Assisted Intervention–MICCAI 2014: 17th International Conference, Boston, MA, USA, September 14–18, 2014, Proceedings, Part I 17, pp. 186–193. Springer, Cham (2014). https://doi.org/10.1007/978-3-319-10404-1_24
6. Huang, Z., et al.: Pele scores: pelvic x-ray landmark detection with pelvis extraction and enhancement. Int. J. Comput. Assist. Radiol. Surg. **19**(5), 939–950 (2024)
7. Huang, Z., Wang, S., Hu, H., Xu, Y.: RetiGAN: a hybrid image enhancement method for medical images. In: 2024 5th International Conference on Computer Vision, Image and Deep Learning (CVIDL), pp. 25–29. IEEE (2024)
8. Jacobs, R.A., Jordan, M.I., Nowlan, S.J., Hinton, G.E.: Adaptive mixtures of local experts. Neural Comput. **3**(1), 79–87 (1991)
9. LeCun, Y., Bengio, Y., Hinton, G.: Deep learning. Nature **521**(7553), 436–444 (2015)
10. Liu, S., Huang, D., et al.: Receptive field block net for accurate and fast object detection. In: Proceedings of the European Conference on Computer Vision (ECCV), pp. 385–400 (2018)
11. Liu, X., Wang, J., Liu, F., Zhou, S.K.: Universal undersampled MRI reconstruction. In: de Bruijne, M., et al. (eds.) International Conference on Medical Image Computing and Computer-Assisted Intervention, pp. 211–221. Springer, Cham (2021). https://doi.org/10.1007/978-3-030-87231-1_21
12. Lu, G., Zhang, Y., Kong, Y., Zhang, C., Coatrieux, J.L., Shu, H.: Landmark localization for cephalometric analysis using multiscale image patch-based graph convolutional networks. IEEE J. Biomed. Health Inform. **26**(7), 3015–3024 (2022)

13. Miao, J., Chen, C., Zhang, K., Chuai, J., Li, Q., Heng, P.A.: FM-OSD: foundation model-enabled one-shot detection of anatomical landmarks. In: Linguraru, M.G., et al. (eds.) International Conference on Medical Image Computing and Computer-Assisted Intervention, pp. 297–307. Springer, Cham (2024). https://doi.org/10.1007/978-3-031-72120-5_28
14. Oktay, O., et al.: Stratified decision forests for accurate anatomical landmark localization in cardiac images. IEEE Trans. Med. Imaging **36**(1), 332–342 (2016)
15. Ronneberger, O., Fischer, P., Brox, T.: U-Net: convolutional networks for biomedical image segmentation. In: Navab, N., Hornegger, J., Wells, W., Frangi, A. (eds.) Medical Image Computing and Computer-Assisted Intervention–MICCAI 2015: 18th International Conference, Munich, Germany, October 5–9, 2015, Proceedings, Part III 18, pp. 234–241. Springer, Cham (2015). https://doi.org/10.1007/978-3-319-24574-4_28
16. Schmidhuber, J.: Deep learning in neural networks: an overview. Neural Netw. **61**, 85–117 (2015)
17. Shao, S., Yuan, X., Huang, Z., Qiu, Z., Wang, S., Zhou, K.: Diffuseexpand: expanding dataset for 2D medical image segmentation using diffusion models. arXiv preprint arXiv:2304.13416 (2023)
18. Simonyan, K.: Very deep convolutional networks for large-scale image recognition. arXiv preprint arXiv:1409.1556 (2014)
19. Tang, H., Liu, J., Zhao, M., Gong, X.: Progressive layered extraction (PLE): a novel multi-task learning (MTL) model for personalized recommendations. In: Proceedings of the 14th ACM Conference on Recommender Systems, pp. 269–278 (2020)
20. Wang, C.W., et al.: A benchmark for comparison of dental radiography analysis algorithms. Med. Image Anal. **31**, 63–76 (2016)
21. Wu, H., et al.: Cephalometric landmark detection across ages with prototypical network. In: Linguraru, M.G., et al. (eds.) International Conference on Medical Image Computing and Computer-Assisted Intervention, pp. 155–165. Springer, Cham (2024). https://doi.org/10.1007/978-3-031-72086-4_15
22. Yan, K., et al.: Sam: self-supervised learning of pixel-wise anatomical embeddings in radiological images. IEEE Trans. Med. Imaging **41**(10), 2658–2669 (2022)
23. Yang, D., Zhang, S., Yan, Z., Tan, C., Li, K., Metaxas, D.: Automated anatomical landmark detection ondistal femur surface using convolutional neural network. In: 2015 IEEE 12th International Symposium on Biomedical Imaging (ISBI), pp. 17–21. IEEE (2015)
24. Yao, Q., Quan, Q., Xiao, L., Kevin Zhou, S.: One-shot medical landmark detection. In: de Bruijne, M., et al. (eds.) Medical Image Computing and Computer Assisted Intervention–MICCAI 2021: 24th International Conference, Strasbourg, France, September 27–October 1, 2021, Proceedings, Part II 24, pp. 177–188. Springer, Cham (2021). https://doi.org/10.1007/978-3-030-87196-3_17
25. Yin, Z., Gong, P., Wang, C., Yu, Y., Wang, Y.: One-shot medical landmark localization by edge-guided transform and noisy landmark refinement. In: Avidan, S., Brostow, G., Cissé, M., Farinella, G.M., Hassner, T. (eds.) European Conference on Computer Vision, pp. 473–489. Springer (2022). https://doi.org/10.1007/978-3-031-19803-8_28
26. Zhang, J., Liu, M., An, L., Gao, Y., Shen, D.: Alzheimer's disease diagnosis using landmark-based features from longitudinal structural MR images. IEEE J. Biomed. Health Inform. **21**(6), 1607–1616 (2017)
27. Zhang, Y., Yang, Q.: A survey on multi-task learning. IEEE Trans. Knowl. Data Eng. **34**(12), 5586–5609 (2021)

28. Zhou, X., Huang, Z., Zhu, H., Yao, Q., Zhou, S.K.: Hybrid attention network: an efficient approach for anatomy-free landmark detection. arXiv preprint arXiv:2412.06499 (2024)
29. Zhu, H., Quan, Q., Yao, Q., Liu, Z., Zhou, S.K.: UOD: universal one-shot detection of anatomical landmarks. In: Greenspan, H., et al. (eds.) International Conference on Medical Image Computing and Computer-Assisted Intervention, pp. 24–34. Springer, Cham (2023). https://doi.org/10.1007/978-3-031-43907-0_3

Federated In-Context Prompt Selection for Multi-modal 3D Dental Imaging: A Theoretical Framework with Privacy-Preserving Guarantees

Ushashi Bhattacharjee[1] and Tirtho Roy[2(✉)]

[1] Bioinformatics and Computational Biology, Iowa State University, Ames, IA, USA
ushashi@iastate.edu

[2] Department of Computer Science, Iowa State University, Ames, IA, USA
tirtho@iastate.edu

Abstract. Vision-language models show remarkable capabilities in medical imaging analysis, yet their deployment in federated healthcare environments faces key challenges in privacy preservation, data heterogeneity, and adversarial robustness. We present FedDental3D-ICL, a theoretical framework for federated in-context prompt learning that enables privacy-preserving collaboration across healthcare institutions without sharing sensitive patient data or model parameters. Our framework introduces four core algorithmic contributions: Multi-Modal Prompt Space (MMPS) abstraction unifying visual and textual prompt representations across 2D and 3D medical imaging modalities; Cross-Modal Prompt Alignment (CMPA) ensuring semantic consistency through information-theoretic contrastive objectives; Hierarchical Multi-Modal Optimization (HMMO) providing theoretical convergence guarantees for non-convex federated objectives; and Byzantine-Resilient Cross-Modal Aggregation (BRCMA) with differential privacy bounds. Our theoretical analysis suggests potential convergence rates of $O(1/\sqrt{T})$, theoretical communication complexity bounds of $O(K \log |P|)$ compared to traditional $O(K \cdot d)$, and (ε, δ)-differential privacy guarantees with optimal composition bounds. While this work establishes comprehensive mathematical foundations, empirical validation and practical implementation remain important directions for future research.

Keywords: Federated learning · Vision-language models · Medical imaging · Privacy preservation · Multi-modal learning · Prompt engineering · Differential privacy · Byzantine resilience

1 Introduction

Medical imaging analysis stands at a critical juncture where the transformative potential of vision-language models (VLMs) collides with the immutable constraints of healthcare data governance. While recent advances in VLMs have

F. Bolelli et al. (Eds.): ODIN 2025, LNCS 16473, pp. 76–88, 2026.
https://doi.org/10.1007/978-3-032-20711-1_8

demonstrated unprecedented capabilities in multimodal medical reasoning [1,2], their deployment in real-world healthcare environments exposes a fundamental contradiction: the models that show the greatest promise require precisely the type of large-scale, cross-institutional data sharing that regulatory frameworks explicitly prohibit [3–5]. This paradox represents more than a technical challenge—it constitutes a systemic barrier that prevents the medical community from leveraging the full potential of modern AI while maintaining the privacy guarantees essential to patient trust and regulatory compliance [6].

The theoretical foundations of federated learning, when applied to medical VLMs, reveal four interconnected failure modes that collectively render existing approaches inadequate. The privacy-utility contradiction creates an irreconcilable tension where meaningful privacy protection fundamentally undermines model performance, while supposedly secure gradient-sharing mechanisms remain vulnerable to sophisticated reconstruction attacks that can recover sensitive patient information [7–10]. Statistical heterogeneity across medical institutions violates the fundamental assumptions underlying federated optimization, creating convergence pathologies that no existing aggregation method can adequately address [11,12]. Communication constraints impose prohibitive overhead costs that scale quadratically with model size, rendering federated training of large VLMs computationally infeasible within realistic healthcare network environments [13,14]. Byzantine robustness requirements introduce additional complexity layers that existing defenses cannot handle without sacrificing the cross-modal learning capabilities that make VLMs valuable for medical applications [15–17].

To demonstrate the versatility and practical applicability of our approach, we present **FedDental3D-ICL**, a specialized implementation tailored for federated 3D dental imaging analysis that showcases how our framework can be adapted to domain-specific requirements while maintaining its core theoretical guarantees.

2 System Model and Problem Formulation

2.1 Federated Multi-modal Medical Imaging System

The heterogeneity in medical institutions creates unique challenges that distinguish our setting from traditional federated learning scenarios. Different institutions may specialize in different types of dental procedures, use varying imaging equipment, and maintain distinct clinical protocols. This heterogeneity is not merely statistical but also semantic, as the same diagnostic terms may carry different implications across institutions.

As shown in Fig. 1, we consider a federated dental care system comprising K medical institutions $\{C_1, C_2, \ldots, C_K\}$ and a central coordination server S. Each client C_k possesses a private multi-modal dataset $D_k = \{(x_k^{(i)}, y_k^{(i)})\}_{i=1}^{n_k}$ where $x_k^{(i)}$ represents multi-modal dental data and $y_k^{(i)}$ denotes diagnostic labels.

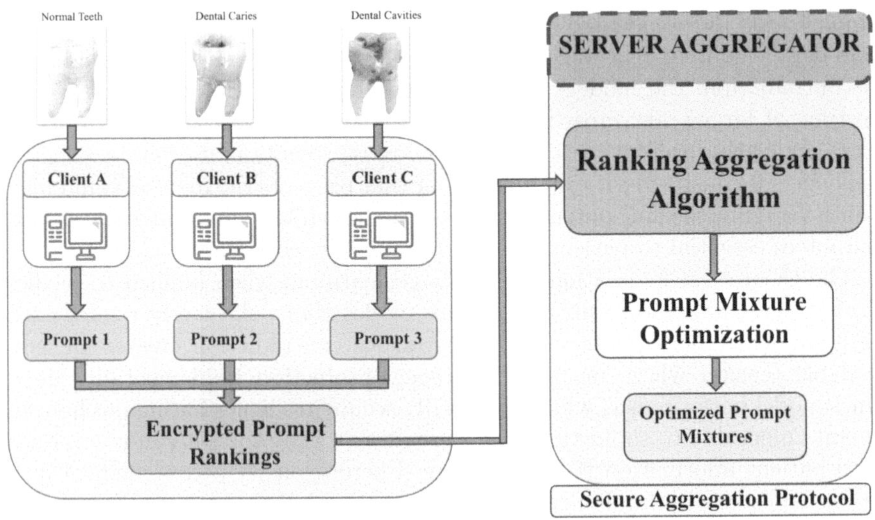

Fig. 1. FedDental3D-ICL System Architecture showing multi-modal data flow across federated dental institutions with privacy-preserving prompt exchange.

2.2 Multi-modal Prompt Space Theory

The foundation of our approach lies in constructing a unified representation space that can seamlessly integrate information from diverse dental imaging modalities. Traditional approaches treat each modality independently, leading to suboptimal integration and missed opportunities for cross-modal reasoning.

Definition 1 (Multi-Modal Prompt Space). *The prompt space* $\mathcal{P} = \mathcal{P}_v \times \mathcal{P}_t \times \mathcal{P}_{3D}$ *where:*

- $\mathcal{P}_v$*: Visual prompt space for 2D/3D teeth images*
- $\mathcal{P}_t$*: Textual prompt space for clinical descriptions*
- $\mathcal{P}_{3D}$*: Specialized prompt space for 3D volumetric analysis*

For each modality $m \in \{v, t, 3D\}$, we define embedding functions $\phi_m : \mathcal{P}_m \rightarrow \mathbb{R}^d$ mapping raw prompts to a common d-dimensional space. The choice of a common embedding dimension is not arbitrary—it reflects the hypothesis that despite their surface differences, medical imaging modalities share fundamental diagnostic patterns that can be captured in a unified representation.

[Lipschitz Continuity] Each embedding function ϕ_m is L-Lipschitz continuous:

$$\|\phi_m(p_1) - \phi_m(p_2)\| \leq L\|p_1 - p_2\| \tag{1}$$

Definition 2 (Multi-Modal Medical Data). *The input space* $\mathcal{X} = \mathcal{X}_{2D} \times \mathcal{X}_{3D} \times \mathcal{X}_{text}$ *where:*

- $\mathcal{X}_{2D}$*: 2D medical images (X-ray)*

- $\mathcal{X}_{3D}$: *3D volumetric data (CBCT images)*
- $\mathcal{X}_{text}$: *Clinical notes and structured reports*

Each client accesses a shared, frozen pre-trained vision-language model $M : \mathcal{X} \times \mathcal{P} \rightarrow \mathcal{Y}$ with parameters Θ that remain fixed throughout federated learning.

Definition 3 (Multi-Modal Prompt Embedding). *For prompt combination (p_v, p_t, p_{3D}), the multi-modal embedding is:*

$$\psi(p_v, p_t, p_{3D}) = F(\varphi_v(p_v), \varphi_t(p_t), \varphi_{3D}(p_{3D})) \tag{2}$$

where $F : \mathbb{R}^d \times \mathbb{R}^d \times \mathbb{R}^d \rightarrow \mathbb{R}^d$ is a fusion function preserving both modality-specific and cross-modal information.

Definition 4 (Fusion Function Implementation). *The fusion function $F : \mathbb{R}^d \times \mathbb{R}^d \times \mathbb{R}^d \rightarrow \mathbb{R}^d$ is implemented as:*

$$F(z_v, z_t, z_{3D}) = \sigma(W_1[z_v; z_t; z_{3D}] + b_1) \tag{3}$$

where $W_1 \in \mathbb{R}^{d \times 3d}$, $b_1 \in \mathbb{R}^d$ are learnable parameters and σ is the ReLU activation function.

Theorem 1 (Universal Approximation for MMPS). *For any target prompt combination (p_v^*, p_t^*, p_{3D}^*) and approximation error $\varepsilon > 0$, there exists a fusion function F with $O(\varepsilon^{-d})$ parameters such that:*

$$\|F(\phi_v(p_v), \phi_t(p_t), \phi_{3D}(p_{3D})) - \psi^*(p_v^*, p_t^*, p_{3D}^*)\| \leq \varepsilon \tag{4}$$

for appropriately chosen prompts (p_v, p_t, p_{3D}).

Proof. By the universal approximation theorem for neural networks, the fusion function F can approximate any continuous mapping between the concatenated embeddings and the target representation with arbitrary precision, provided sufficient network capacity.

Corollary 1 (Stability of MMPS Embeddings). *MMPS embeddings are stable with respect to small perturbations in input prompts:*

$$\|\psi(p_v + \delta_v, p_t + \delta_t, p_{3D} + \delta_{3D}) - \psi(p_v, p_t, p_{3D})\| \leq 3L\|F\|_{Lip}(\|\delta_v\| + \|\delta_t\| + \|\delta_{3D}\|) \tag{5}$$

where $\|F\|_{Lip}$ is the Lipschitz constant of the fusion function F.

2.3 Federated Prompt Optimization Problem

Building upon the multi-modal prompt space foundation, we now formulate the central optimization problem that drives collaborative learning across institutions.

Definition 5 (Federated Multi-Modal Prompt Optimization). *Find optimal prompt parameters* $\theta^* = \{p_v^*, p_t^*, p_{3D}^*\}$ *that minimize:*

$$\min_{\theta} L(\theta) = \sum_{k=1}^{K} w_k L_k(\theta; D_k) \tag{6}$$

where $w_k \geq 0$ *are client weights with* $\sum_{k=1}^{K} w_k = 1$*, and the local loss function incorporates:*

$$L_k(\theta; D_k) = L_k^{task}(\theta; D_k) + \lambda L_k^{align}(\theta; D_k) + \gamma L_k^{reg}(\theta) \tag{7}$$

where L_k^{task} *is the primary diagnostic task loss,* L_k^{align} *is the cross-modal alignment loss, and* L_k^{reg} *is the regularization term.*

3 Proposed Algorithms

3.1 Multi-Modal Prompt Space Construction

Algorithm 1. Multi-Modal Prompt Space Construction (MMPS)

Require: Raw prompts P_v, P_t, P_{3D}; contrastive parameters (τ, batch_size)
Ensure: Unified embeddings $\psi(p_v, p_t, p_{3D})$, learned fusion function F
Initialize embedding functions ϕ_v, ϕ_t, ϕ_{3D} with random weights
Initialize fusion network F with Xavier initialization
▷ Phase 1: Individual modality embedding learning
for each modality $m \in \{v, t, 3D\}$ **do**
  for epoch $= 1$ to E_1 **do**
    Sample batch of prompts $\{p_m^{(i)}\}$
    Compute embeddings $z_m^{(i)} = \phi_m(p_m^{(i)})$
    Update ϕ_m via contrastive loss minimization
  end for
end for
▷ Phase 2: Cross-modal fusion learning
for epoch $= 1$ to E_2 **do**
  Sample multi-modal triplets $(p_v^{(i)}, p_t^{(i)}, p_{3D}^{(i)})$
  Compute modality embeddings $z_v^{(i)} = \phi_v(p_v^{(i)})$, $z_t^{(i)} = \phi_t(p_t^{(i)})$, $z_{3D}^{(i)} = \phi_{3D}(p_{3D}^{(i)})$
  Compute fused embedding $\psi^{(i)} = F(z_v^{(i)}, z_t^{(i)}, z_{3D}^{(i)})$
  Update F via contrastive loss on $\psi^{(i)}$
end for
return $\psi(p_v, p_t, p_{3D})$, F

3.2 Cross-Modal Prompt Alignment (CMPA) Framework

Information-Theoretic Foundation

Definition 6 (Cross-Modal Mutual Information). *For visual and textual representations Z_v and Z_t:*

$$I(Z_v; Z_t) = \mathbb{E}\left[\log \frac{p(z_v, z_t)}{p(z_v)p(z_t)}\right] \tag{8}$$

We employ the InfoNCE lower bound to make optimization tractable:

$$I(Z_v; Z_t) \geq \mathbb{E}\left[\log \frac{e^{f(z_v, z_t)}}{\mathbb{E}[e^{f(z_v, z_t')}]}\right] \tag{9}$$

where $f(z_v, z_t)$ is a critic function (cosine similarity).

Theorem 2 (Temperature Sensitivity Bounds). *For temperature $\tau > 0$, the alignment quality satisfies:*

$$\frac{\partial \mathcal{L}_{InfoNCE}}{\partial \tau} = -\frac{1}{\tau^2}\mathbb{E}\left[f(z_v, z_t) - \log \sum_{z_t'} e^{f(z_v, z_t')/\tau}\right] \tag{10}$$

$$\left|\frac{\partial^2 \mathcal{L}_{InfoNCE}}{\partial \tau^2}\right| \leq \frac{C_{align}}{\tau^3} \tag{11}$$

where C_{align} is the alignment constant bounded by the maximum similarity score.

3.3 Hierarchical Multi-Modal Optimization (HMMO) Framework

Theoretical Framework We formulate federated prompt optimization as a hierarchical problem:

- **Upper Level (Global):** Optimize global prompt mixture distribution
- **Lower Level (Local):** Evaluate prompts on local data and generate rankings

Definition 7 (Hierarchical Optimization Problem). *The global objective:*

$$\min_{\theta} L(\theta) = \sum_{k=1}^{K} w_k L_k(\theta; \arg\min_{\varphi_k} G_k(\varphi_k, \theta)) \tag{12}$$

where $G_k(\varphi_k, \theta)$ is the local evaluation function and φ_k are client-specific parameters.

Convergence Analysis. [Smoothness] Each local objective L_k is L-smooth: $\|\nabla L_k(\theta_1) - \nabla L_k(\theta_2)\| \leq L\|\theta_1 - \theta_2\|$.

[Bounded Variance] Stochastic gradients have bounded variance: $\mathbb{E}[\|\nabla L_k(\theta) - \nabla \hat{L}_k(\theta)\|^2] \leq \sigma^2$.

Theorem 3 (HMMO Convergence). *Under Assumptions 3.1–3.2, HMMO achieves convergence rate:*

$$\mathbb{E}[\|\nabla L(\theta^T)\|^2] \leq \frac{C_1}{\sqrt{T}} + \frac{C_2}{T} + \frac{L\sigma^2}{p_{min}\sqrt{T}} \tag{13}$$

where C_1, C_2 are constants depending on client heterogeneity and p_{min} is minimum participation probability.

Algorithm 2. Hierarchical Multi-Modal Optimization (HMMO)

```
Require: Global prompt candidates P_global, participation probability p_m
Ensure: Optimal prompt distribution θ, client adaptations {θ_k}
Initialize global prompt parameters θ^(0)
for round t = 1 to T do
    Select subset of clients S_t ⊆ [K] with probability p_m
    for each client k ∈ S_t do
        Evaluate prompt candidates on local data: q_k(p) = quality(M(x_k, p), y_k) for p ∈ P_global
        Generate local prompt ranking: r_k = argsort(q_k, descending = True)
        Compute alignment statistics: a_k = cross_modal_alignment(r_k)
        Send encrypted (r_k, a_k) to server
    end for
    Aggregate rankings via Byzantine-resilient mechanism: θ^(t) = BRCMA({r_k, a_k}_{k∈S_t})
end for
return θ^(T), {θ_k^(T)}
```

3.4 Byzantine-Resilient Cross-Modal Aggregation (BRCMA) Framework

Byzantine Threat Model

Definition 8 (Byzantine-Resilient Multi-Modal Aggregation). *Given prompt rankings from K clients where up to $f < K/3$ are Byzantine, compute a global ranking maintaining convergence guarantees for honest clients.*

Theorem 4 (Byzantine Resilience). *Under the assumption that $f < K/3$ clients are Byzantine, BRCMA maintains convergence with rate:*

$$\mathbb{E}[\|\nabla L(\theta^T)\|^2] \leq \frac{C_1}{\sqrt{T}} + \frac{C_2}{T} + \frac{L\sigma^2}{(K-f)\sqrt{T}} + \frac{C_f}{T} \tag{14}$$

where C_f is a constant depending on Byzantine attack magnitude.

Privacy-Preserving Multi-Modal Selection (PMMS)

Definition 9 (Multi-Modal Quality Function). *For prompt combination* $p = (p_v, p_t, p_{3D})$ *and dataset* D*:*

$$q(D, p) = accuracy(M(x, p), y) + \lambda \cdot alignment(p) \tag{15}$$

Theorem 5 (PMMS Privacy Guarantee). *The PMMS mechanism satisfies* (ε, δ)*-differential privacy with:*

$$\varepsilon = \frac{2\Delta q}{n} \cdot \log |P| + \sqrt{\frac{2\log(1/\delta)}{n}} \tag{16}$$

where Δq *is the global sensitivity of the quality function.*

Algorithm 3. Byzantine-Resilient Cross-Modal Aggregation with Privacy-Preserving Selection (BRCMA-PMMS)

Require: Client rankings $\{r_k\}$, privacy parameters (ε, δ), prompt set P
Ensure: Aggregated prompt parameters θ, privacy-preserving selection
Initialize global prompt parameters $\theta^{(0)}$
for round $t = 1$ to T **do**
  Collect client rankings $\{r_k^{(t)}\}$ and quality scores $\{q_k^{(t)}\}$
  Apply exponential mechanism to select top prompts:
    $p_{\text{select}}(p) \propto \exp\left(\frac{\varepsilon \cdot q(D,p)}{2\Delta q}\right)$
  Filter out Byzantine clients using cross-modal consistency check:
    $S_t^{\text{valid}} = \{k : \text{consistency}(r_k, \{r_j\}_{j \neq k}) > \tau_{\text{byz}}\}$
  Aggregate valid client rankings using median-based robust estimator
  Add calibrated Gaussian noise for (ε, δ)-differential privacy
  Update global prompt distribution: $\theta^{(t)} = \text{weighted\_aggregate}(S_t^{\text{valid}})$
end for
return $\theta^{(T)}$

---

4 Comprehensive Theoretical Analysis

4.1 Extended Byzantine Tolerance

We relax the standard $f < K/3$ assumption:

Theorem 6 (Adaptive Byzantine Resilience). *Under adaptive adversary model where Byzantine clients can coordinate, BRCMA maintains convergence if:*

$$f < \min\left(\frac{K}{3}, \frac{K \cdot \rho_{honest}}{2 + \rho_{honest}}\right) \tag{17}$$

$$\textit{where } \rho_{honest} = \frac{\min_k \|\nabla L_k(\theta^*)\|}{\max_k \|\nabla L_k(\theta^*)\|} \tag{18}$$

Lemma 1 (Imbalance-Aware Prompt Scoring). *For dataset $\mathcal{D}_k$ with class distribution $\pi_k = (\pi_{k,1}, \ldots, \pi_{k,C})$, the bias-corrected prompt quality is:*

$$q_k^{corrected}(p) = q_k(p) - \lambda_{bias} \sum_{c=1}^{C} \pi_{k,c} \log \pi_{k,c} \cdot \mathbb{I}[prompt\ p\ favors\ class\ c]$$

4.2 Communication Complexity Analysis

Theorem 7 (Optimal Prompt Pool Size). *The optimal prompt pool size minimizes the total error:*

$$|P|^* = \arg\min_{|P|} [\varepsilon_{approx}(|P|) + \varepsilon_{comm}(|P|)] \tag{19}$$

$$where\ \varepsilon_{approx}(|P|) = \frac{C_{approx}}{|P|^{1/d}} \quad (approximation\ error) \tag{20}$$

$$\varepsilon_{comm}(|P|) = \frac{C_{comm}|P| \log |P|}{B} \quad (communication\ error) \tag{21}$$

and B is the available bandwidth per round.

Theorem 8 (Communication Complexity). *The FedDental3D-ICL framework achieves communication complexity of $O(K \log |P|)$ per round, compared to $O(K \cdot d)$ for traditional federated learning.*

Proof. In traditional federated learning, each client sends gradient updates of size d (typically 10^9 parameters). Our approach only requires:

- Prompt rankings: $O(|P| \log |P|)$ bits per client
- Alignment statistics: $O(1)$ bits per client
- Quality scores: $O(|P|)$ bits per client

Total per client: $O(|P| \log |P|)$ bits. Since $|P| \ll d$, this represents significant reduction.

4.3 Privacy Analysis

Theorem 9 (Composition-Based Privacy). *Running FedDental3D-ICL for T rounds with parameters $(\varepsilon_t, \delta_t)$ per round satisfies $(\varepsilon_{total}, \delta_{total})$-differential privacy where:*

$$\varepsilon_{total} = \sum_{t=1}^{T} \varepsilon_t + \sqrt{2T \log(1/\delta_{total})} \sum_{t=1}^{T} \varepsilon_t^2 \tag{22}$$

$$\delta_{total} = \sum_{t=1}^{T} \delta_t \tag{23}$$

[Bounded Correlation] Prompt updates across rounds satisfy:

$$\max_{t,t'} |\mathrm{Corr}(r_k^{(t)}, r_k^{(t')})| \leq \rho < 1$$

Theorem 10 (Correlated Composition Privacy). *Under bounded correlation assumption, the total privacy cost after T rounds is:*

$$\varepsilon_{total} \leq \sum_{t=1}^{T} \varepsilon_t + \sqrt{2T\log(1/\delta)}\sqrt{\sum_{t=1}^{T} \varepsilon_t^2 \cdot (1+\rho)} \tag{24}$$

$$\delta_{total} \leq \sum_{t=1}^{T} \delta_t \cdot (1+\rho T) \tag{25}$$

4.4 Convergence Rate Analysis

Theorem 11 (Global Convergence Rate). *The FedDental3D-ICL framework achieves the following convergence rate:*

$$\mathbb{E}[L(\theta^T) - L^*] \leq \frac{C_1}{\sqrt{T}} + \frac{C_2\sigma^2}{KT} + \frac{C_3\zeta^2}{T} + \frac{C_4 f}{T} \tag{26}$$

where the constants are defined as:

$$C_1 = L\sqrt{2(L(\theta^0) - L^*)} \tag{27}$$

$$C_2 = 2\eta^2 L^2 \tag{28}$$

$$C_3 = 4\eta L \tag{29}$$

$$C_4 = 4\eta L \Delta^2 \tag{30}$$

and the problem parameters are:

$$\sigma^2 = \max_k \mathbb{E}[\|\nabla L_k(\theta) - \nabla \hat{L}_k(\theta)\|^2] \tag{31}$$

$$\zeta^2 = \max_k \mathbb{E}[\|\nabla L_k(\theta^*) - \nabla L(\theta^*)\|^2] \tag{32}$$

$$\Delta^2 = \max_{i,j} \|\nabla L_i(\theta) - \nabla L_j(\theta)\|^2 \tag{33}$$

$$f < \frac{K}{3} \tag{34}$$

Proof. The proof follows from the convergence analysis of hierarchical multi-modal optimization with Byzantine resilience. The first term $\frac{C_1}{\sqrt{T}}$ captures the standard convergence rate for non-convex optimization, the second term $\frac{C_2\sigma^2}{KT}$ reflects the benefit of averaging across K clients, the third term $\frac{C_3\zeta^2}{T}$ accounts for data heterogeneity across institutions, and the final term $\frac{C_4 f}{T}$ quantifies the impact of Byzantine adversaries.

5 Architectural Framework

5.1 Dental System Architecture

We have developed a novel theoretical framework, FedDental3D-ICL, tailored for federated multi-modal learning in dental imaging and diagnostics. Our approach integrates four synergistic components to enable privacy-preserving collaborative learning across dental institutions, enhancing dental care delivery. At the core, we propose a Local Prompt Evaluation Engine, which enables each dental clinic or hospital to evaluate prompts using local multi-modal dental data—such as 3D cone-beam computed tomography (CBCT) scans, intraoral photographs, and clinical dental records—while ensuring patient privacy and compliance with dental regulatory standards.

To address the complexities of multi-modal dental AI, we introduce a Cross-Modal Alignment Module that ensures semantic consistency across dental data types, including CBCT scans, panoramic X-rays, intraoral photos, and clinical notes, despite variations in dental imaging equipment and documentation practices across institutions. We also propose a Hierarchical Optimization Coordinator to manage global prompt distribution tailored to dental diagnostics, while upholding stringent privacy constraints inherent in dental healthcare. Additionally, we introduce a Byzantine-Resilient Aggregator, leveraging dental-specific cross-modal validation to defend against malicious participants.

5.2 Dental Privacy-Preserving Architecture

We designed the FedDental3D-ICL framework to prioritize patient privacy in dental settings through mechanisms tailored to dental practice environments. Our approach ensures that raw dental imaging data, patient records, and clinical notes never leave institutional boundaries, addressing critical privacy and regulatory concerns in dental healthcare. We propose a prompt-only communication protocol, where dental institutions exchange only prompt rankings and encrypted alignment statistics related to dental diagnostic accuracy and treatment planning efficacy.

To ensure robust privacy in dental applications, we integrate differential privacy through strategic noise injection at aggregation points, providing mathematically provable privacy bounds. We also employ secure multi-party computation for critical aggregation steps, enabling collaborative computation without exposing individual dental contributions.

5.3 Scalability Considerations

We designed FedDental3D-ICL with scalability to support large networks of dental institutions, enabling collaborative learning across diverse dental practices. Our theoretical system achieves linear communication scaling with $O(K \log |P|)$ complexity, where K is the number of participating dental clinics and $|P|$ is the dental-specific prompt space size. We include adaptive participation mechanisms that dynamically select dental clients based on computational capacity and data quality.

5.4 Implementation Gap: From Theory to Practice

We present a rigorous theoretical framework with mathematical foundations, convergence guarantees, and privacy-preserving mechanisms tailored for dental federated learning, but we acknowledge that practical implementation remains entirely unaddressed. Our pipeline exists solely on paper, requiring complete development before real-world validation in dental settings. We acknowledge that our components are purely theoretical constructs, each requiring extensive software development, testing, and optimization for deployment in dental environments.

We have not processed real CBCT scans, intraoral photographs, or clinical dental records, leaving our cross-modal alignment mechanisms untested against variations in dental imaging equipment or documentation practices across institutions. Our differential privacy guarantees and secure multi-party computation protocols require implementation in cryptographic libraries and validation against real attack vectors. Our framework lacks validation across all dental aspects, with theoretical privacy guarantees unaudited against dental healthcare privacy regulations.

6 Conclusion and Future Directions

We have established foundational mathematical frameworks for federated multimodal learning in dental AI applications, but we lack any implementation roadmap, development timeline, or practical steps toward a working dental system. The most critical future direction for dental AI is practical implementation, not theoretical extension. We need proof-of-concept development to build a minimal working system demonstrating feasibility in dental settings, pilot studies with real dental data, and incremental validation to test each component separately before full system integration.

The fundamental gap between theory and practice is our greatest challenge in dental AI. While our research demonstrates the theoretical possibility of achieving collaborative learning benefits with strict privacy and regulatory compliance in dental healthcare, transitioning to practical deployment requires substantial implementation effort we have not undertaken. We are actively collaborating with dental care institutions across South Asian countries to collect CBCT scans along with panoramic X-rays, intraoral photographs, and clinical notes. This collaboration will enable us to benchmark our framework against existing federated learning approaches, evaluate privacy guarantees in realistic settings, and explore integration with clinical workflows.

Acknowledgments. We gratefully acknowledge the support and guidance received during our COM S 4590X: Security and Privacy in Cloud Computing final project at Iowa State University, which made this work possible. We would also like to express our appreciation to the Translational AI Center as a token of gratitude for their encouragement and support throughout this research.

Disclosure of Interests. The authors have no competing interests to declare that are relevant to the content of this article.

References

1. Zhang, Z., et al.: BioMedGPT: unified and Generalist Biomedical Foundation Model Bridging Vision, Language, and Multimodal Tasks. arXiv preprint arXiv:2305.17153 (2023)
2. Eslami, M., et al.: PubMedCLIP: A Contrastive Vision-Language Pre-training for Biomedical Vision-Language Processing. arXiv preprint arXiv:2112.10683 (2021)
3. HIMSS: What is Federal Health IT Policy? HIMSS Knowledge Center (2024)
4. ONC: Federal Health IT Strategic Plan 2020-2025. Office of the National Coordinator for Health IT (2023)
5. Sheller, M.J., et al.: Federated learning in medicine: facilitating multi-institutional collaborations without sharing patient data. Sci. Rep. **10**(1), 12598 (2020)
6. Radford, A., et al.: Learning Transferable Visual Models from Natural Language Supervision. arXiv preprint arXiv:2103.00020 (2021)
7. Abadi, M., et al.: Deep learning with differential privacy. In: Proceedings of the 2016 ACM SIGSAC Conference on Computer and Communications Security, pp. 308–318 (2016)
8. Zhu, L., et al.: Deep leakage from gradients. Adv. Neural Inf. Process. Syst. **32** (2019)
9. Melis, L., Song, C., De Cristofaro, E., Shmatikov, V.: Exploiting unintended feature leakage in collaborative learning. In: 2019 IEEE Symposium on Security and Privacy (SP), pp. 691–706 (2019)
10. Geyer, R.C., Klein, T., Nabi, M.: Differentially private federated learning: a client level perspective. arXiv preprint arXiv:1712.07557 (2017)
11. Li, T., Sahu, A.K., Talwalkar, A., Smith, V.: Federated learning: challenges, methods, and future directions. IEEE Signal Process. Mag. **37**(3), 50–60 (2020)
12. Li, X., et al.: federated learning on non-IID data silos: an experimental study. In: International Conference on Learning Representations (2022)
13. Kairouz, P., et al.: Advances and open problems in federated learning. J. Mach. Learn. Res. **22**(1), 1–210 (2021)
14. Sattler, F., Wiedemann, S., Müller, K.R., Samek, W.: Robust and communication-efficient federated learning from non-I.I.D. data. IEEE Trans. Neural Netw. Learn. Syst. **31**(9), 3400–3413 (2019)
15. Blanchard, P., el Mhamdi, E.M., Guerraoui, R., Stainer, J.: Machine learning with adversaries: byzantine tolerant gradient descent. Adv. Neural Inf. Process. Syst. **30** (2017)
16. Yin, D., Chen, Y., Kannan, R., Bartlett, P.: Byzantine-Robust Distributed Learning: Towards Optimal Statistical Rates. arXiv preprint arXiv:1803.01498 (2018)
17. Bagdasaryan, E., et al.: How To backdoor federated learning. In: International Conference on Artificial Intelligence and Statistics, pp. 2938–2948 (2020)

Tooth-Diffusion: Guided 3D CBCT Synthesis with Fine-Grained Tooth Conditioning

Said Djafar Said[1], Torkan Gholamalizadeh[2], and Mostafa Mehdipour Ghazi[1(✉)]

[1] Pioneer Centre for AI, Department of Computer Science, University of Copenhagen, Copenhagen, Denmark
ghazi@di.ku.dk
[2] Research and Development, 3Shape A/S, Copenhagen, Denmark

Abstract. Despite the growing importance of dental CBCT scans for diagnosis and treatment planning, generating anatomically realistic scans with fine-grained control remains a challenge in medical image synthesis. In this work, we propose a novel conditional diffusion framework for 3D dental volume generation, guided by tooth-level binary attributes that allow precise control over tooth presence and configuration. Our approach integrates wavelet-based denoising diffusion, FiLM conditioning, and masked loss functions to focus learning on relevant anatomical structures. We evaluate the model across diverse tasks, such as tooth addition, removal, and full dentition synthesis, using both paired and distributional similarity metrics. Results show strong fidelity and generalization with low FID scores, robust inpainting performance, and SSIM values above 0.91 even on unseen scans. By enabling realistic, localized modification of dentition without rescanning, this work opens opportunities for surgical planning, patient communication, and targeted data augmentation in dental AI workflows. The codes are available at: https://github.com/djafar1/tooth-diffusion.

Keywords: CBCT Scan Synthesis · Tooth Inpainting · 3D Generative Modeling · Conditional Diffusion · FiLM

1 Introduction

Cone-beam computed tomography (CBCT) has become indispensable in dental and maxillofacial imaging, offering high-resolution 3D representations of dentition. However, it remains challenged by inherent limitations such as noise, metal artifacts, and a restricted field of view [1,2]. Deep learning methods have demonstrated strong potential in segmentation and reconstruction tasks, yet they often struggle with the anatomical variability of teeth, the presence of missing teeth, and the limited capacity to control or correct for structural artifacts.

F. Bolelli et al. (Eds.): ODIN 2025, LNCS 16473, pp. 89–98, 2026.
https://doi.org/10.1007/978-3-032-20711-1_9

Teeth segmentation from CBCT has achieved high accuracy using convolutional neural networks (CNNs), U-Net variants, and attention-based architectures [3–5]. However, these methods are primarily deterministic and do not support conditional generation for treatment planning, such as simulating missing teeth, implants, bridges, or fillings. Generative models based on generative adversarial networks (GANs) and denoising diffusion probabilistic models (DDPMs) have been explored for image enhancement tasks in CBCT-to-CT and MRI-to-CBCT synthesis [6–8], yet prior work on generating synthetic dentition conditioned on user-specified tooth-level attributes remains scarce. To the best of our knowledge, no prior approach enables fine-grained control over individual tooth presence or absence in 3D CBCT, which is a key novelty of this study.

DDPMs have emerged as a robust framework for image synthesis due to their stability and ability to model complex distributions [9]. Recent medical imaging adaptations include CBCT-to-CT translation [7], limited-angle CBCT reconstruction [10], and medical image denoising [11]. However, these approaches have not been extended to the generation of anatomically accurate, condition-driven dental CBCTs. Such generative capabilities are clinically valuable for simulating anatomical variations, including missing or restored teeth, essential for planning personalized treatments such as implants or orthodontic interventions. Moreover, this can enhance data augmentation, address missing data scenarios, and support the training of robust models in low-resource or imbalanced datasets.

In this work, we propose a novel method to generate synthetic CBCT volumes of dentition with explicit, user-defined tooth configurations. We train a wavelet-based latent diffusion model conditioned on tooth presence, encoded via Feature-wise Linear Modulation (FiLM) embeddings [12]. By employing a masked L2 loss focused on tooth regions during training, and simulating tooth removal or addition through augmentation, the model achieves precise localization and reconstruction of dental structures. Beyond improving generative controllability, the ability to insert or remove specific teeth enables realistic pre/post-treatment simulations, supporting surgical planning, patient communication, and multidisciplinary case discussion, while also providing a targeted source of variation for augmenting datasets in tasks such as segmentation and detection.

The contributions of this paper are as follows. (1) We introduce an efficient generative framework for guided CBCT dentition synthesis, enabling explicit control over tooth presence at inference time. (2) We incorporate FiLM conditioning and a masked L2 loss to emphasize anatomically realistic reconstruction in tooth regions while suppressing background influence. (3) By simulating tooth removal and addition, we train the model to operate in two distinct modes, completion and removal, enabling scan-aware generation for clinically relevant editing (e.g., implant planning) or robust model training via data augmentation. (4) We conduct comprehensive quantitative and qualitative evaluations, including fairness across tooth positions and fidelity of reconstructed teeth, demonstrating the high realism, variability, and flexibility of the proposed model.

2 Related Work

Deep learning has improved automatic tooth segmentation, with convolutional models achieving average Dice scores above 0.9 across maxillary and mandibular scans [13]. A meta-analysis of 29 studies confirms these high accuracies and robustness across datasets [3]. However, segmentation remains inherently limited; it does not support image generation or editing, and performance is often degraded by metal artifacts, scanner variability, and background dominance [14].

Despite growing interest in synthetic medical imaging using deep learning models, generative models have been sparsely applied to dental data. PanoGAN [15] uses a Wasserstein GAN [16] to synthesize 2D panoramic radiographs for augmentation, but it cannot capture full 3D anatomical structure. GANs also suffer from well-documented drawbacks such as mode collapse and difficulty preserving structural consistency, especially in volumetric settings.

DDPMs have emerged as a powerful alternative with greater stability and diversity in image synthesis [9]. They have been applied to CBCT denoising and CT translation, improving quality and downstream tasks like segmentation or dosimetry [7,8]. Recent variants, including DiffDenoise [11] and cycle-consistent diffusion models [10], further enhance reconstruction from sparse or artifact-prone scans. Yet, these methods treat the image volume holistically, lacking mechanisms for localized anatomical control such as tooth editing or generation.

Conditional diffusion frameworks have enabled controllable image synthesis in other domains via latent diffusion modeling (LDM) [17], cross-modal conditioning, and feature-wise transformations like FiLM. While such mechanisms support attribute-driven generation, no existing work addresses conditional 3D CBCT synthesis with anatomically precise, tooth-level guidance.

3 Methods

3.1 Guided Wavelet Diffusion Model

We employ a wavelet denoising diffusion model (WDM) [18] tailored for 3D CBCT volume synthesis. As illustrated in Fig. 1, the proposed framework follows a conditional generation paradigm, where the model is guided by binary attribute vectors representing tooth presence and a 3D CBCT scan to be edited. This conditional design enables the generation and editing of 3D scans with precise control over dental configurations.

To alleviate the high computational demands and accelerate training and inference, we replace standard Gaussian noise perturbation in pixel space with a wavelet-domain formulation. Specifically, we apply a 3D Haar wavelet transform to decompose the signal into multi-scale frequency components, and inject Gaussian noise into these components. The diffusion model then learns to iteratively denoise in the wavelet domain, operating on representations with half the original spatial resolution. This latent formulation significantly reduces memory and compute requirements while preserving semantic fidelity (e.g., global volume structure) and enhancing detail reconstruction (e.g., tooth boundaries).

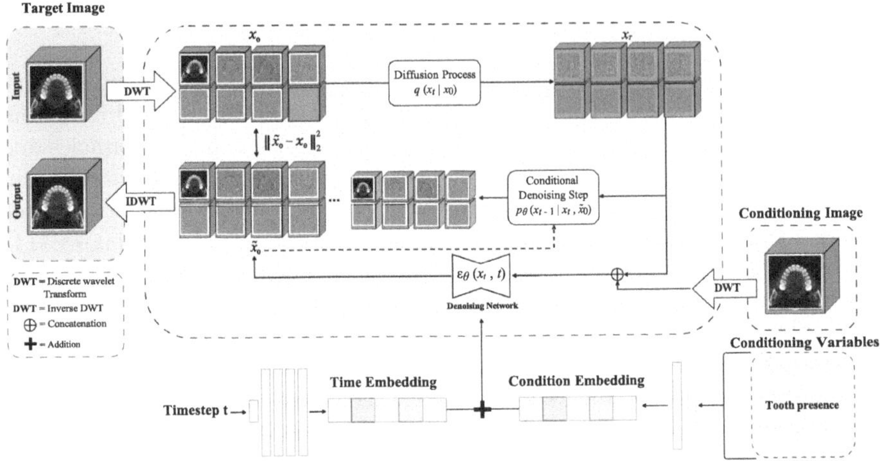

Fig. 1. Overview of the proposed framework. A guided diffusion model is used for 3D CBCT scan generation with editable tooth configurations.

3.2 Condition Embedding

Each scan is associated with a binary vector of length 32, indicating the presence or absence of individual teeth. This vector is passed through a linear layer to produce a learned conditioning embedding with the same dimensionality as the time embedding, which is obtained using a two-layer multilayer perceptron. These embeddings are combined within each residual block via FiLM [12], implemented as a SiLU activation followed by a linear projection, and integrated into the U-Net architecture. FiLM enables the network to modulate intermediate feature activations by applying learned, condition-dependent scaling and shifting, thereby allowing dynamic control based on the desired tooth configuration. During training, the model is conditioned on a real scan and optimized to reconstruct a version consistent with the specified tooth attributes.

3.3 Tooth Augmentation

In addition to standard training, where conditions are derived from reconstructing the input scan to match its original dental configuration, we introduce augmentation strategies to promote robustness. Specifically, we simulate two complementary scenarios by modifying the conditioning and target images: tooth addition and tooth removal. In the addition scenario, up to 50% of the teeth are randomly masked in the conditioning image, while the target remains the original, unaltered scan. The conditioning vector guides the model to plausibly reconstruct the missing structures, and the loss is computed against the original label to penalize inaccurate synthesis. In the removal scenario, up to 50% of teeth are removed from the target image, while the conditioning image retains the full dental configuration. The model learns to suppress specified regions, with supervision still applied relative to the original, unaltered label. These augmentations simulate clinically relevant use cases, such as handling missing or implanted teeth in surgical planning or restorative workflows.

To ensure that missing teeth appear realistic in the simulated training data, we avoid naive zeroing or masking of the region. Instead, we employ an image-based inpainting strategy to fill the masked tooth cavity with anatomically plausible content. Specifically, we first dilate the tooth mask to accommodate boundary uncertainty and define a broader region for removal. This expanded mask is used to set the corresponding region in the CBCT scan to missing values. Next, we apply the Manhattan (city-block) distance transform to the binary mask, indicating missing regions as zeros. The resulting distance map identifies the nearest valid voxels, whose intensity values are then propagated to fill the cavity. This approach allows the reconstructed region to reflect plausible anatomical structure, such as gradients between air and jawbone intensities near the crown and root, rather than introducing artificial holes to which the model could overfit. Finally, we apply Gaussian smoothing to the inpainted region to eliminate abrupt transitions and promote spatial coherence.

To further increase the effective training sample size, we apply a simple yet effective data augmentation by horizontally flipping the scans and their corresponding label maps (left-to-right). Given the approximate bilateral symmetry of human dentition, we adjust the tooth label values post-flip to preserve anatomical correctness. For the upper jaw (labels 1 to 16), each label is reassigned as $17 - t$, and for the lower jaw (labels 17 to 32), as $49 - t$, where t is the original tooth label. This transformation ensures consistency in leftright orientation and tooth identity, thereby augmenting the dataset without introducing semantic noise.

3.4 Loss Function

Given the high background-to-signal ratio in CBCT scans, we introduce a masked L2 loss to concentrate learning on tooth-bearing regions. During training, a soft spatial mask M is derived from the ground truth tooth segmentation by applying a Gaussian blur around tooth boundaries. This mask emphasizes regions near the teeth while down-weighting the less informative background. The masked L2 reconstruction loss is defined as:

$$\mathcal{L}_{\text{Masked}} = \|M \odot (x - \hat{x})\|_2^2, \tag{1}$$

where x is the ground truth scan, $\hat{x}$ is the generated output, M is the soft mask, and $\odot$ denotes element-wise multiplication. This loss penalizes discrepancies, specifically in regions affected by tooth additions or removals, encouraging anatomically faithful reconstructions. The masked loss is then combined with the primary WDM reconstruction loss after the denoising process to yield the total training objective:

$$\mathcal{L}_{\text{Total}} = \mathcal{L}_{\text{WDM}} + \lambda \, \mathcal{L}_{\text{Masked}}, \tag{2}$$

where λ is a weighting factor, empirically set to 10 in our experiments.

4 Experiments and Results

4.1 Data

We utilize a curated dataset of CBCT scans with ground truth dental segmentation[1] for our study, originally introduced in [19–21]. From the initial set of 150 CBCT volumes, we exclude 50 scans from a different cohort acquired at higher resolution (0.2 mm^3 voxel size) for subsequent analysis. Additionally, we discard two scans with missing segmentation maps and two segmentation volumes without corresponding scans. The resulting 98 volumes are manually relabeled according to the Universal Numbering System (tooth numbers 1–32), excluding supernumerary teeth present in two of the scans. For missing teeth annotations, we provide manual annotations where applicable. Notably, the dataset includes patients with multiple CBCT acquisitions at different treatment stages, enabling analysis of longitudinal consistency and anatomical changes.

All CBCT scans are spatially standardized to a fixed volume size of $256 \times 256 \times 256$ voxels by cropping or padding based on the tooth annotations. This ensures full dentition coverage while preserving the original voxel resolution of 0.4 mm^3, and reduces memory usage by excluding excessive background regions. Intensity values are normalized to the $[-1, 1]$ range for stable training. For each scan, binary labels are generated for individual teeth and are used both as supervision during training and for computing the masked reconstruction loss.

4.2 Experimental Setup

To scale training across multiple GPUs, we adapted the diffusion model using Distributed Data Parallel framework along with a Distributed Sampler for efficient data loading. The model was trained for 100,000 iterations with 1,000 diffusion time steps using a linear noise schedule. Optimization was performed using Adam optimizer with an initial learning rate of 1×10^{-5}, scaled linearly with the number of GPUs. A batch size of 1 per GPU was used to accommodate the memory constraints of volumetric data. During evaluation, we test the model on real CBCT scans, both with and without artificially removed/added teeth, and compare reconstructions against the corresponding ground truth volumes.

Out of the 98 available scans, we reserve 8 unique patient scans for testing, selected to represent edge cases such as complete dentition, partial dentition with only a few remaining teeth, or the presence of artifacts like brackets, braces, and mini-screws. The remaining 90 scans are used for training/validation. Although the dataset appears limited in size, each scan encompasses 32 distinct tooth states, creating a combinatorial space of present/missing patterns. Combined with data augmentation during training, this allows diverse testing scenarios in generative settings, where variability rather than sample count is critical.

We evaluate model performance using standard quality metrics for visual fidelity, including the Structural Similarity Index Measure (SSIM) for paired

---

[1] https://github.com/ErdanC/Tooth-and-alveolar-bone-segmentation-from-CBCT.

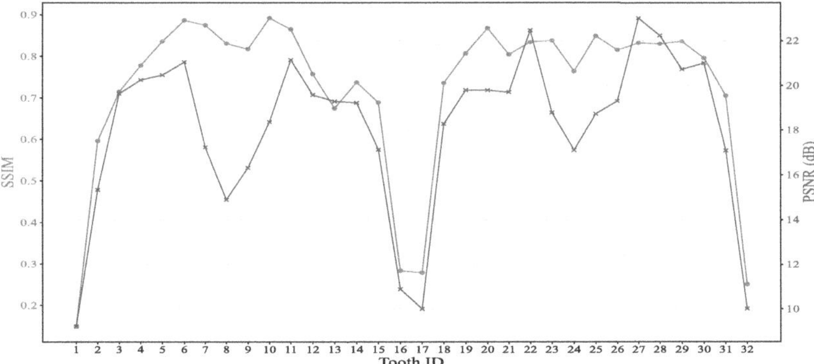

Fig. 2. Similarities between the original and reconstructed tooth when individually removed and regenerated by the model. Lower similarity is observed for wisdom teeth, likely due to their anatomical variability and data scarcity.

comparisons and the Fréchet Inception Distance (FID) for distributional comparison, both computed in 3D between real and generated volumes. In addition, we assess fairness in generation using per-tooth similarity analysis to identify potential bias in reconstruction fidelity, particularly in scans with a full dental set used for simulated tooth removal and addition scenarios.

4.3 Results

Reconstruction Synthesis. We first assess the model's ability to reconstruct full CBCT scans from conditioning vectors reflecting the original dentition. Quantitative evaluation is conducted using FID between training-validation and training-test splits, providing insight into both overfitting and generalization. The FID score on the test set is notably low (40.27), indicating high-quality image generation relative to the real training samples. It also suggests that the model does not overfit or memorize the training distribution. The relatively higher FID scores for the validation set (88.81) may be attributed to the smaller number of samples (2 vs. 8) used during validation.

Tooth Addition Synthesis. To evaluate single-tooth completion, we simulate missing teeth by masking individual teeth in test scans with complete dentition. The model is then tasked with reconstructing the missing tooth based on the remaining context. We compute the SSIM and PSNR between the reconstructed and ground-truth teeth on a per-tooth basis. The average SSIM scores per tooth are visualized in Fig. 2, highlighting variation across tooth positions. As can be seen, the tooth addition results demonstrate fairly accurate synthesis across most teeth, except for the molars and wisdom teeth (i.e., tooth IDs 1, 16, 17, and 32), which are typically scarce in the training datasets and exhibit greater anatomical variability in size, shape, and orientation.

Table 1. Comparison of FID scores between test-time generated scans with removed teeth and training scans exhibiting matching tooth absence.

Missing Teeth	[1, 16]	[1, 16, 17, 32]	[16, 17, 18, 19]
FID Score	75.20	74.36	80.03

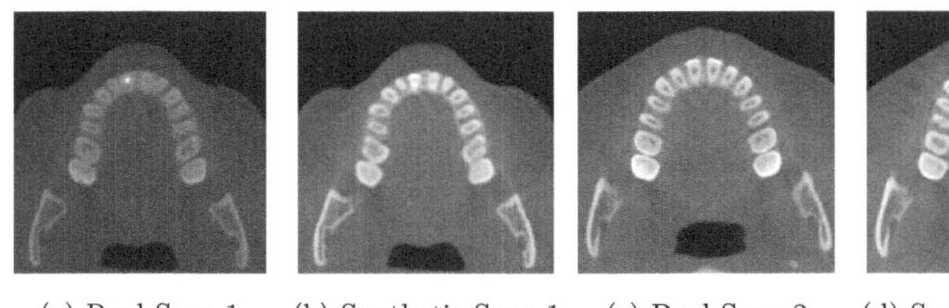

(a) Real Scan 1 (b) Synthetic Scan 1 (c) Real Scan 2 (d) Synthetic Scan 2

Fig. 3. Qualitative comparison between generated CBCT scans and their corresponding real scans with complete dentition.

Tooth Removal Synthesis. We assess the model's capacity to synthesize realistic scans with specific teeth removed. For this, we define common patterns of tooth absence and apply them to scans with full dentition in the test set. The model generates corresponding scans with these teeth removed. We then compare the generated scans to real samples from the matching tooth-absence groups using FID. Table 1 reports the FID scores for different target tooth-absence patterns. As shown in the table, the results yield low FID scores across different missing-tooth groups compared to the corresponding generated samples, demonstrating the model's ability to successfully inpaint missing teeth.

Full Dental Synthesis. As a final experiment, we evaluate the model's performance on generating a complete dentition in scans with no teeth present. This assesses the model's ability to synthesize anatomically plausible full dental structures from the conditioning vector. Figure 3 presents qualitative results comparing the generated samples to real scans with complete dentition. The visual comparison demonstrates a strong alignment between the real and synthetic inpainted regions. Quantitative evaluation supports this observation, with an average SSIM of 0.9123 and an average PSNR of 18.35 computed over the inpainted areas, despite the model not having seen the test samples during training.

5 Conclusion

We proposed a guided diffusion framework for controllable synthesis of 3D CBCT dental scans, enabling realistic generation, addition, and removal of teeth based on per-tooth attributes. Our approach integrated a wavelet-based denoising diffusion backbone with FiLM conditioning and masked reconstruction loss alongside tooth augmentations to guide the generative process toward anatomically plausible outputs. Experimental results demonstrated high visual fidelity and generalization performance, with low FID scores in reconstruction and inpainting tasks, and consistent SSIM values across most teeth. The model successfully handles complex cases, such as missing dentition or the presence of artifacts, and shows potential for clinically oriented simulation tasks such as visualizing treatment outcomes or testing AI models under diverse dentition patterns.

While we focused on per-tooth conditioning, broader clinical factors such as implants, crowns, and bridges remain challenging and represent promising directions for future work. Moreover, although our dataset was limited in size, each scan enabled extensive variability via combinatorial tooth presence patterns, supporting robust generative evaluation. Scaling to larger public datasets, such as ToothFairy[2], and assessing impact on downstream segmentation or detection tasks will be important future steps toward clinical deployment. This study highlights the feasibility of fine-grained, tooth-level controllable generation and provides a tool for simulation, targeted data augmentation, and the development of more customizable and interpretable generative models in dental imaging.

Acknowledgments. This project is supported by the Pioneer Centre for AI, funded by the Danish National Research Foundation (grant number P1).

Disclosure of Interests. The authors have no competing interests in the paper.

References

1. Scarfe, W.C., Farman, A.G.: What is cone-beam CT and how does it work? Dent. Clin. North Am. **52**(4), 707–730 (2008)
2. Pauwels, R., Araki, K., Siewerdsen, J., Thongvigitmanee, S.S.: Technical aspects of dental CBCT: state of the art. Dentomaxillofacial Radiol. **44**(1), 20140224 (2015)
3. Sadr, S., et al.: Deep learning for tooth identification and numbering on dental radiography: a systematic review and meta-analysis. Dentomaxillofacial Radiol. **53**(1), 5–21 (2024)
4. Singh, N.K., Raza, K.: Progress in deep learning-based dental and maxillofacial image analysis: a systematic review. Expert Syst. Appl. **199** (2022)
5. Bolelli, F., et al.: Segmenting maxillofacial structures in CBCT volumes. In: Proceedings of the Computer Vision and Pattern Recognition Conference, pp. 5238–5248 (2025)
6. Choi, H., Yun, J.P., Lee, A., Han, S.S., Kim, S.W., Lee, C.: Deep learning synthesis of cone-beam computed tomography from zero echo time magnetic resonance imaging. Sci. Rep. **13**(1), 6031 (2023)
7. Hu, C., Cao, N., Li, X., He, Y., Zhou, H.: CBCT-to-CT synthesis using a hybrid U-Net diffusion model based on transformers and information bottleneck theory. Sci. Rep. **15**(1), 10816 (2025)
8. Zhang, Y., et al.: Texture-preserving diffusion model for CBCT-to-CT synthesis. Med. Image Anal. **99**, 103362 (2025)
9. Ho, J., Jain, A., Abbeel, P.: Denoising diffusion probabilistic models. Adv. Neural. Inf. Process. Syst. **33**, 6840–6851 (2020)

[2] https://ditto.ing.unimore.it/toothfairy3/.

10. Gao, Y., et al.: Limited-angle CBCT reconstruction via geometry-integrated cycle-domain denoising diffusion probabilistic models. arXiv:2506.13545 (2025)
11. Demir, B., et al.: DiffDenoise: self-supervised medical image denoising with conditional diffusion models. arXiv preprint arXiv:2504.00264 (2025)
12. Perez, E., Strub, F., De Vries, H., Dumoulin, V., Courville, A.: FiLM: visual reasoning with a general conditioning layer. In: Proceedings of the AAAI Conference on Artificial Intelligence, Vol. 32 (2018)
13. Polizzi, A., Qet al.: Tooth automatic segmentation from CBCT images: a systematic review. Clin. Oral Invest. **27**(7), 3363–3378 (2023)
14. Dot, G., et al.: DentalSegmentator: robust open source deep learning-based CT and CBCT image segmentation. J. Dent. **147**, 105130 (2024)
15. Pedersen, S., Jain, S., Chavez, M., Ladehoff, V., de Freitas, B.N., Pauwels, R.: Pano-GAN: a deep generative model for panoramic dental radiographs. J. Imaging **11**(2), 41 (2025)
16. Arjovsky, M., Chintala, S., Bottou, L.: Wasserstein generative adversarial networks. In: International Conference on Machine Learning, PMLR, pp. 214–223 (2017)
17. Rombach, R., Blattmann, A., Lorenz, D., Esser, P., Ommer, B.: High-resolution image synthesis with latent diffusion models. In: Proceedings of the IEEE/CVF Conference on Computer Vision and Pattern Recognition, pp. 10684–10695 (2022)
18. Friedrich, P., Wolleb, J., Bieder, F., Durrer, A., Cattin, P.C.: WDM: 3D wavelet diffusion models for high-resolution medical image synthesis. In: Mukhopadhyay, A., Oksuz, I., Engelhardt, S., Mehrof, D., Yuan, Y. (eds.). MICCAI Workshop on Deep Generative Models, vol. 15224, pp. 11–21. Springer, Cham (2024). https://doi.org/10.1007/978-3-031-72744-3_2
19. Cui, Z., Li, C., Wang, W.: ToothNet: automatic tooth instance segmentation and identification from cone beam CT images. In: Proceedings of the IEEE/CVF Conference on Computer Vision and Pattern Recognition, pp. 6368–6377 (2019)
20. Cui, Z., et al.: Hierarchical morphology-guided tooth instance segmentation from CBCT images. In: Feragen, A., Sommer, S., Schnabel, J., Nielsen, M. (eds.) Information Processing in Medical Imaging: 27th International Conference, Virtual Event, pp. 150–162. June 28–June 30, 2021, Proceedings 27, Springer, Cham (2021). https://doi.org/10.1007/978-3-030-78191-0_12
21. Cui, Z., et al.: A fully automatic AI system for tooth and alveolar bone segmentation from cone-beam CT images. Nat. Commun. **13**(1) (2022)

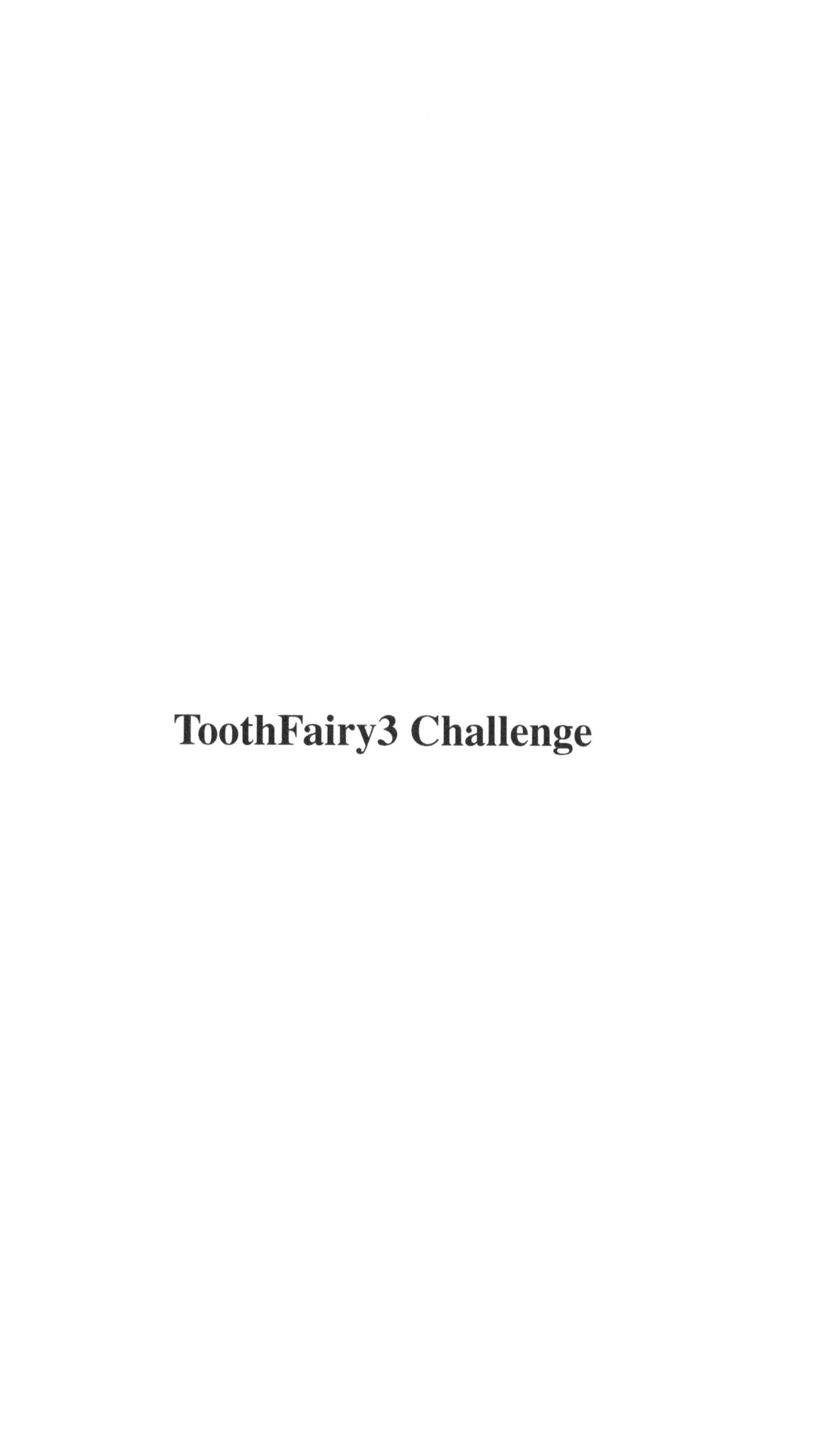

ToothFairy3 Challenge

Efficient CBCT Segmentation via nnU-Net with Structure-Aware Post-processing and Interactive Refinement

Changkai Ji, Yusheng Liu, Yuxian Jiang, and Lisheng Wang(✉)

School of Automation and Intelligent Sensing, Shanghai Jiao Tong University, Shanghai 200240, People's Republic of China
{changkaiji,lswang}@sjtu.edu.cn

Abstract. Accurate segmentation of anatomical structures from cone-beam computed tomography (CBCT) is essential for clinical applications in dentistry, maxillofacial surgery, and orthodontics. The ToothFairy3 Challenge has a comprehensive 77-class segmentation task, emphasizing both accuracy and computational efficiency. In this work, we present a method based on the nnU-Net framework, enhanced with a Structure Aware Post-processing (SAP) strategy. nnU-Net serves as a backbone for multi-class segmentation, while SAP refines predictions by introducing individualized thresholds for each anatomical structure, thereby mitigating noise and preserving clinically important fine structures. To further improve efficiency, we disabled mirroring augmentation during training and employed inference acceleration strategies, including the removal of test-time augmentation and optimized interpolation on floating-point tensors. Experimental results validate the effectiveness of our approach in balancing segmentation accuracy with computational efficiency. To further ensure robustness in challenging clinical scenarios, we also utilize an interactive refinement module based on nnInteractive. This strategy allows clinicians to correct local segmentation errors with minimal user guidance, providing a safety net for complex anatomical variations.

Keywords: nnU-Net · Structure Aware Post-processing · Computational efficiency

1 Introduction

Cone-beam computed tomography (CBCT) has become an indispensable imaging modality in dentistry, maxillofacial surgery, and orthodontics due to its short acquisition time, low radiation dose, and high spatial resolution for hard tissues [1,13]. Accurate delineation of anatomical structures from CBCT is essential for surgical planning, risk assessment, and clinical decision-making. Building on the success of previous ToothFairy challenges, the ToothFairy3 – MICCAI 2025 competition pushes the boundaries of multi-class segmentation with an

F. Bolelli et al. (Eds.): ODIN 2025, LNCS 16473, pp. 101–112, 2026.
https://doi.org/10.1007/978-3-032-20711-1_10

expanded dataset encompassing 77 anatomical categories, including newly introduced structures such as the pulp cavity, incisive nerve, and lingual foramen. This task emphasizes not only segmentation accuracy but also computational efficiency, reflecting the growing demand for real-time, reliable clinical tools.

Traditionally, the identification and delineation of anatomical structures in CBCT images have relied heavily on manual segmentation by experienced radiologists and dental professionals. The process requires substantial expertise and can take considerable time per case, making it impractical for routine clinical workflows where rapid decision-making is essential [5,16]. Moreover, the subjective nature of manual segmentation can lead to inconsistent results across different practitioners, potentially affecting treatment planning reliability.

In recent years, artificial intelligence techniques, particularly deep learning-based approaches using convolutional neural networks (CNNs), have demonstrated remarkable success in medical image segmentation tasks [9,10,15,17]. These automated methods have shown promising results in various dental imaging applications, offering the potential to significantly reduce processing time while maintaining or even improving segmentation accuracy. Deep learning frameworks have proven particularly effective at learning complex patterns and features from medical images, enabling robust identification of anatomical structures across diverse patient populations and imaging conditions [2,8,11].

Despite these advances, significant challenges remain for the ToothFairy3 task. First, the large number of categories (77) introduces class imbalance, as certain anatomical structures are underrepresented compared to larger, more prominent ones such as the mandible. This imbalance risks biasing the model toward dominant classes. Second, fine-scale structures like the incisive nerve or lingual foramen are difficult to segment reliably, requiring high-resolution features without overwhelming memory usage. Third, efficiency must be considered alongside accuracy: prolonged inference times or excessive memory consumption may render otherwise accurate models impractical for real-world clinical use [6,7]. Striking a balance between precision and computational efficiency is therefore essential.

To address these challenges, we propose a solution based on nnU-Net, enhanced with Structure Aware Post-processing (SAP) [4,14]. nnU-Net provides a strong backbone for multi-class segmentation, automatically adapting to the CBCT dataset's characteristics, while SAP refines predictions by removing spurious regions and ensuring anatomical plausibility. This approach aims to achieve high segmentation accuracy across 77 classes while maintaining computational efficiency, aligning with the dual objectives of the ToothFairy3 challenge. Despite the high performance of automated models, purely automatic segmentation may still falter in cases with severe artifacts or ambiguous boundaries (e.g., discontinuous inferior alveolar canals). To address this, we incorporate an interactive segmentation paradigm as a complementary refinement step. By leveraging user provided point prompts, this module enables precise correction of difficult targets, ensuring that the system meets the rigorous reliability standards required for surgical planning. The contributions of our work can be summarized as follows:

- We employed an automated segmentation framework based on nnU-Net with SAP to address the multi-class segmentation challenge in CBCT images.
- The proposed approach optimizes the trade-off between segmentation quality and computational efficiency, ensuring both clinical accuracy and practical feasibility.
- Our approach achieved top-three performance in the ToothFairy3 Challenge validation phase, demonstrating its effectiveness for comprehensive dental and maxillofacial structure segmentation.

2 Proposed Method

2.1 Framework Overview

As shown in Fig. 1, we propose a segmentation approach for CBCT images, leveraging nnU-Net as the foundational architecture with disabled mirroring augmentation, combined with a SAP strategy. Disabling mirroring augmentation preserves the inherent left-right anatomical asymmetry of oral structures, enabling the model to learn structure-specific positional features. Structure Aware Thresholds provide adaptive morphological optimization, thereby minimizing false positives across diverse oral tissues.

2.2 Data Preprocessing

We employed nnU-Net's automated preprocessing pipeline to optimize data handling and network configuration for our multi-structure segmentation task. The preprocessing stage involved comprehensive dataset validation to ensure annotation consistency and data integrity across all CBCT volumes. The framework automatically determined optimal patch sizes, spacing parameters, and intensity normalization strategies based on the inherent characteristics of the dataset. This automated approach eliminates manual hyperparameter tuning while ensuring that preprocessing parameters are specifically tailored to the morphological and intensity characteristics of CBCT imaging data.

Additionally, the preprocessing pipeline established network topology and memory allocation strategies optimized for 3D volumetric segmentation of high-resolution CBCT images. The intensity normalization was performed using dataset-specific statistics computed from foreground regions, ensuring consistent intensity distributions across the training cohort.

2.3 Model Training Strategy

Model training was conducted using the 3D full-resolution configuration to preserve high spatial resolution critical for accurate delineation of fine anatomical

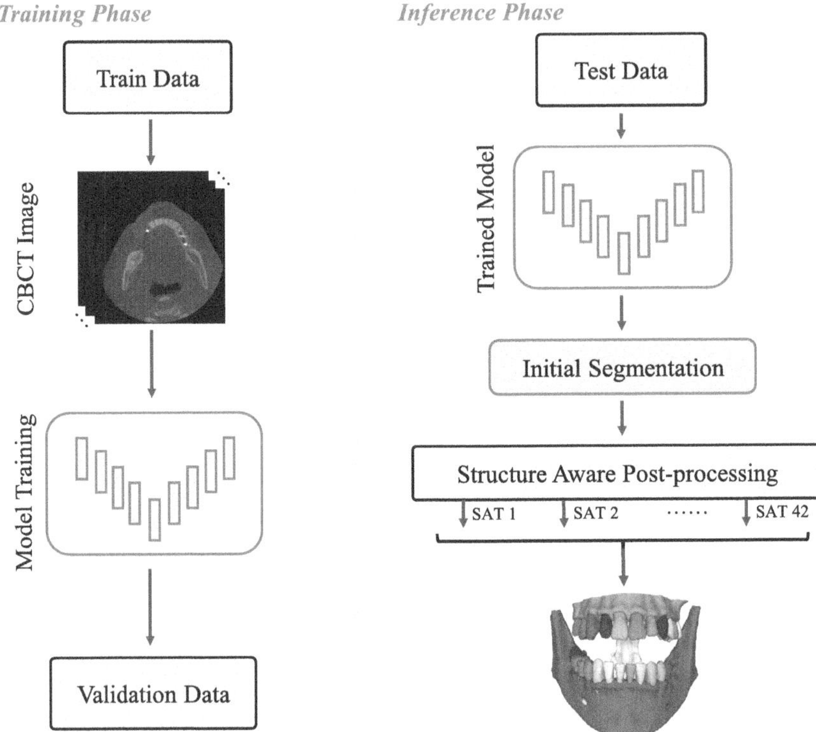

Fig. 1. Overview of the proposed framework. The training procedure utilized nnU-Net with disabled mirroring augmentation to enhance structure-specific learning. During inference, initial segmentation outputs were refined through Structure Aware Post-processing, wherein predetermined Structure Aware Thresholds were applied to target anatomical structures for morphological optimization.

structures. During the training phase, we selectively disabled mirroring-based data augmentation techniques. This approach addresses the inherent positional specificity of oral anatomical structures, where spatial location serves as one of the fundamental identifying characteristics. For instance, the left and right inferior alveolar canals, while morphologically similar, are distinguished primarily by their anatomical position. Similarly, FDI numbering assignment for teeth would be compromised by mirroring augmentation. Applying mirroring augmentation would artificially transpose these position-dependent structures, compromising the model's ability to learn spatial-anatomical relationships essential for accurate structure identification and increasing classification difficulty between bilaterally symmetric yet distinct anatomical entities.

2.4 Structure Aware Post-processing

Traditional post-processing approaches for medical image segmentation typically employ fixed filtering parameters across all anatomical structures, such as removing connected components smaller than a predetermined volume threshold or retaining only the largest connected component for each structure. However, this "one-size-fits-all" strategy presents significant limitations: overly conservative thresholds may preserve noise and erroneous segmentations, while aggressive thresholds risk eliminating clinically important small structures.

To address these limitations, we propose a Structure Aware Post-processing method that computes individualized Structure-aware Thresholds (SAT) for each anatomical structure, rather than applying uniform criteria across all structures. The core insight is that different anatomical structures exhibit distinct morphological characteristics and volume distributions, necessitating structure-specific optimization strategies.

Let $\mathcal{S} = \{S_1, S_2, \ldots, S_K\}$ denote the set of K target anatomical structures. For each structure S_i, we define a SAT τ_i that specifies the minimum volume required for a connected component to be considered valid. The collection of thresholds is represented as $\mathbf{T} = \{\tau_1, \tau_2, \ldots, \tau_K\}$. Given an initial segmentation prediction $\mathbf{P}$, the structure-aware post-processing procedure consists of four sequential steps.

1. Connected Component Analysis. For each structure S_i, we extract all connected components from the corresponding segmentation mask:

$$\mathcal{C}_i = \{c_{i,1}, c_{i,2}, \ldots, c_{i,n_i}\},$$

where n_i denotes the number of connected components predicted for structure S_i, and each pair of components is disjoint, i.e., $c_{i,a} \cap c_{i,b} = \varnothing$ for $a \neq b$.

2. Volume Computation. For each connected component $c_{i,j}$, we compute its volume $v_{i,j}$. In the general case with voxel volume $V_{\text{vox}}(x, y, z)$, the volume is:

$$v_{i,j} = \sum_{(x,y,z) \in c_{i,j}} V_{\text{vox}}(x, y, z).$$

3. Threshold-based Filtering. Each connected component is retained only if its volume exceeds the corresponding threshold:

$$c_{i,j}^{\text{filtered}} = \begin{cases} c_{i,j}, & \text{if } v_{i,j} \geq \tau_i, \\ \varnothing, & \text{otherwise,} \end{cases}$$

where $\varnothing$ denotes the empty set, i.e., the component is discarded.

4. Final Reconstruction. The refined segmentation for structure S_i is obtained by the union of all retained components:

$$\hat{S}_i = \bigcup_{j:\, v_{i,j} \geq \tau_i} c_{i,j}.$$

The complete post-processed segmentation is given by

$$\hat{\mathbf{P}} = \{\hat{S}_1, \hat{S}_2, \ldots, \hat{S}_K\},$$

which can be further represented as a labeled mask for downstream evaluation or visualization.

This approach enables differentiated treatment of anatomical structures with varying size characteristics. For instance, large structures such as jawbones can utilize higher thresholds to effectively eliminate substantial noise regions, while smaller structures like nerve canals employ lower thresholds to preserve their inherently compact morphology. The structure-aware post-processing thus provides a framework for balancing the trade-off between noise removal and structure preservation in multi-class anatomical segmentation tasks.

To determine the optimal values for the structure-aware thresholds (τ_{vol}), we analyze the volumetric distribution of each anatomical class within the training dataset. The filtering strategy is empirically tailored to the scale of the target structures. For the pharynx, we retain only the largest connected component. For other structures, thresholds are stratified by anatomical size: massive bone structures like the lower jawbone and upper jawbone utilize high thresholds ($10,000$ and $5,000$ voxels, respectively) to filter out major misclassifications. Medium-sized prosthetics employ a threshold of $2,000$ voxels. Specific subsets of teeth are assigned a threshold of $1,500$ voxels. Fine-grained structures, including the inferior alveolar canals, use a lower threshold of 500 voxels. The detailed configuration is presented in our Github.

2.5 Interactive Refinement Module

While the proposed nnU-Net with SAP achieves efficient automated segmentation, we introduce an interactive refinement module, nnInteractive, to handle corner cases requiring human expertise. This module adopts a "human-in-the-loop" workflow where clinicians can iteratively refine segmentation results using point prompts.

Network Architecture: Unlike methods using separate image and prompt encoders (e.g., SAM), nnInteractive employs an early prompt strategy. User-provided prompts (e.g., foreground/background clicks) are encoded as Gaussian heatmaps and concatenated with the original image and the current segmentation mask along the channel dimension. The network input consists of eight channels: the original image, the previous mask, and six channels representing different interaction types (points, scribbles, bounding boxes).

AutoZoom Mechanism: To handle small, fine-grained structures like the inferior alveolar canal within large FOV CBCT scans, the module incorporates an

AutoZoom mechanism. This dynamic strategy automatically crops and resamples the Region of Interest (ROI) around the user's interaction points, allowing the model to focus on local details at higher resolution without losing context. This ensures that even subtle anatomical structures can be precisely corrected with minimal user interaction (1–5 clicks).

3 Experiments and Results

3.1 Dataset and Assessment Metrics

The dataset used in Task 1 of the ToothFairy3 challenge is composed of CBCT scans annotated with 77 anatomical classes, encompassing not only large bony structures such as the mandible and maxilla, but also fine-grained elements such as pulp cavities, incisive canals, and the lingual foramen [2,3,12]. The volumes are provided in NIfTI format with intensity values in Hounsfield units. Across all scans, the maximum spatial dimensions are $(298, 512, 512)$, the minimum are $(170, 272, 345)$, and the median shape is $(168, 362, 371)$.

For evaluation, we adopt two widely used metrics in medical image segmentation: the Dice Similarity Coefficient (DSC) and the 95th percentile Hausdorff Distance (HD95). Both metrics are computed for each class on each test volume, followed by averaging across all volumes. DSC quantifies the voxel-wise overlap between the predicted segmentation and the ground truth, while HD95 assesses the boundary-level agreement by measuring the distance between surfaces. Together, these metrics capture both volumetric and geometric accuracy.

Although our analysis in this work focuses on DSC and HD95, it is worth noting that computational efficiency plays a crucial role in the challenge design. Inference runtime and maximum memory usage are also recorded and will contribute to the final ranking of submitted methods, reflecting their practical applicability in clinical settings.

3.2 Implementation Details

Environments and Requirements. The training of our method was conducted for a total of 1000 epochs. The details of the computational environment and dependencies are summarized in Table 1.

Inference Acceleration. Since runtime was an important factor in the challenge evaluation, we applied several strategies to accelerate inference. First, we disabled test-time augmentation in nnU-Net, which substantially reduced the computational burden while maintaining competitive accuracy. Second, we optimized the handling of multi-class predictions by refining the interpolation step. Instead of relying on conventional integer-based resampling methods that are computationally demanding, we leveraged PyTorch's `interpolate` function on floating-point tensors. This choice preserves numerical precision while improving throughput in large-scale volumetric segmentation. Together, these strategies enabled efficient inference across the entire test set.

Table 1. System Configuration

Ubuntu version	Ubuntu 24.04 LTS
CPU	Intel(R) Xeon(R) Platinum 8352S CPU @ 2.20GHz
RAM	503 GB
GPU	1 NVIDIA GeForce RTX 4090 (24G)
CUDA version	12.4
Programming language	Python 3.9.19
Deep learning framework	PyTorch (torch 1.12.1, torchvision 0.19.1)
Code will available at	https://github.com/duola-wa/Toothfairy3

3.3 Results and Analysis

Quantitative Performance. The quantitative results for both the debug and test phases are summarized in Table 2. We report the Dice similarity coefficient and the HD95, with the former reflecting overlap accuracy and the latter assessing boundary alignment. Higher Dice and lower HD95 values indicate better performance.

Table 2. Evaluation results across debug and test phases. Dice similarity coefficient and HD95 are reported.

Metric	Statistic	Debug Phase	Test Phase
Dice Average	Min	0.9090	0.5671
	25%	0.9371	0.7340
	50%	0.9653	0.7821
	75%	0.9695	0.8329
	Max	0.9737	0.8670
	Mean	0.9493	0.7705
	Std	0.0352	0.0754
HD95 Average	Min	11.13	54.58
	25%	11.16	77.29
	50%	11.18	93.36
	75%	28.13	122.91
	Max	45.07	206.55
	Mean	22.46	104.59
	Std	19.58	37.21

In the debug phase, which included only three cases, our method demonstrated high segmentation accuracy with an average Dice score of 0.949 and a relatively low HD95 of 22.46. However, the larger-scale test phase presented more challenging scenarios, where the average Dice dropped to 0.770, and the mean HD95 increased to 104.59. This performance gap highlights the difficulty of generalization from a limited validation set to a more diverse and comprehensive test set. Nevertheless, the results remain competitive and validate the robustness of our approach under varying anatomical and imaging conditions.

Qualitative Results. To provide visual insight into the segmentation performance, Fig. 2 presents representative examples from the debug phase. These three cases illustrate the method's ability to accurately delineate anatomical structures across different imaging conditions and patient anatomies. Each row displays the input CBCT image (left), the predicted segmentation result (center), and the corresponding ground truth annotation (right). The visual comparison demonstrates the accuracy of our segmentation results on debug data, with predicted boundaries closely matching the expert annotations across multiple anatomical regions.

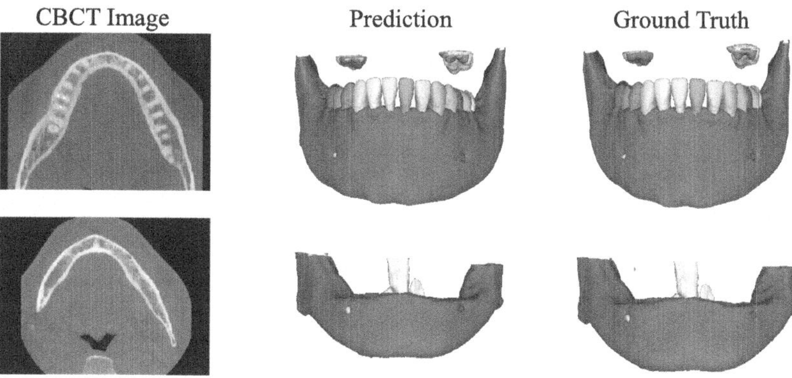

Fig. 2. Representative segmentation results from debug phase cases. Each row shows (from left to right): input CBCT image, predicted segmentation result, and ground truth. The results demonstrate accurate delineation of anatomical structures across different patient anatomies and imaging conditions on debug data.

As shown in Fig. 3, we provide a visual comparison of the segmentation results for nnInteractive with the introduction of 3 and 5 interaction points, respectively. This visualization highlights the impact of increasing the number of user interactions on the segmentation accuracy. Due to the limited number of submissions in the competition, we did not include metric-based results in this analysis, focusing instead on the visual comparison of the segmentation outputs.

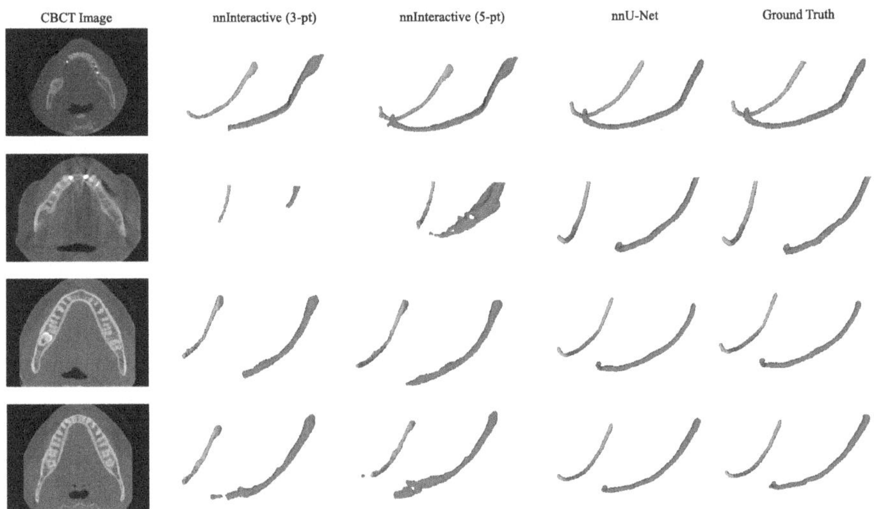

Fig. 3. The nnInteractive method is evaluated with 3 and 5 interaction points, highlighting the effect of prompt refinement on segmentation accuracy.

4 Conclusion

In this paper, we presented a segmentation framework for multi-class CBCT images, designed for the ToothFairy3 Challenge. Our approach leverages nnU-Net as a backbone and introduces SAP to account for the morphological variability of different anatomical structures. The proposed strategy enables differentiated handling of large and fine-scale structures, thereby reducing false positives while preserving clinically relevant details. Experiments demonstrated that our method achieves consistently high accuracy in the debug phase. Importantly, by optimizing interpolation strategies, we achieved notable improvements in inference efficiency. Furthermore, the integration of the interactive refinement module demonstrates a viable path for clinical deployment. It bridges the gap between fully automated processing and the need for meticulous precision in complex surgical cases, effectively balancing algorithmic efficiency with clinical reliability.

References

1. Acar, B., Kamburoğlu, K.: Use of cone beam computed tomography in periodontology. World J. Radiol. **6**(5), 139 (2014)
2. Bolelli, F., et al.: Segmenting the inferior alveolar canal in cbcts volumes: the toothfairy challenge. IEEE Trans. Med. Imaging (2024)

3. Bolelli, F., et al.: Segmenting maxillofacial structures in cbct volumes. In: Proceedings of the Computer Vision and Pattern Recognition Conference, pp. 5238–5248 (2025)
4. Isensee, F., et al.: nnu-net: self-adapting framework for u-net-based medical image segmentation. arXiv preprint arXiv:1809.10486 (2018)
5. Ji, C., et al.: Mammo-net: Integrating gaze supervision and interactive information in multi-view mammogram classification. In: Greenspan, H., et al. (eds.) International Conference on Medical Image Computing and Computer-Assisted Intervention, pp. 68–78. Springer, Cham (2023). https://doi.org/10.1007/978-3-031-43990-2_7
6. Ji, C., Liu, Y., He, L., Jiang, Y., Huang, C., Wang, L.: Two-stage semi-supervised nnu-net framework for tooth segmentation in cbct images. In: Wang, Y., et al. (eds.) International Conference on Medical Image Computing and Computer-Assisted Intervention, pp. 100–109. Springer, Cham (2024). https://doi.org/10.1007/978-3-031-88977-6_10
7. Ji, C., Liu, Y., He, L., Jiang, Y., Huang, C., Wang, L.: A two-stage semi-supervised nnu-net model for automated tooth segmentation in panoramic x-ray images. In: Wang, Y., et al. (eds.) International Conference on Medical Image Computing and Computer-Assisted Intervention, pp. 91–99. Springer, Cham (2024). https://doi.org/10.1007/978-3-031-88977-6_9
8. Jiang, Y., Liu, Y., Ji, C., Wang, L.: Enhanced multi-structure segmentation in cbct images with adaptive structure optimization. In: Wang, Y., et al. (eds.) International Conference on Medical Image Computing and Computer-Assisted Intervention, pp. 30–40. Springer, Cham (2024). https://doi.org/10.1007/978-3-031-88977-6_4
9. Lin, Z., Liu, Y., Wu, J., Wang, D.H., Zhang, X.Y., Zhu, S.: Multi-modal pre-post treatment consistency learning for automatic segmentation and evaluation of the circle of willis. Comput. Med. Imaging Graph. **122**, 102521 (2025)
10. Liu, Y., Xin, R., Yang, T., Wang, L.: Inferior alveolar nerve segmentation in cbct images using connectivity-based selective re-training. In: Wang, Y., et al. (eds.) International Conference on Medical Image Computing and Computer-Assisted Intervention. pp. 3–12. Springer, Cham (2024). https://doi.org/10.1007/978-3-031-88977-6_1
11. Liu, Y., Zhao, Z., Wang, L.: A cnn-based multi-stage framework for renal multi-structure segmentation. In: Xiao, Y., Yang, G., Song, S. (eds.) MICCAI Challenge on Correction of Brainshift with Intra-Operative Ultrasound, pp. 18–26. Springer, Cham (2022). https://doi.org/10.1007/978-3-031-27324-7_3
12. Lumetti, L., Pipoli, V., Bolelli, F., Ficarra, E., Grana, C.: Enhancing patch-based learning for the segmentation of the mandibular canal. IEEE Access **12**, 79014–79024 (2024)
13. Patel, S., Durack, C., Abella, F., Shemesh, H., Roig, M., Lemberg, K.: Cone beam computed tomography in e ndodontics-a review. Int. Endod. J. **48**(1), 3–15 (2015)
14. Ronneberger, O., Fischer, P., Brox, T.: U-net: Convolutional networks for biomedical image segmentation. In: Navab, N., Hornegger, J., Wells, W., Frangi, A. (eds.) International Conference on Medical image computing and computer-assisted intervention, pp. 234–241. Springer, Cham (2015). https://doi.org/10.1007/978-3-319-24574-4_28
15. Shen, D., Wu, G., Suk, H.I.: Deep learning in medical image analysis. Annu. Rev. Biomed. Eng. **19**(1), 221–248 (2017)

16. Wang, S., Ouyang, X., Liu, T., Wang, Q., Shen, D.: Follow my eye: using gaze to supervise computer-aided diagnosis. IEEE Trans. Med. Imaging **41**(7), 1688–1698 (2022)
17. Yang, T., Yu, X., Tao, R., Li, H., Zhou, J.: Blood glucose prediction for type 2 diabetes using clustering-based domain adaptation. Biomed. Signal Process. Control **105**, 107629 (2025)

Efficient and Robust CBCT Segmentation of Oral and Maxillofacial Structures

Fan Xiao[1], Xinrui Huang[2], Anqi Gao[1,3], Dongming He[1], Xiaofan Zhang[2], and Xudong Wang[1,3,4,5,6,7,8](✉)

[1] Department of Oral Craniomaxillofacial, Shanghai Ninth People's Hospital, Shanghai Jiao Tong University School of Medicine, Shanghai, China
xudongwang70@hotmail.com

[2] School of Electronic Information and Electrical Engineering, Shanghai Jiao Tong University, Shanghai, China
{huangxr,xiaofan.zhang}@sjtu.edu.cn

[3] College of Stomatology, Shanghai Jiao Tong University, Shanghai, China

[4] National Center for Stomatology, Shanghai, China

[5] National Clinical Medical Research Center for Oral Diseases, Shanghai, China

[6] Shanghai Key Laboratory of Stomatology, Shanghai, China

[7] Shanghai Research Institute of Stomatology, Shanghai, China

[8] Research Unit of Oral and Maxillofacial Regenerative Medicine, Chinese Academy of Medical Science, Shanghai, China

Abstract. In dental practice, accurate segmentation of oral and maxillofacial structures from cone-beam computed tomography (CBCT) images is essential for diagnostic and treatment planning purposes. However, manual segmentation is time-consuming and labor-intensive. Although numerous deep learning-based methods have been proposed to automate this process, most rely on a single model architecture, which struggles to handle the complex and diverse nature of oral anatomical structures. To address this limitation, we propose a hybrid framework integrating nnUNet and VISTA models for automated and interactive segmentation of oral and maxillofacial structures. Our approach employs a class-wise ensemble strategy to improve inference efficiency and accuracy, and incorporates post-processing techniques such as threshold-based small object removal and disconnected region filtering to enhance robustness. The proposed method achieved third place in Task 1 and second place in Task 2 of the ToothFairy3 Challenge. Code and model weights are available at https://github.com/ff741333/toothfairy3_blcakmyth.

Keywords: CBCT image · Oral and maxillofacial structures segmentation · Interactive segmentation

1 Introduction

In dental practice, obtaining accurate oral and maxillofacial structures is essential for disease diagnosis and treatment. Cone-beam computed tomography

F. Bolelli et al. (Eds.): ODIN 2025, LNCS 16473, pp. 113–121, 2026.
https://doi.org/10.1007/978-3-032-20711-1_11

(CBCT), as a commonly used imaging modality, is frequently applied in dentistry and related fields due to its advantages of short acquisition time, low radiation dose, and high resolution for hard tissues. The oral and maxillofacial structures that can be obtained from CBCT images are illustrated in Fig. 1, including teeth (and dental attachments such as bridges, crowns, and implants), jawbone, maxillary sinus, pharynx, inferior alveolar canal (IAC), mandibular incisive canal, lingual canal, and others. These anatomical structures are critical for clinical applications such as surgical planning in implantology [6] and maxillofacial surgery [9], as well as tooth alignment in orthodontics. However, manually segmenting these structures from CBCT images is time-consuming and labor-intensive.

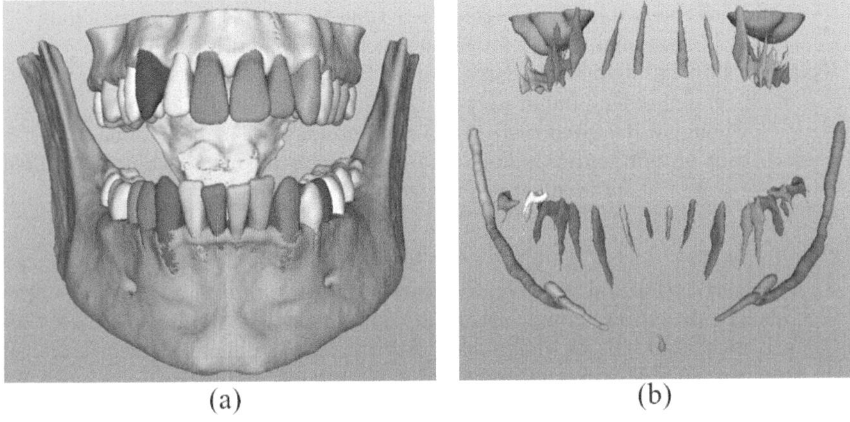

Fig. 1. Visualization of Oral and Maxillofacial Structures in CBCT: (a) Jawbone, Teeth, Pharynx; (b) Inferior Alveolar Canal, Mandibular Incisive Canal, Lingual Canal, Maxillary Sinus, Pulp.

In recent years, numerous studies [2,4,5,8,16] have focused on achieving automatic segmentation of oral and maxillofacial structures. Cui et al. [4] proposed a two-stage deep network leveraging hierarchical tooth morphology for precise tooth segmentation and a filter-enhanced network enhancing intensity contrasts for accurate alveolar bone segmentation. Dot et al. [5] has developed an open-source tool for robust segmentation of oral and maxillofacial structures on CBCT and CT images, including the maxilla, mandible, teeth, and mandibular canal. Bolelli et al. [2] constructed a dataset consisting of 42 different types of CBCT maxillofacial structure segmentation, and employed various strategies to optimize the performance of existing excellent segmentation models [3,10–12,14,15,18]. The existing segmentation models for oral and maxillofacial structures are usually based on a single architecture, which is insufficient for their complex and diverse nature. Each tooth is of a similar size, yet they vary in morphology and position. Additionally, the jawbone has a relatively large volume and contains numerous neural structures. Different model architectures possess varying receptive fields and exhibit differences in segmenting diverse oral and maxillofacial structures. Therefore, designing diverse model architectures is highly beneficial for the segmentation of oral and maxillofacial structures.

In this work, we propose an algorithm for segmenting different oral and maxillofacial structures in CBCT images based on the nnUNet [10] and VISTA [7] framework, which also supports interactive segmentation of the IAC. To balance inference efficiency and accuracy, we designed multiple strategies to optimize the algorithm's inference process. Additionally, we employed post-processing techniques such as custom threshold-based small label removal and non-connected region filtering to further enhance robustness. Finally, we validated our algorithm in the ToothFairy3 Challenge, achieving **3**rd place on Task 1 and **2**nd place on Task 2.

2 Method

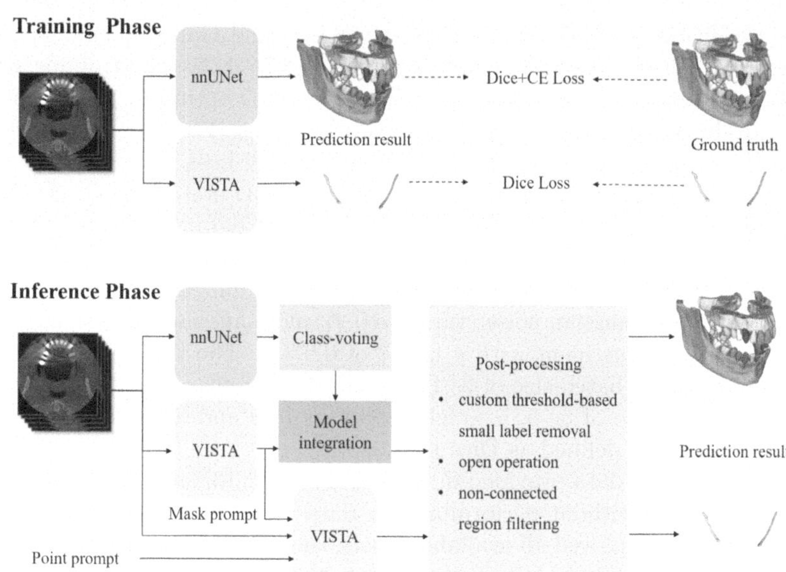

Fig. 2. The framework of our proposed method. An nnUNet model is trained for oral and maxillofacial segmentation and a VISTA model for interactive IAC segmentation. Inference combines the models with a class-voting ensemble and a two stage automatic and point-based refinement for interactive segmentation. Outputs of both models are post-processed to improve robustness.

Our proposed method is illustrated in Fig. 2. We first separately train an nnUNet-based model for oral and maxillofacial structures segmentation and a

VISTA-based model for interactive IAC segmentation. Considering computational efficiency, we adopt a class-voting ensemble strategy to reduce memory usage and improve inference speed. To take advantage of the differences in various oral and maxillofacial structures, we integrate the two models to enhance segmentation accuracy. For the interactive segmentation task, we adopt a two-stage strategy: an automatic segmentation stage is first applied to obtain an initial result, followed by a point-based prompt refinement stage to further enhance the segmentation accuracy. Finally, we apply post-processing techniques such as custom threshold-based small label removal and non-connected region filtering to the outputs of both models to further enhance robustness.

2.1 Model Training

For nnUNet model training phase, we chose nnUNet ResEnc L as backbone network. Since all data share the same spacing [0.3, 0.3, 0.3], no resampling was performed on any data. The data were cropped into patches of size 128×224×224 and augmented using techniques including rotation within the range of $-30°$ to $30°$, scaling with a factor of 0.7–1.4, anterior–posterior and superior–inferior mirroring, addition of Gaussian noise (variance 0.1) and Gaussian blur (sigma 0.5–1.0), and contrast adjustment with a factor of 0.75–1.25. The training proceeded for 1500 epochs with a batch size of 2. The SGD optimizer was adopted with an initial learning rate of 0.01 and a Poly scheduler [17]. The loss function was defined as the sum of Dice Loss and Cross-Entropy Loss.

For VISTA model training phase, we chose VISTA3D pretrained checkpoint. No resampling was also performed on any data. The data were cropped into patches of size 96×160×160 and augmented using techniques including scaling with a factor of 0.8–1.2, simulation of low resolution images with a factor of 0.3–1.0, addition of Gaussian noise (variance 0.2) and Gaussian blur (sigma 0.5–1.0), and contrast adjustment with a factor of 0.9–1.1. The training proceeded for 200 epochs with a batch size of 2. The AdamW optimizer was adopted with an initial learning rate of 5e-5, a weight decay of 1e-5 and a cosine scheduler. The loss function was defined as Dice Loss.

We utilized all the data provided in Toothfairy3 [1,2,13] as both the training set and the test set, without performing any data partitioning. However, while the nnUNet model employed all available labels, the VISTA model only used the labels corresponding to the IAC.

2.2 Ensemble Strategy

Class-Voting. The sliding window inference process of the nnU-Net model is highly memory-intensive. To achieve efficient segmentation, we adopt a class-voting strategy. Specifically, for each patch S_i, the predicted logits are converted into one-hot encoded vectors, which are then aggregated through summation. The final predicted label is determined by selecting the class with the maximum accumulated value. The formulation is as follows:

$$\hat{y} = \arg \max_{c \in 1,\cdots,C} \sum_{i=1}^{N} \mathbb{I}_c \left(\arg\max f(S_i)\right) \tag{1}$$

where $\hat{y}$ denotes the final predicted label, C represents the total number of classes, N is the total number of sliding window patches that cover the spatial location, $f(S_i)$ denotes the predicted logits for patch S_i, $\mathbb{I}_c(\cdot)$ is the indicator function that outputs 1 if the argument equals class c and 0 otherwise, $\arg\max f(S_i)$ obtains the predicted class label for patch S_i. The outer arg max operation selects the class with the highest vote count.

Model Integration. The VISTA model demonstrated superior performance compared to the nnUNet model in segmenting the IAC. Therefore, we integrated the nnUNet model with the VISTA model. Specifically, we first removed the IAC segmentation labels predicted by the nnUNet model and then replaced them with the corresponding labels generated by the VISTA model. This approach allowed us to substitute the relatively inaccurate IAC labels from nnUNet with more precise ones.

2.3 Interactive Segmentation

To achieve better interactive segmentation results, we employ a method that combines automatic segmentation with point-prompt-based interactive segmentation. Specifically, we first use the automatic segmentation decoder from the VISTA model to obtain the automatic segmentation mask of the IAC, and then apply the point-prompt decoder to generate the point-prompt-based segmentation mask. We then add or remove only the connected component regions that contain the point clicks to avoid unexpected modifications. This refinement of the automatic segmentation results using point-prompt-based segmentation significantly improves the overall performance.

2.4 Post-processing Techniques

The post-processing techniques employed in our pipeline are designed to enhance segmentation accuracy and robustness by incorporating both morphological operations and prior anatomical knowledge. These techniques include custom threshold-based small label removal, morphological open operations, and non-connected region filtering. Specifically, we first perform label size filtering to remove anatomically implausible labels whose pixel area falls within predefined ranges (e.g., 320–1,819 pixels for certain upper teeth and 970–6,140 pixels for wisdom teeth), as determined from the training set distribution. This step helps to suppress spurious predictions and reduce false positives associated with small, isolated regions.

Next, a morphological open operation is applied to the upper jawbone and pharynx regions to address potential boundary ambiguities and to smooth jagged edges in the predicted segmentation masks. The open operation, which consists of an erosion followed by a dilation, effectively removes small noise while preserving the overall structure of the anatomical regions.

Finally, non-connected region filtering is performed on the lower jawbone, pharynx, and tooth labels. This step leverages prior anatomical knowledge by retaining only the largest connected components for each label, thereby eliminating isolated or incorrectly segmented regions that are inconsistent with realistic anatomical structures. By combining these post-processing steps, our framework not only improves the visual consistency of the segmentations but also enhances quantitative metrics by reducing both false positives and false negatives in critical regions.

3 Experiment

3.1 Implementation Details

The training of the nnUNet model was conducted on two NVIDIA GeForce RTX 4090 GPUs, while all other training and experiments were performed on a single NVIDIA GeForce RTX 4090 GPU. The metrics used in the experiment include Dice, HD95, and inference time.

Table 1. Comparison with other models. Prediction time refers to the time taken by the model to predict a single CBCT.

Models	Patch size	Dice	Prediction time(s)
nnWnet L	$96 \times 160 \times 160$	0.7886	27.7
nnWnet M	$96 \times 160 \times 160$	0.7868	21.3
nnWnet S	$96 \times 160 \times 160$	0.7774	13.7
nnUNet ResEnc L	$96 \times 160 \times 160$	0.8037	5.0
U-mamba	$128 \times 224 \times 224$	**0.8535**	7.7
nnUNet ResEnc L	$128 \times 224 \times 224$	0.8312	**4.7**

Comparison with Other Models. In consideration of the balance between efficiency and accuracy of the algorithm, we compared several existing models, such as U-Mamba [14] and nnWNet [19]. As shown in Table 1, the Dice score of nnUNet ResEnc L ($96 \times 160 \times 160$) reaches 0.8037, which is higher than that of all nnWNet (ranging from 0.7774 to 0.7886), but lower than nnUNet ResEnc L ($128 \times 224 \times 224$) with Dice score of 0.8312. This indicates that enlarging the patch size contributes to performance improvement, as nnUNet ResEnc L with patches ($128 \times 224 \times 224$) outperform their counterparts trained on smaller patches ($96 \times 160 \times 160$). In terms of inference speed, nnUNet ResEnc L demonstrates the best efficiency, requiring only 4.7 s per CBCT, which is faster than all other models including U-Mamba (7.7 s). These results suggest that nnUNet ResEnc L achieves a favorable trade-off, delivering the fastest inference while maintaining competitive segmentation accuracy.

Table 2. Ablation study on debugging phase. Inference time denotes the complete duration required for processing a single CBCT during inference.

Class-voting	Model integration	Post-processing	Dice	HD95	Inference time(s)
×	✓	✓	**0.9575**	**18.66**	51.0
✓	×	✓	0.9563	18.67	25.5
✓	✓	×	0.8772	55.88	**25.2**
✓	✓	✓	0.9573	**18.66**	35.0

Ablation Study. To further investigate the contributions of different components, we conducted an ablation study, as summarized in Table 2. When only model integration and post-processing were employed, the framework achieved the highest Dice score of 0.9575, with an HD95 of 18.66, albeit at the cost of the longest inference time (51.0 s). By contrast, applying class-voting with post-processing but without model integration reduced the Dice score slightly to 0.9563 while improving efficiency (25.5 s). Removing post-processing led to a substantial degradation in accuracy, with the Dice dropping to 0.8772 and HD95 increasing to 55.88, although this configuration achieved the fastest inference (25.2 s). Incorporating all three components (class-voting, model integration, and post-processing) yielded a balanced performance, with a Dice of 0.9573, HD95 of 18.66, and moderate inference time (35.0 s). These results highlight the critical role of post-processing for maintaining segmentation accuracy and demonstrate that combining ensemble strategies can effectively balance accuracy and efficiency.

Table 3. Final result on test phase leaderboards.

Task	Team	Dice	HD95
Multi-class Segmentation	Black_Myth	$\mathbf{0.7981 \pm 0.0640}$	$\mathbf{88.7228 \pm 32.3250}$
	TAIR Lab	0.7917 ± 0.0652	93.1873 ± 30.4327
	sjtu_eiee_2-426lab	0.7705 ± 0.0754	104.5936 ± 37.2139
	ring821	0.7684 ± 0.0969	104.4004 ± 47.9841
	DLaBella29	0.7386 ± 0.0708	97.7059 ± 33.2051
IAC Interactive Segmentation	Black_Myth	$\mathbf{0.8642 \pm 0.0507}$	$\mathbf{2.2675 \pm 1.7112}$
	TAIR Lab	0.8519 ± 0.0752	7.3863 ± 20.4354
	DLaBella29	0.7465 ± 0.0724	4.7094 ± 3.4713
	sjtu_eiee_2-426lab	0.7683 ± 0.1896	32.2318 ± 85.8957
	gagaha	0.7220 ± 0.2554	76.8298 ± 159.1321

Finally, our final results are presented in Table 3. We achieved the best performance on both the Multi-class Segmentation leaderboard and the IAC Interactive Segmentation test phase leaderboard of the MICCAI Toothfairy3 Challenge. However, due to considerations regarding algorithmic runtime and computational cost, our final official standings were third place on Task 1 and second place on Task 2.

4 Discussion

This work presents a segmentation framework that integrates nnUNet and VISTA for accurate delineation of oral and maxillofacial structures in CBCT images. The complementary strengths of the two architectures–nnUNet for large-volume structures and VISTA for the fine-grained IAC–enabled superior performance compared with single-model approaches. The use of class-voting, interactive segmentation, and post-processing further enhanced efficiency and robustness, which was reflected in our third place result in Task 1 and second place result in Task 2 of the ToothFairy3 Challenge.

Nevertheless, the method was trained and validated only on the challenge dataset, and its generalizability to multi-center or clinical data remains to be verified. Future work will explore multi-institutional validation, lightweight deployment strategies, and extension to pathological segmentation for broader clinical applicability.

Acknowledgments. This study was funded by National Key R&D Program of China (2023YFC2414100), National Natural Science Foundation of China (82370905, 82071096), Shanghai Professional Service Platform of Oral-Cranio-Maxillofacial Digital Technology Research and Application (21DZ2294600), National Clinical Key Specialty (Z155080000004), Shanghai's Top Priority Research Center (2022ZZ01017), and CAMS Innovation Fund for Medical Sciences (CIFMS, 2019-I2M-5-037).

References

1. Bolelli, F., et al.: Segmenting the inferior alveolar canal in cbcts volumes: the ToothFairy challenge. IEEE Trans. Med. Imaging 1–17 (2024). https://doi.org/10.1109/TMI.2024.3523096
2. Bolelli, F., et al.: Segmenting maxillofacial structures in CBCT volume. In: IEEE/CVF Conference on Computer Vision and Pattern Recognition (CVPR), pp. 1–10. IEEE (2025)
3. Chen, J., et al.: Transunet: transformers make strong encoders for medical image segmentation. arXiv preprint arXiv:2102.04306 (2021)
4. Cui, Z., et al.: A fully automatic ai system for tooth and alveolar bone segmentation from cone-beam ct images. Nat. Commun. **13**(1), 2096 (2022)
5. Dot, G., et al.: Dentalsegmentator: robust open source deep learning-based ct and cbct image segmentation. J. Dent. **147**, 105130 (2024)
6. Elgarba, B.M., Van Aelst, S., Swaity, A., Morgan, N., Shujaat, S., Jacobs, R.: Deep learning-based segmentation of dental implants on cone-beam computed tomography images: a validation study. J. Dent. **137**, 104639 (2023)
7. He, Y., et al.: Vista3d: versatile imaging segmentation and annotation model for 3d computed tomography. CoRR (2024)

8. Huang, X., He, D., Li, Z., Zhang, X., Wang, X.: Iossam: label efficient multi-view prompt-driven tooth segmentation. In: International Conference on Medical Image Computing and Computer-Assisted Intervention, pp. 632–642. Springer, Heidelberg (2024)
9. Huang, X., He, D., Li, Z., Zhang, X., Wang, X.: Maxillofacial bone movements-aware dual graph convolution approach for postoperative facial appearance prediction. Med. Image Anal. **99**, 103350 (2025)
10. Isensee, F., Jaeger, P.F., Kohl, S.A., Petersen, J., Maier-Hein, K.H.: nnu-net: a self-configuring method for deep learning-based biomedical image segmentation. Nat. Methods **18**(2), 203–211 (2021)
11. Liu, J., et al.: Swin-umamba: mamba-based unet with imagenet-based pretraining. In: International Conference on Medical Image Computing and Computer-Assisted Intervention, pp. 615–625. Springer, Heidelberg (2024)
12. Y, L., et al.: Vmamba: visual state space model. Adv. Neural. Inf. Process. Syst. **37**, 103031–103063 (2024)
13. Lumetti, L., Pipoli, V., Bolelli, F., Ficarra, E., Grana, C.: Enhancing patch-based learning for the segmentation of the mandibular canal. IEEE Access 1–12 (2024). https://doi.org/10.1109/ACCESS.2024.3408629
14. Ma, J., Li, F., Wang, B.: U-mamba: enhancing long-range dependency for biomedical image segmentation. arXiv preprint arXiv:2401.04722 (2024)
15. Shaker, A., Maaz, M., Rasheed, H., Khan, S., Yang, M.H., Khan, F.S.: Unetr++: delving into efficient and accurate 3d medical image segmentation. IEEE Trans. Med. Imaging **43**(9), 3377–3390 (2024)
16. Wang, Y., et al.: Root canal treatment planning by automatic tooth and root canal segmentation in dental cbct with deep multi-task feature learning. Med. Image Anal. **85**, 102750 (2023)
17. Zhang, T., Li, W.: kdecay: just adding k-decay items on learning-rate schedule to improve neural networks. arXiv preprint arXiv:2004.05909 (2020)
18. Zhou, H.Y., et al.: nnformer: volumetric medical image segmentation via a 3d transformer. IEEE Trans. Image Process. **32**, 4036–4045 (2023)
19. Zhou, Y., Li, L., Lu, L., Xu, M.: nnwnet: rethinking the use of transformers in biomedical image segmentation and calling for a unified evaluation benchmark. In: Proceedings of the IEEE/CVF Conference on Computer Vision and Pattern Recognition (CVPR), pp. 20852–20862 (2025)

U-Mamba2: Scaling State Space Models for Dental Anatomy Segmentation in CBCT

Zhi Qin Tan[1(✉)], Xiatian Zhu[2], Owen Addison[1], and Yunpeng Li[1,2]

[1] Centre for Oral, Clinical and Translational Sciences, King's College London, London, UK
{zhi_qin.tan,owen.addison,yunpeng.li}@kcl.ac.uk

[2] Surrey Institute for People-Centred AI, University of Surrey, Guildford, UK
{yunpeng.li, xiatian.zhu}@surrey.ac.uk

Abstract. Cone-Beam Computed Tomography (CBCT) is a widely used 3D imaging technique in dentistry, providing volumetric information about the anatomical structures of jaws and teeth. Accurate segmentation of these anatomies is critical for clinical applications such as diagnosis and surgical planning, but remains time-consuming and challenging. In this paper, we present U-Mamba2, a neural network architecture designed for multi-anatomy CBCT segmentation in the context of the ToothFairy3 challenge. U-Mamba2 integrates the Mamba2 state space models into the U-Net architecture, enforcing stronger structural constraints for higher efficiency without compromising performance. In addition, we integrate interactive click prompts with cross-attention blocks, pre-train U-Mamba2 using self-supervised learning, and incorporate dental domain knowledge into the model design to address key challenges of dental anatomy segmentation in CBCT. Extensive experiments, including independent tests, demonstrate that U-Mamba2 is both effective and efficient, securing first place in both tasks of the Toothfairy3 challenge. In Task 1, U-Mamba2 achieved a mean Dice of 0.84, HD95 of 38.17 with the held-out test data, with an average inference time of 40.58 s. In Task 2, U-Mamba2 achieved the mean Dice of 0.87 and HD95 of 2.15 with the held-out test data. The code is publicly available at https://github.com/zhiqin1998/UMamba2.

Keywords: U-Mamba2 · CBCT Imaging · Dental Anatomy Segmentation · Deep Learning · ToothFairy3 Challenge

1 Introduction

Cone-Beam Computed Tomography (CBCT) is a widely used imaging modality in dentistry. It provides comprehensive 3D volumetric information and excellent visualization of the orofacial region, including jaws, teeth, nerves [14]. Accurate segmentation of individual anatomical structures in CBCT images is crucial in

F. Bolelli et al. (Eds.): ODIN 2025, LNCS 16473, pp. 122–132, 2026.
https://doi.org/10.1007/978-3-032-20711-1_12

applications such as dental diagnosis, treatment, and surgical planning [13,19, 25]. However, manual segmentation of CBCT scans requires specialized domain expertise and is extremely time-consuming due to their three-dimensional nature [3]. Thus, there is a strong demand for robust and efficient CBCT segmentation algorithms to improve the accuracy and efficiency of dental care and ultimately lead to better patient outcomes.

Generally, network architectures for semantic segmentation can be categorized into three: 1) Convolutional neural networks (CNN) such as U-Net [10,21] and DeepLab [4] with translation-invariant convolutions that can effectively capture hierarchical image features and are parameter-efficient with their shared kernel weights; 2) Transformers [27] such as SETR [29] and SwinTransformer [15] that treat images as a sequence of patches instead of extracting image features hierarchically to capture the global information better; and 3) Hybrid CNN-Transformer architectures such as nnFormer [30] and SwinUNETR [23] that attempt to exploit the best of both worlds by combining their architectures.

While the hybrid architectures have improved the global feature capabilities of CNNs, transformers are highly resource-intensive due to the attention mechanism which scales quadratically with input size. This limitation reduces their suitability for healthcare applications, which often involve high-resolution 3D data and constrained computational resources in real-world settings. Recently, structured state space sequence models [8], particularly the Mamba [7] model, have emerged as an efficient and effective alternative to the transformer model. By selectively capturing relevant input features and scaling linearly with input size, Mamba outperforms transformers across multiple modalities [7,12,18]. U-Mamba [17] presented the first work to leverage Mamba for image segmentation, achieving superior performance and surpassing transformer-based networks in a range of medical image segmentation tasks. More recently, Dao *et al.* [6] proposed Mamba2, based on the structured state-space duality (SSD) framework, which dramatically improves speed without weakening its performance.

In this paper, we propose U-Mamba2, a hybrid CNN-SSD architecture for 3D image segmentation. U-Mamba2 extends the previous U-Mamba model [7] by leveraging the Mamba2 SSD framework that simplifies the Mamba architecture with stronger constraints imposed on the hidden space structure. Mamba2 introduced several architectural changes to enable tensor and sequence parallelism, providing a significant speedup without compromising performance. Similar to U-Mamba, U-Mamba2 can effectively extract local spatial features via CNN and capture global long-range dependencies with Mamba2. We implement interactive click prompts with cross-attention blocks and incorporate several domain knowledge to address key challenges of dental anatomy segmentation in CBCT. Our extensive experiments demonstrate the superior performance of U-Mamba2 for CBCT segmentation, outperforming previous alternatives and achieving first place for Tasks 1 and 2 of the ToothFairy3 challenge.

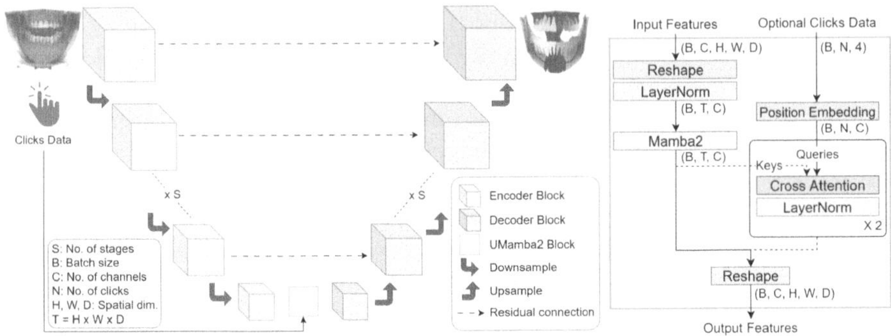

Fig. 1. (Left): Overall architecture of the U-Mamba2 model. U-Mamba2 employs the encoder-decoder framework with residual connections between each stage and the U-Mamba2 block in the bottleneck. The number of stages is configurable depending on the dataset input size. (Right): The U-Mamba2 block contains the SSD-based Mamba2 and an optional click position encoder and cross-attention blocks. The output of Mamba2 follows the solid line for tasks without interactive clicks, while it follows the dashed line when clicks are present.

2 Method

This section describes our method, designed in the scope of the two tasks of the ToothFairy3 [2,3,16] challenges. Task 1 extends the previous ToothFairy2 challenge by adding segmentation of pulps, incisive nerves, and the lingual foramen to the existing 42 anatomy classes (*e.g.* jaws, sinuses, and 32 teeth), and includes inference time to the evaluation criteria. The dataset contains 532 CBCT scans with shapes ranging from $(170, 272, 345)$ to $(298, 512, 512)$, along with the segmentation labels of 46 anatomy classes. On the other hand, Task 2 focuses on the interactive segmentation of the inferior alveolar nerves, allowing interactive user clicks as prompts to segment the inferior alveolar nerves. Figure 1 shows the overall structure of the U-Mamba2 model and the details of the U-Mamba2 block.

2.1 U-Mamba2: Integrating Mamba2 to U-Net

Inspired by U-Mamba [17], we propose U-Mamba2, which integrates the strengths of U-Net and Mamba2 to efficiently capture global information. As shown in Fig. 1, U-Mamba2 follows a structure similar to U-Net, with a symmetric encoder-decoder architecture that extracts image features across multiple scales. Residual connections between the encoder and decoder blocks at each stage facilitate the fusion of low-level and high-level features. As convolutional operations are inherently localized, we leverage Mamba2 to enhance the vanilla U-Net's limited capability to model global long-range dependencies in images by treating the features as long sequences. Similar to Mamba, Mamba2 scales linearly with sequence length but leverages the SSD framework to constrain the internal recurrent structure and uses matrix multiplication instead of selective scan, thereby improving efficiency through parallelism.

The encoder blocks consist of two consecutive Residual blocks [9], followed by a strided downsampling convolution, while the decoder blocks are composed of Residual blocks and transposed convolutions for upsampling. In the U-Mamba2 block, image features of shape (B, C, H, W, D) are reshaped and transposed to (B, T, C) where B denotes the batch size, C the number of channels, and H, W, D are the spatial dimensions, with $T = H \times W \times D$. Then, Layer Normalization [1] is applied to the features before they are passed to Mamba2 to capture the global contexts. The output features are then reshaped and transposed back to (B, C, H, W, D). We apply the U-Mamba2 block exclusively in the bottleneck stage, as it results in the best empirical performance for 3D computed tomography modality, consistent with Ma *et al.* [17]. Finally, Softmax is applied to the final decoder feature to produce the segmentation class probabilities, and U-Mamba2 is trained with a combination of cross entropy loss and Dice loss.

2.2 Cross-Attention with Point Encoder

We introduce an optional interactive branch to enable the model to incorporate user-provided clicks to refine the output of U-Mamba2, improve accuracy, and support human-in-the-loop collaboration. Following the SAM2 framework [20], this branch employs a position embedding and two cross-attention blocks, as illustrated in Fig. 1. The optional clicks data contain a varying number of N clicks consisting of the X, Y, Z coordinates, and class labels. These clicks are first encoded with a learnable position embedding depending on their spatial positions and class labels. Next, the embedded click prompts and the output features of Mamba2 are fused through two-way cross-attention blocks as queries and keys, respectively. The cross-attention blocks, followed by Layer Normalization, are repeated twice to allow the model to integrate click information with the image features. The final output of the cross-attention block is then reshaped and transposed back to the original spatial dimensions.

2.3 Pre-training with Self-Supervised Learning

Recent studies [24,26] have shown that pre-training models on large datasets with self-supervised learning (SSL) produces stronger models that can extract meaningful feature representations, leading to improved performance of downstream segmentation tasks, particularly when there is limited labeled data.

In addition to the 532 scans of ToothFairy3, we utilize the STS-3D-Tooth [28] dataset consisting of 371 unlabeled CBCT scans to pre-train U-Mamba2 with the disruptive autoencoder (DAE) [26] framework. DAE aims to reconstruct the original 3D volume after it is corrupted by several low-level perturbations. Specifically, we corrupt the input volume by randomly applying local masks, downsampling, and adding Gaussian noise to the input. The disrupted input is then passed through the U-Mamba2 to learn to reconstruct the original image with an L1 loss function. The pre-trained weights are then used to initialize U-Mamba2 (except for the weights of the optional interactive branch and the final segmentation layer) for effective downstream training.

2.4 Domain Knowledge for Dental Anatomy Segmentation

Label Smoothing of Related Anatomies. Anatomies in the orofacial region are not always distinct and often share similar shapes and properties. For instance, similar tooth types (incisor, canine, molar, premolar) between left-right counterparts, as well as the inferior alveolar and incisive nerves, exhibit close structural relationships. Therefore, to guide the model in recognizing similar classes and their spatial relationship, we introduce label smoothing for related anatomies instead of learning with hard one-hot labels. For each pixel with class k, we set the k-th class's target probability to 0.9 and distribute the remaining 0.1 evenly across the related classes. Specifically, for each voxel with a ground truth class label, k, and a set of related classes, S_r, we first initialize a zero vector, p, as the soft label, then set $p_k = 0.9$ and $p_r = \frac{0.1}{|S_r|}, \forall r \in S_r$. We apply this strategy to all anatomies with left-right counterparts, neighboring teeth, and to the inferior alveolar and incisive nerves.

Weighted Loss for Tiny Structures. ToothFairy3 introduced three additional classes corresponding to the left and right incisive nerves and the lingual foramen, which house thin, sensitive nerves in the mandible. These structures are considerably smaller than other anatomies in the dataset. We account for the volume differences by applying a class weight of 10 to these three tiny classes, so that their contribution to the overall loss is not overshadowed by larger anatomies.

Left-Right Mirroring Augmentation. The findings of the previous ToothFairy2 challenge [3,11] showed that left-right mirroring augmentation can degrade the model's capability to reliably differentiate the left/right orientation. In dentistry, even dentists may struggle to identify a horizontally-flipped 2D image reliably without visual cues [5], due to the structural symmetry between left/right anatomies in the sagittal plane. However, we can exploit this anatomical symmetry with careful pre-processing and post-processing, enabling left-right mirroring augmentation without reducing model performance. We propose to swap the class labels of anatomies opposite to the sagittal plane whenever left-right mirroring occurs during data augmentation (*e.g.* 'Upper left canine' and 'Upper right canine'). Additionally, we also switch the predicted logits of the corresponding left/right anatomies if the image is mirrored in the left-right axis during test-time augmentation (TTA). With proper processing during training and inference, the number of possible axes combinations for mirroring augmentation is expanded from 3 to 7, substantially increasing the generalization capabilities and performance of U-Mamba2.

Post-processing. We incorporate anatomical priors of the orofacial region that voxels belonging to the same anatomy should be connected and not separated into blobs, as a post-processing step. Unlike the first-place solution [11] of the previous ToothFairy2 challenge, we perform post-processing to remove small predictions that are likely false positives based on the volume of the computed connected components [22] instead of the total volume of each class. Specifically,

Table 1. Validation set evaluation metrics. † indicates applying post-processing.

Model	Task 1					Task 2				
	Dice	HD95	Dice†	HD95†	Time	Dice	HD95	Dice†	HD95†	Time
SwinUNETR [23]	0.858	48.86	0.874	40.09	7.23	–	–	–	–	–
nnU-Net ResE [10]	0.861	45.28	0.887	32.05	**6.20**	0.901	1.98	0.905	1.71	**5.06**
U-Mamba [17]	0.865	42.06	0.896	25.88	6.98	0.903	1.65	**0.913**	1.58	5.88
U-Mamba2 (ours)	**0.873**	**41.08**	**0.908**	**21.35**	6.81	**0.905**	**1.63**	**0.913**	**1.57**	5.70

we select the threshold as the 0.5th percentile of the connected components' volume computed using the ground truth for each class. Importantly, this threshold is determined through the statistics of the ground truth rather than model predictions, ensuring that it is not model-specific. The threshold for each class is pre-computed using the entire ToothFairy3 training dataset.

3 Experiment Results

We implement U-Mamba2 with the nnU-Net [10] framework. We perform a 9:1 stratified train-validation split on the ToothFairy3 dataset to ensure the same proportion of data sources (with different fields of view and imaging machines) in the train and validation datasets. All models are pre-trained with SSL (Sect. 2.3) following the original training configuration of DAE [26]. Each model employs seven encoder-decoder stages, an input patch size of $128 \times 256x256$, the native voxel spacing of 0.3mm^3 (leading to no downsampling or upsampling during model training and inference), and a batch size of 1. During training, we disable left/right mirroring augmentation for all models except U-Mamba2, while during inference, we use sliding window inference with a tile size of 0.5 and disable left/right mirroring in TTA for all models, including U-Mamba2, for fair comparison. Other hyperparameters follow the default values of nnU-Net. Model training and time computation are performed on an RTX4090 GPU. We evaluate the models with the Dice coefficient, the Hausdorff Distance at the 95th percentile (HD95), and the average inference time in seconds, where lower is better for all metrics except Dice.

3.1 Quantitative Results

Table 1 compares the proposed U-Mamba2 with nnU-Net ResE [10], U-Mamba [17] which utilizes the original Mamba layer [7], and SwinUNETR [23] on the ToothFairy3 dataset. For Task 2, we incorporate a point prompt encoder to nnU-Net ResE and U-Mamba at the bottleneck stage, similar to U-Mamba2. U-Mamba2 outperforms all benchmark models, achieving the best mean Dice score of 0.873 and 0.905 for Tasks 1 and 2, respectively. After applying post-processing, U-Mamba2 further improves to a mean Dice score of 0.908 and 0.913 for Tasks

Table 2. Ablation Study of U-Mamba2 for the validation set of Task 1. ILN indicates the metrics for the left and right incisive nerves and the lingual nerve.

Label Smoothing	Weighted Loss	L/R Mirroring	Dice	HD95	Dice (ILN)	HD95 (ILN)
×	×	×	0.867	42.36	0.617	38.41
✓	×	×	0.872	40.74	0.628	38.15
×	✓	×	0.870	41.31	0.635	37.99
×	×	✓	0.871	41.20	0.642	36.48
✓	✓	✓	**0.873**	**41.08**	**0.646**	**35.21**

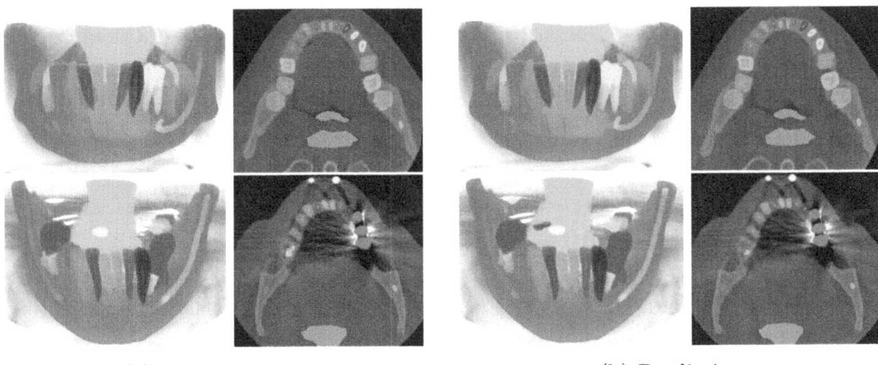

(a) Ground Truth (b) Prediction

Fig. 2. Qualitative results of U-Mamba2 on the validation set of Task 1. The 3D render and a representative 2D slice are shown for: (Top) the best scoring case and (Bottom) the worst scoring case.

1 and 2, respectively. U-Mamba2 delivers the best performance with an average inference time of 6.81 and 5.70 s per scan for the two tasks, demonstrating a slight speedup over U-Mamba.

Furthermore, we perform an ablation study on U-Mamba2 by individually applying the dental domain knowledge introduced in Sect. 2.4, excluding the post-processing step (See Table 1 for post-processing results). Table 2 shows that these techniques lead to small performance improvements. In particular, the weighted loss and left/right mirroring techniques improve the mean Dice score on the three tiny structures, *i.e.* the left and right incisive nerves and the lingual nerve (ILN) from 0.617 to 0.635 and 0.642, respectively. When all three techniques are applied, U-Mamba2 achieves the best performance, with a mean Dice score of 0.873 and 0.646 for all classes and the ILN classes, respectively.

3.2 Qualitative Results

Figure 2 visualizes the qualitative comparison between the ground truth and our model's predictions of the scans with the highest and lowest Dice score in the validation set, in the top and bottom rows, respectively. We observe that in most cases, U-Mamba2 produces precise segmentation predictions, showcasing the effectiveness of incorporating dental domain knowledge into the model design. Furthermore, we observe that U-Mamba2 can accurately localize the three tiny structures (ILN), producing visually acceptable segmentations. In the worst-case scenario, although the scan is imperfect due to image artifacts caused by metallic objects, false positives are primarily confined around the image edge or confusion between the actual tooth and the crown or implant, underscoring U-Mamba2's robustness under noisy conditions.

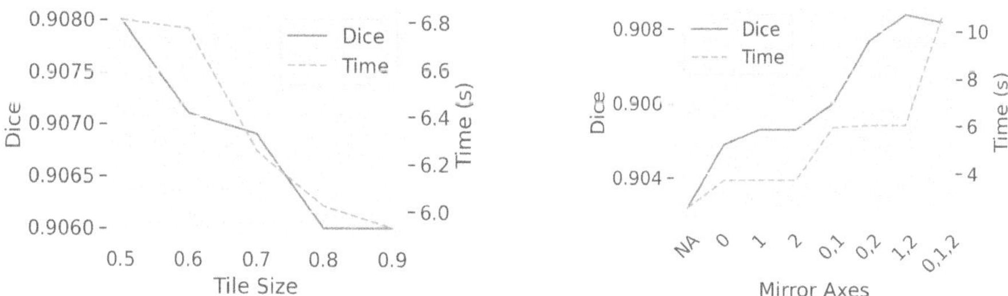

Fig. 3. (Left): Effect of the tile size on the metrics with '0,1' mirror axes in TTA. (Right): Effect of various mirror axes combinations in TTA on the metrics when tile size is set to 0.9. Axis definition: '0' is superior/inferior, '1' is anterior/posterior, and '2' is left/right.

3.3 Optimizing Speed in Sliding Window Inference

As the inference time is an important metric in the ToothFairy 3 challenge, we optimize the sliding window inference parameters to improve speed without significantly deteriorating model accuracy. Specifically, we optimize the tile size parameter, where a larger value results in less border overlap during sliding window inference, and the mirror axes combinations in TTA. Figure 3 shows the tradeoff between Dice score and inference time for different tile sizes and mirror axes combinations in TTA. By setting the tile size to 0.9, we can reduce the inference time by 12.9% with a negligible drop of only 0.002 Dice score. Moreover, Fig. 3 also demonstrates that the optimal mirror axes combination is '1,2', representing anterior/posterior and left/right, offering the best Dice score with an average inference time of only 6.02 s. We believe this is due to the larger spatial dimension in these axes containing more information.

3.4 Final Challenge Submission

For the final submission, we extended training to 1500 epochs using all available data with a batch size of 2 and increased the input patch size to $160 \times 288x288$. During inference, we use a sliding window inference with a tile size of 0.9 and enable mirroring in the anterior/posterior and left/right axes during TTA. The final U-Mamba2 model achieved a mean Dice of 0.84, HD95 of 38.17, with an average inference time of 40.58 s, computed on the Grand Challenge platform using a T4 GPU, securing first place in Task 1 of the ToothFairy3 challenge with a 3.1 overall ranking while obtaining first place in Task 2 with a mean Dice, HD95 and overall rank of 0.87, 2.15 and 1.66, respectively, on the hidden test set.

4 Conclusion

We presented a new architecture, U-Mamba2, designed for multi-anatomy segmentation of CBCT images in the scope of the ToothFairy3 challenge. U-Mamba2 integrates the Mamba2 SSD framework into the U-Net backbone, achieving higher efficiency without compromising performance compared to U-Mamba. By incorporating domain-specific knowledge of dental anatomy, we improved the model's performance on multi-anatomy segmentation of CBCT scans. Both the validation and independent test results demonstrate the effectiveness and efficiency of U-Mamba2, securing first place in both Tasks 1 and 2 of the ToothFairy3 challenge.

References

1. Ba, J.L., Kiros, J.R., Hinton, G.E.: Layer normalization. arXiv:1607.06450 (2016)
2. Bolelli, F., et al.: Segmenting the inferior alveolar canal in CBCTs volumes: the toothfairy challenge. IEEE Trans. Med. Imag. 1–17 (2024). https://doi.org/10.1109/TMI.2024.3523096
3. Bolelli, F., et al.: Segmenting maxillofacial structures in CBCT volume. In: Proceedings of IEEE Conference on Computer Vision and Pattern Recognition (CVPR), Nashville, Tennessee, USA, pp. 5238–5248 (2025)
4. Chen, L.C., Zhu, Y., Papandreou, G., Schroff, F., Adam, H.: Encoder-decoder with atrous separable convolution for semantic image segmentation. In: Proceedings of European Conference on Computer Vision (ECCV), Munich, Germany (2018)
5. Chiam, S.L.: A note on digital dental radiography in forensic odontology. J. Forensic Dent. Sci. **6**(3), 197–201 (2014)
6. Dao, T., Gu, A.: Transformers are SSMs: generalized models and efficient algorithms through structured state space duality. In: Proceedings of International Conference on Machine Learning (ICML), Vienna, Austria (2024)
7. Gu, A., Dao, T.: Mamba: linear-time sequence modeling with selective state spaces. arXiv:2312.00752 (2023)
8. Gu, A., Goel, K., Ré, C.: Efficiently modeling long sequences with structured state spaces. In: Proceedings of International Conference on Learning Represention (ICLR) (2022)
9. He, K., Zhang, X., Ren, S., Sun, J.: Deep residual learning for image recognition. In: Proceedings of IEEE Conference Computer Vision and Pattern Recognition (CVPR), Las Vegas, NV, USA (2016)
10. Isensee, F., Jaeger, P.F., Kohl, S.A.A., Petersen, J., Maier-Hein, K.H.: nnu-net: a self-configuring method for deep learning-based biomedical image segmentation. Nat. Methods **18**(2), 203–211 (2021). https://doi.org/10.1038/s41592-020-01008-z

11. Isensee, F., Kirchhoff, Y., Kraemer, L., Rokuss, M., Ulrich, C., Maier-Hein, K.H.: Scaling nnu-net for cbct segmentation. In: Supervised and Semi-supervised Multi-structure Segmentation and Landmark Detection in Dental Data, MICCAI, pp. 13–20 (2024)
12. Islam, M.M., Bertasius, G.: Long movie clip classification with state-space video models. In: Proceedings of European Conferenc on Computer Vision (ECCV), Tel Aviv, Israel, pp. 87–104 (2022). https://doi.org/10.1007/978-3-031-19833-5_6
13. Jaju, P.P., Jaju, S.P.: Clinical utility of dental cone-beam computed tomography: current perspectives. Clin. Cosmet. Investig. Dent. **6**, 29–43 (2014)
14. Kaasalainen, T., Ekholm, M., Siiskonen, T., Kortesniemi, M.: Dental cone beam ct: an updated review. Physica Med. **88**, 193–217 (2021). https://doi.org/10.1016/j.ejmp.2021.07.007
15. Liu, Z., et al.: Swin transformer: hierarchical vision transformer using shifted windows. In: Proceedings of IEEE International Conference on Computer Vision (ICCV) (2021)
16. Lumetti, L., Pipoli, V., Bolelli, F., Ficarra, E., Grana, C.: Enhancing patch-based learning for the segmentation of the mandibular canal. IEEE Access 1–12 (2024)
17. Ma, J., Li, F., Wang, B.: U-mamba: enhancing long-range dependency for biomedical image segmentation. arXiv:2401.04722 (2024)
18. Nguyen, E., et al.: S4nd: modeling images and videos as multidimensional signals using state spaces. In: Proceedings of Advances Neural Information and Processing Systems (NeurIPS), New Orleans, LA, USA, pp. 2846–2861 (2022)
19. Patel, S., Durack, C., Abella, F., Shemesh, H., Roig, M., Lemberg, K.: Cone beam computed tomography in endodontics – a review. Int. Endod. J. **48**(1), 3–15 (2015). https://doi.org/10.1111/iej.12270
20. Ravi, N., et al.: Sam 2: segment anything in images and videos. arXiv preprint arXiv:2408.00714 (2024)
21. Ronneberger, O., Fischer, P., Brox, T.: U-net: convolutional networks for biomedical image segmentation. In: Navab, N., Hornegger, J., Wells, W.M., Frangi, A.F. (eds.) Proceedings of Medical Image Computing and Computer-Assisted Intervention (MICCAI), Munich, Germany, pp. 234–241 (2015)
22. Silversmith, W.: cc3d: connected components on multilabel 3d & 2d images (2021). https://doi.org/10.5281/zenodo.5719536
23. Tang, Y., et al.: Self-supervised pre-training of swin transformers for 3d medical image analysis. In: Proceedings of IEEE Conference on Computer Vision and Pattern Recognition (CVPR), New Orleans, LA, USA, pp. 20730–20740 (2022)
24. Tang, Y., et al.: Self-supervised pre-training of swin transformers for 3d medical image analysis. In: Proceedings of IEEE Conference on Computer Vision and Pattern Recognition (CVPR), New Orleans, LA, USA, pp. 20698–20708 (2022)
25. Tyndall, D.A., Price, J.B., Tetradis, S., Ganz, S.D., Hildebolt, C., Scarfe, W.C.: Position statement of the American academy of oral and maxillofacial radiology on selection criteria for the use of radiology in dental implantology with emphasis on cone beam computed tomography. Oral Surg. Oral Med. Oral Pathol. Oral Radiol. **113**(6), 817–826 (2012)
26. Valanarasu, J.M.J., et al.: Disruptive autoencoders: leveraging low-level features for 3d medical image pre-training. In: Proceedings of International Conference on Medical Imaging with Deep Learning, vol. 250, pp. 1553–1570 (2024)
27. Vaswani, A., et al.: Attention is all you need. In: Proceedings of Advances Neural Information and Processing Systems (NeurIPS), Long Beach, CA, USA, vol. 30 (2017)

28. Wang, Y., et al.: A multi-modal dental dataset for semi-supervised deep learning image segmentation. Sci. Data **12**(1), 117 (2025). https://doi.org/10.1038/s41597-024-04306-9
29. Zheng, S., et al.: Rethinking semantic segmentation from a sequence-to-sequence perspective with transformers. In: Proceedings of IEEE Conference on Computer Vision and Pattern Recognition (CVPR) (2021)
30. Zhou, H.Y., et al.: nnformer: volumetric medical image segmentation via a 3d transformer. Trans. Imag. Proc. **32**, 4036–4045 (2023). https://doi.org/10.1109/TIP.2023.3293771

Optimizing the CBCT Segmentation Pipeline with Intuition-Guided Processing

Qingyu Kuang[1,2](✉)

[1] Institute of Automation, Chinese Academy of Sciences, Beijing, China
kuangqingyu23@mails.ucas.ac.cn

[2] School of Artificial Intelligence, University of Chinese Academy of Sciences, Beijing, China

Abstract. In the past, general medical image models attracted considerable research interest. However, since medical imaging modalities vary widely and often fundamentally differ from RGB images, applying a general segmentation framework to specific tasks usually requires further optimization to achieve satisfactory performance. Cone-beam computed tomography (CBCT) is a commonly used medical imaging technique in dentistry. Optimizing the segmentation process for CBCT images can greatly enhance the effectiveness of computer-aided diagnostic systems in dental applications. In this work, we analyzed the ToothFairy3 dataset and proposed improvements to the nnU-Net framework. While preserving the auto-configuration capabilities of nnU-Net, we introduced targeted optimizations across the data preprocessing pipeline, network architecture, inference process, and postprocessing strategies to enhance performance for the CBCT multi-class segmentation task. Furthermore, the trained multi-class segmentation model can be integrated with user click prompts to train an interactive segmentation model. These modifications collectively reduced inference time, improved model effectiveness, and increased practical applicability. Code is available at https://github.com/kaoquanyu-for/formedseg.git.

Keywords: CBCT Segmentation · Deep Learning · Medical Images

1 Introduction

Over the past decade, digital dentistry has advanced rapidly, with its key focus being the acquisition and segmentation of complete three-dimensional dental models and related structures. Currently, the mainstream technologies for obtaining 3D dental models mainly include intraoral scanning (IOS) or desktop scanning, and CBCT. Among these, intraoral or desktop scanning can conveniently capture the geometric morphology of the teeth crown surface but is limited to recording the external structure of teeth [6,8]. In contrast, CBCT not only provides teeth surface information but also acquires internal 3D data such as jawbones, dental roots, and surrounding bone structures, offering greater

F. Bolelli et al. (Eds.): ODIN 2025, LNCS 16473, pp. 133–144, 2026.
https://doi.org/10.1007/978-3-032-20711-1_13

advantages in clinical diagnosis and complex treatment planning [3]. As a result, it is widely used in oral and maxillofacial examinations and dental diagnostics [10]. However, manual segmentation of CBCT images is time-consuming and demands specialized expertise and experience. Therefore, training deep learning-based models to automatically segment structures such as the maxillofacial bones and teeth in CBCT images can significantly streamline the process of diagnosis, evaluation, and surgical planning for dentists, while also providing critical references for applications such as dental crown design and the fabrication of surgical guides [9,11].

However, current segmentation methods still face challenges due to variations in oral cavity opening states caused by different examination purposes, as well as considerable variations in morphological characteristics across different structures, which adversely affect segmentation accuracy and robustness. Examples of images with different oral cavity states from the public dataset ToothFairy3 [1,2,7] are illustrated in Fig. 1. Furthermore, the practical application of these models is limited by computational resources and time constraints, underscoring the gap that remains between theoretical research and clinical deployment.

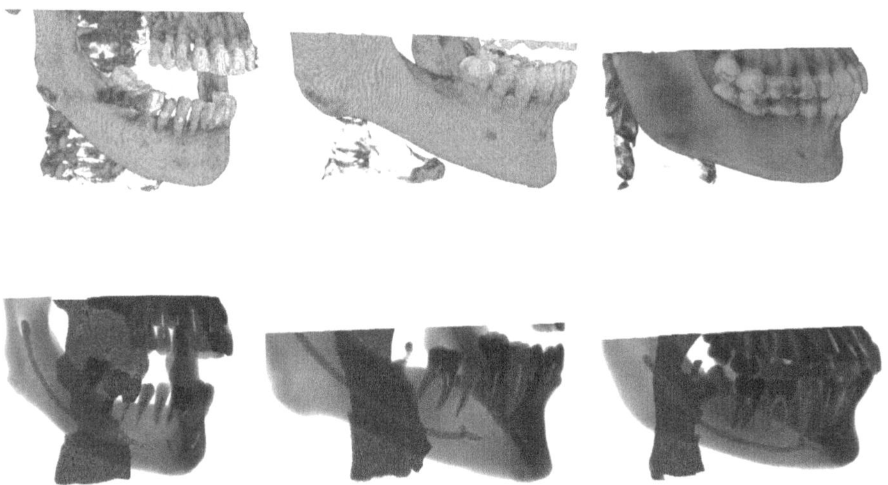

Fig. 1. The CBCT images and annotations in the Toothfairy3 dataset are shown in the figure. The top row displays the images under different oral cavity opening states, and the bottom row shows the corresponding annotated label images.

To address these issues, we re-examined the fundamental differences between CBCT images and RGB images. Inspired by human perceptual intuition for segmentation, we developed a novel processing pipeline for CBCT volume segmentation based on the nnU-Net [4] framework.

The main contributions of our work can be summarized as follows:

- Based on the nnU-Net framework, we introduced several modifications to enhance segmentation accuracy. These include adjusting the type and depth of deep supervision loss computation, and adding category prediction heads to supervise the encoding process, thereby encouraging the extraction of more discriminative features.
- Furthermore, the trained multi-class segmentation model can be integrated with user click prompts to train a single-class segmentation model, enabling interactive prompt-based segmentation.
- The rules for constraining flip augmentation were adjusted to mitigate mis-segmentation caused by symmetrically similar structures in the images. And a novel augmentation method termed "tooth eraser" was introduced to increase data diversity.
- New designed post processing workflow was optimized to align with the structural features of the segmentation output, balancing trade-offs between accuracy and inference time. And to enable large-patch inference, we optimized the inference process.

2 Methods

2.1 Overview

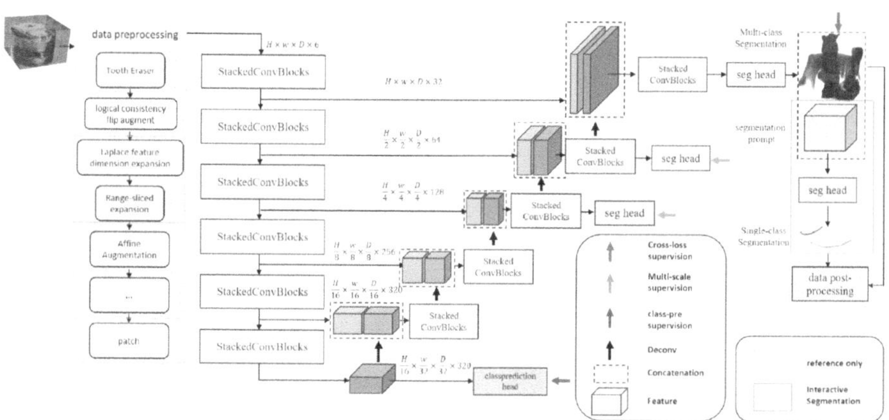

Fig. 2. Overview of the segmentation processing pipeline, illustrating the key stages and components of both the training and inference processes.

We have revisited the entire training and inference pipeline for medical image segmentation. Building upon the nnU-Net framework, we further improved a multi-class segmentation pipeline tailored for CBCT images, as illustrated in Fig. 2.

For the segmentation task on the ToothFairy3 dataset, the network utilized the architecture configuration derived from nnU-Net's automated parameter configuration, including the network depth and feature dimensionality across different layers. Building on this foundation, we introduced modifications to the data preprocessing pipeline, network architecture, postprocessing strategies, and inference procedure to enhance its performance specifically for the ToothFairy3 segmentation task.

2.2 Dataset

The ToothFairy3 dataset comprises a large collection of 3D-annotated CBCT scans covering 77 anatomical structures that are highly relevant to orthodontics. In addition, the associated challenge not only focuses on segmentation accuracy but also incorporates inference efficiency as an evaluation metric and introduces an interactive segmentation task for the Inferior Alveolar Canal, addressing both automation and clinical needs. These features make ToothFairy3 particularly suitable for developing and evaluating segmentation models with strong clinical applicability.

The dataset contains 532 images, each with an isotropic resolution of 0.3 along all axes, but we manually selected 507 samples, discarding some extreme cases. The dataset contains three different sets, and their corresponding images are shown in Fig. 1.

2.3 Data Preprocessing

Tooth Eraser. Based on image characteristics, given that missing teeth are always present in the images, we randomly remove complete lower teeth without crowns in the images to enhance image diversity. Its effects are shown in Fig. 3.

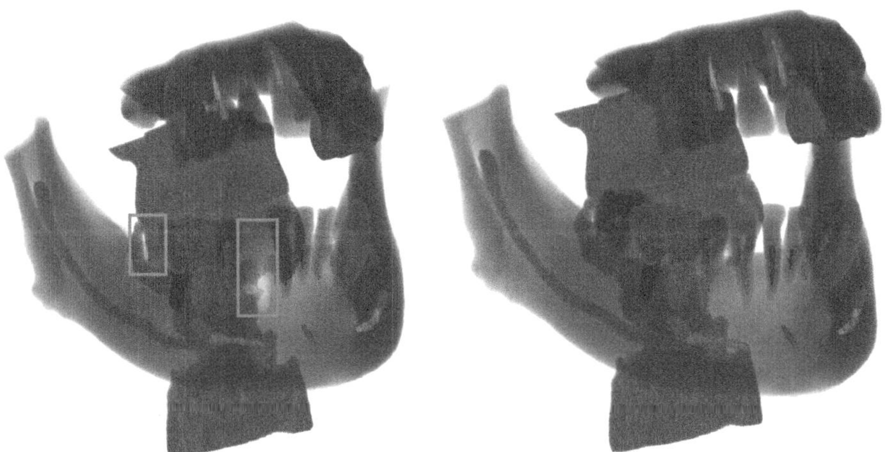

Fig. 3. The visualization shows the processing effects of manually removing teeth according to image features.

Logical Consistency Flip Augment. Flipping augmentation of 3D images is commonly employed as a standard processing step to enhance data diversity. However, as noted in the article [5], when the segmentation targets include symmetrically similar structures, applying flipping augmentation without appropriate restrictions may cause confusion between these symmetrical parts in the images. This issue is particularly prominent in CBCT data, where multiple anatomical structures such as teeth and the inferior alveolar canal (IAC) display inherent symmetry. Moreover, when working with small patches, it becomes difficult to distinguish between upper and lower teeth based on structural features alone.

This issue is seldom encountered when processing images of other body parts, primarily for two reasons. First, most anatomical regions possess sufficient structural features with low morphological similarity between distinct structure. Second, in many cases there is no clinical need to differentiate between symmetric categories.

Intuitively, to mitigate the mis-segmentation caused by symmetrical structures, we diverged from the experimental setup described in article by retaining the flipping augmentation operation but imposing a key constraint: the number of flipping operations must always be even. When allowing flips along the x, y, and z axes, this means either performing no flips or flipping across an even number of axes.

The intuition behind this is straightforward: an odd number of flips results in a completely symmetrical version of the image, which can disrupt the perception of anatomical orientation. When the model is sufficiently complex, it may still learn to distinguish such flipped samples. However, both the model and human observers are likely to struggle when dealing with inherently symmetrical anatomical regions. The effects of applying different numbers of flipping operations are illustrated in Fig. 4.

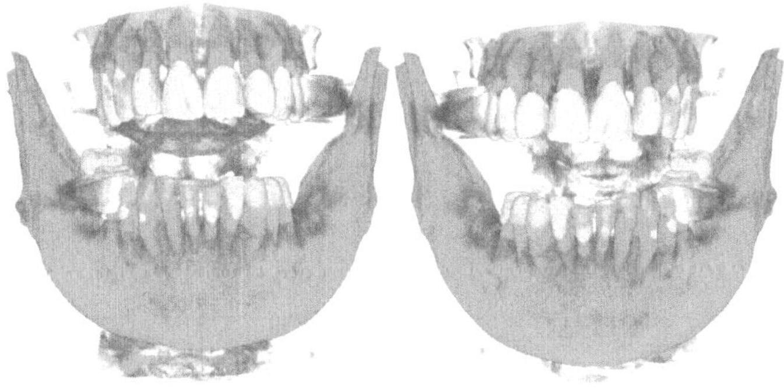

Fig. 4. The left figure shows the results of an even number of flipping operations, while the right figure displays the visualizations generated by an odd number of flipping operations.

Dimension Expansion. The imaging principle of CBCT differs significantly from that of RGB images, as its pixel values carry specific physical meanings. Since the ToothFairy3 dataset used in this study extends ToothFairy2 with additional annotation categories, we randomly sampled points across each category and recorded their Hounsfield Unit (HU) values in the ToothFairy2 dataset and visualized the statistics in Fig. 5. Based on this analysis, we divided the intensity values into multiple channels using the following intervals: [−600, 0], [0, 1000], [0, 2000], [1000, 3000], and [3000, maximum]. Different HU values may correspond to different tissue types, and in clinical practice, different intensity ranges are commonly used to capture images of specific tissues. Therefore, we analyzed the data ranges for each anatomical label and established the divisions described above. Given that teeth generally exhibit high HU values, the low-HU regions that are challenging to distinguish were split into multiple channels to provide the model with more detailed information. To enhance edge information, we computed a boundary channel by applying the Laplacian operator to the image restricted to the intensity range [-600, 3000], and incorporated it as an additional channel. At this stage, each channel is individually normalized to [0,1]. This multi-channel partitioning strategy constitutes one key component of our data preprocessing pipeline.

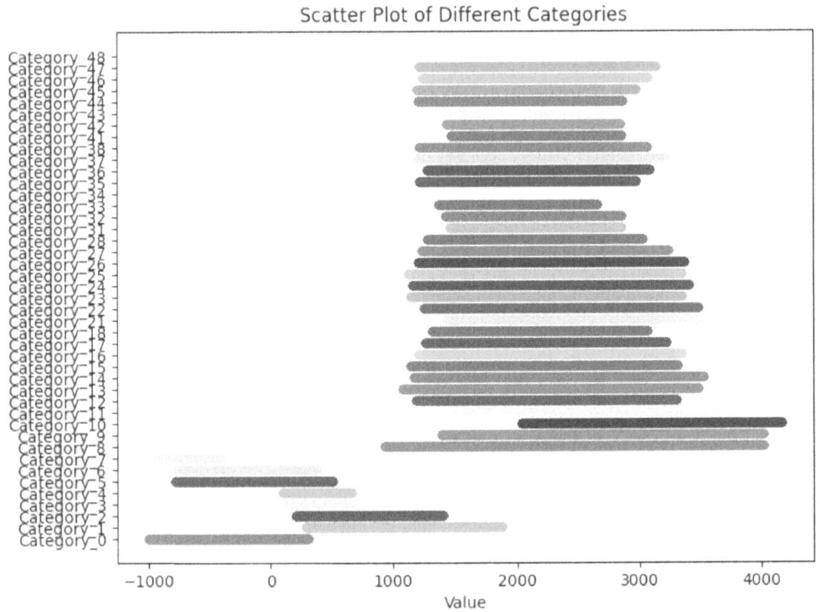

Fig. 5. The figure shows the Hounsfield Unit (HU) value ranges for different anatomical structures.

2.4 Network Architecture.

To enable accurate identification of different segmentation categories, we refined the deep supervision mechanism in the nnU-Net by reducing the number of supervised decoding layers from supervision at each stage to only the final three layers. Additionally, a category prediction head was added to the final encoder layer to perform 77-class prediction for each input image patch in the ToothFairy3 segmentation task. This design enhances discriminative feature learning through explicit category-wise supervision.

For this task, we employed a composite loss function consisting of cross-entropy loss, Dice loss, and focal cross-entropy loss. The i denotes the outputs at different levels of deep supervision. The formulation is as follows:

$$\text{loss} = \left(\sum_{i=0}^{2} \frac{1}{2^i} \left(l_{\text{dice}}^i + l_{\text{fce}}^i \right) \right) + l_{\text{ice}}^{\text{class}} \tag{1}$$

Dice loss and focal cross-entropy loss are computed for the outputs of the decoding stages at different levels, and cross-entropy loss is computed for the output of the category prediction head.

When training a single-class segmentation model with user click prompts, we froze the pretrained multi-class segmentation model and stacked the user click information with the multi-class inference outputs as an additional input channel to train a dedicated single-class segmentation head. When organizing the user click information, we only assign a value of 1 to the positions that the user clicked, and set all other positions to 0. At this stage, the model outputs predictions for only one class.

2.5 Model Training

All experiments were conducted on 4 NVIDIA V100 GPUs (32 GB). During training, 20% of each set was used for validation. The models were trained for 30 epochs, with each epoch corresponding to a full traversal of all training data rather than random patch sampling. The training patch size was set to [160, 192, 192] and the batch size was set to 1. The model achieving the best performance on the validation set was retained.

For nnU-Net, we adopted the defaultUNet L configuration and further customized it. In addition to the preprocessing enhancements described above, RandAffine augmentation was applied. The model was optimized using AdamW with an initial learning rate of 1×10^{-4} and a ReduceLROnPlateau learning rate scheduler. We use a learning rate scheduler with a reduction factor of 0.8. The learning rate will not decrease below 1×10^{-6}, and the scheduler monitors the validation metric at every epoch.

2.6 Inference

Due to the substantial computational requirements of training 3D data and the constraints on inference time and computing resources imposed by the Tooth-

Fairy3 challenge, we intuitively reasoned that increasing the patch size, during training and inference, could serve as an effective way to mitigate mis-segmentation in symmetrically similar structures. Although limited computational resources restricted the training patch size to [160, 192, 192], we re-examined the inference functions in both nnU-Net and MONAI and implemented strict memory management on the GPU during inference. This approach allowed the use of patch sizes consistent with those used in training, reduced the number of patches requiring inference under the same overlap ratio setting, shortened inference time, and ultimately improved the practical usability of the model.

Table 1. Inference time for different image sizes.

Image size	Inference Repeat (%)	Patch Num	Inference time(s) (without argmax and Post-processing)
262, 512, 512(F_001)	25	32	41
170, 352, 370(P_001)	25	18	19
188, 385, 462(S_0001)	25	18	17

Table 1 shows the inference time required on an RTX 4060 GPU (8 GB). By keeping only one patch and the model in GPU memory at a time, memory consumption is relatively low. This enables the use of a larger patch size and significantly reduces the number of patches needed for inference. As tested, the patch size can be increased to [192, 192, 192].

Post-processing and the argmax operation are configured to run on the CPU. As their execution time is strongly affected by system RAM, these steps are excluded from the reported runtime.

2.7 Data Post-processing

Determining the optimal post-processing strategy in nnU-Net requires repeated inference across the entire dataset to evaluate the retention of the largest connected component for each category, which is a highly time-consuming process. Based on the structural characteristics of the data, we employed a hybrid strategy combining projection-based connected region preservation with 3D connected-component labeling.

Compared to nnU-Net's automated strategy, our method requires configuration based on observational analysis of the dataset, but it reduces inference time and avoids repeated post-processing selection across different combination schemes. The specific procedure is shown in Fig. 6.

It can be observed that most segmentation errors in the model's output occur in the maxilla, mandible, and pharyngeal regions. During multi-class segmentation, we first retain the largest 3D connected components of the pharynx and mandible. The labels are then projected along the z-axis, and the two largest connected regions in the projection are preserved. These are back-projected into 3D to remove erroneous segmentation areas outside the main anatomical structures, yielding the final segmentation result after post-processing.

When processing the output of a single-class segmentation, we assign labels to the results based on user prompts, as also illustrated in Fig. 6.

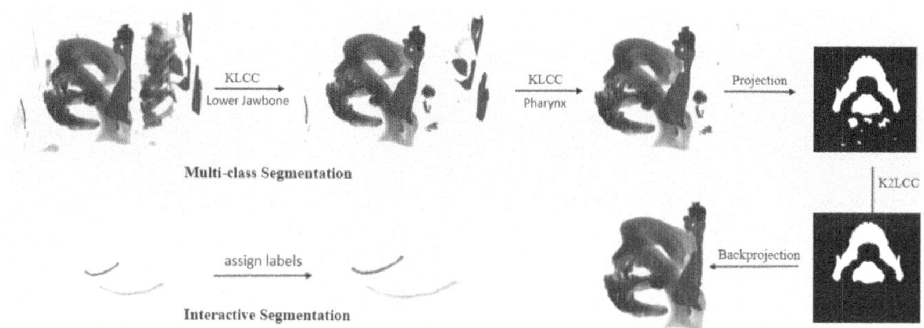

Fig. 6. The figure illustrates the post-processing pipeline for both multi-class and single-class segmentation. KLCC stands for "Keeping the Largest Connected Component".

3 Results

3.1 Validate the Effectiveness of the Flip Constraint

We used a portion of the data as a validation set. For each patch, we performed inference to validate the Dice coefficient, then averaged the results. During training, all models were trained for the same duration, and the best performance results on the test set were recorded. The outcomes are presented in Table 2. Demonstrates the effectiveness of the constraint rules.

Table 2. Results of different constraint rules.

Model	Dice
default	0.9288
constraint	0.9409

3.2 Validation Results

The inference results for the three different sets are presented in Fig. 7.

On the current challenge leaderboard, the results from my final submission show that in the multi-instance segmentation task, the maximum Dice score reached 0.82, while the minimum was 0.14.

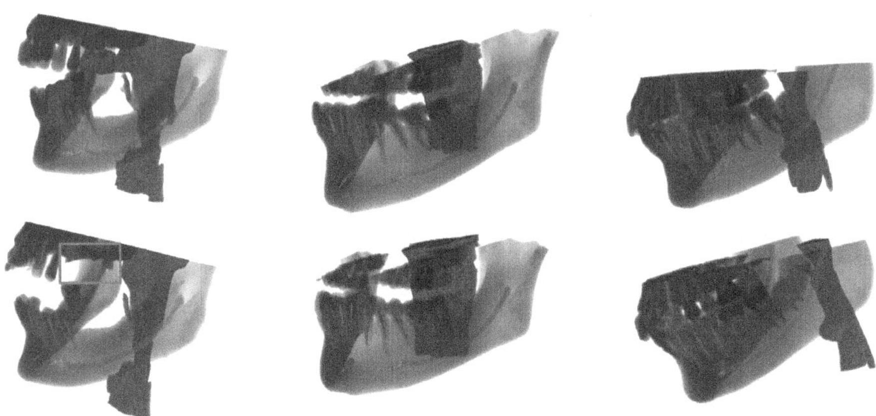

Fig. 7. The top row shows the labels, and the bottom row shows the modeln's inference results, corresponding from left to right to F_001, P_001, and S_0001 in ToothFairy3.

Similarly, for the interactive segmentation task, the highest Dice score achieved was 0.92, although several cases completely failed, producing no segmentation output whatsoever.

The best results of both tasks in the test phase are summarized in Table 3. The overlap ratio in the inference function was set to 25% for the multi-instance

Table 3. Evaluation results of both tasks in test phase. Dice similarity coefficient and HD95 are reported.

Metric	Statistic	Multi-class	Interactive
Dice Average	Min	0.149	0.0
	25%	0.516	0.66
	50%	0.652	0.83
	75%	0.718	0.88
	Max	0.820	0.92
	Mean	0.594	0.72
	Std	0.185	0.25
HD95 Average	Min	78.40	1.0
	25%	107.09	1.73
	50%	142.38	2.80
	75%	185.98	45.11
	Max	358.28	607.86
	Mean	163.31	76.82
	Std	69.14	159.13

segmentation task and 50% for the interactive segmentation task. And our inference speed was ranked second in the interactive segmentation task.

Inspection of the inference results shows that certain data setup errors remain to be resolved, since the model identify the implants and the maxillary sinus. It remains a challenge for the model to accurately distinguish between dental crowns and bridges. In addition, in interactive segmentation tasks, the model may fail when processing certain images. This failure is possibly caused by variations in oral cavity opening states across images or by overfitting, which prevents the model from generalizing to different conditions. However, preliminary experiments have already achieved promising progress in both multi-class segmentation and interactive segmentation, providing valuable insights and ideas for further studies.

Acknowledgements. We would like to express our sincere gratitude to the organizers of the ToothFairy Challenge for their continuous efforts in creating and updating the publicly available CBCT datasets. Their dedicated work has made this study possible.

Disclosure of Interests. The authors have no competing interests to declare that are relevant to the content of this article.

References

1. Bolelli, F., et al.: Segmenting the inferior alveolar canal in CBCTs volumes: the toothfairy challenge. IEEE Trans. Med. Imaging **44**(4), 1890–1906 (2025). https://doi.org/10.1109/TMI.2024.3523096
2. Bolelli, F., et al.: Segmenting maxillofacial structures in CBCT volumes. In: Proceedings of the IEEE/CVF Conference on Computer Vision and Pattern Recognition (CVPR), pp. 5238–5248 (2025)
3. Bornstein, M.M., Scarfe, W.C., Vaughn, V.M., Jacobs, R.: Cone beam computed tomography in implant dentistry: a systematic review focusing on guidelines, indications, and radiation dose risks. Int. J. Oral Maxillofacial Implants **29**(Suppl), 55–77 (2014)
4. Isensee, F., Jaeger, P.F., Kohl, S.A.A., Petersen, J., Maier-Hein, K.H.: nnU-Net: a self-configuring method for deep learning-based biomedical image segmentation. Nat. Methods **18**(2), 203–211 (2021)
5. Isensee, F., Kirchhoff, Y., Kraemer, L., Rokuss, M., Ulrich, C., Maier-Hein, K.H.: Scaling NNU-net for CBCT segmentation. In: Wang, Y., et al. (eds.) MICCAI 2024. LNCS, vol. 15571, pp. 13–20. Springer, Cham (2025). https://doi.org/10.1007/978-3-031-88977-6_2
6. Joda, T., Ferrari, M., Gallucci, G., Wittneben, J., Brägger, U.: Digital technology in fixed implant prosthodontics. Periodontology 2000 **73**(1), 178–192 (2017)
7. Lumetti, L., Pipoli, V., Bolelli, F., Ficarra, E., Grana, C.: Enhancing patch-based learning for the segmentation of the mandibular canal. IEEE Access **12**, 79014–79024 (2024). https://doi.org/10.1109/ACCESS.2024.3408629
8. Mangano, F., Gandolfi, A., Luongo, G., Logozzo, S.: Intraoral scanners in dentistry: a review of the current literature. BMC Oral Health **17**(1), 149 (2017)
9. Revilla-León, M., et al.: Artificial intelligence applications in implant dentistry: a systematic review. J. Prosthet. Dent. **129**(2), 293–300 (2023). https://doi.org/10.1016/j.prosdent.2021.05.008

10. Scarfe, W.C., Angelopoulos, C.: Maxillofacial Cone Beam Computed Tomography: Principles. Techniques and Clinical Applications. Springer, Cham (2018). https://doi.org/10.1007/978-3-319-62061-9
11. Torosdagli, N., Liberton, D.K., Verma, P., Sincan, M., Lee, J.S., Bagci, U.: Deep geodesic learning for segmentation and anatomical landmarking. IEEE Trans. Med. Imaging **38**(4), 919–931 (2019)

Multi-phase Automated Segmentation of Dental Structures in CBCT Using a Lightweight Auto3DSeg and SegResNet Implementation

Dominic LaBella[1(✉)], Keshav Jha[2], Jared Robbins[1], and Esther Yu[1]

[1] Department of Radiation Oncology, Duke University Medical Center, Durham, NC 27710, USA
dominic.labella@duke.edu

[2] Duke University, Durham, NC 27710, USA

Abstract. Cone-beam computed tomography (CBCT) has become an invaluable imaging modality in dentistry, enabling 3D visualization of teeth and surrounding structures for diagnosis and treatment planning. Automated segmentation of dental structures in CBCT can efficiently assist in identifying pathology (e.g., pulpal or periapical lesions) and facilitate radiation therapy planning in head and neck cancer patients. We describe the DLaBella29 team's approach for the MICCAI 2025 ToothFairy3 Challenge, which involves a deep learning pipeline for multi-class tooth segmentation. We utilized the MONAI Auto3DSeg framework with a 3D SegResNet architecture, trained on a subset of the ToothFairy3 dataset (63 CBCT scans) with 5-fold cross-validation. Key preprocessing steps included image resampling to 0.6 mm isotropic resolution and intensity clipping. We applied an ensemble fusion using Multi-Label STAPLE on the 5-fold predictions to infer a Phase 1 segmentation and then conducted tight cropping around the easily segmented Phase 1 mandible to perform Phase 2 segmentation on the smaller nerve structures. Our method achieved an average Dice of 0.87 on the ToothFairy3 challenge out-of-sample validation set. This paper details the clinical context, data preparation, model development, results of our approach, and discusses the relevance of automated dental segmentation for improving patient care in radiation oncology.

Keywords: Radiation Oncology · Hyperbaric Oxygen · Osteoradionecrosis · Automated Segmentation · MONAI · Auto3DSeg · SegResNet

1 Introduction

Cone-beam computed tomography (CBCT) has revolutionized dental imaging over the past two decades, overcoming the limitations of 2D panoramic radiography and providing accurate multiplanar visualization of maxillofacial structures [1–3]. CBCT's ability to produce high-resolution 3D images enables improved detection of dental pathologies. Notably, the most common pathologic conditions involving teeth, inflammatory lesions of the pulp and periapical areas, can be visualized more reliably with CBCT than with

F. Bolelli et al. (Eds.): ODIN 2025, LNCS 16473, pp. 145–158, 2026.
https://doi.org/10.1007/978-3-032-20711-1_14

conventional radiographs [3]. Lesions confined to cancellous bone that might be missed on intraoral X-rays are often evident on CBCT, leading to greater diagnostic accuracy, as shown by Jaju et al., where CBCT detected periapical lesions with ~ 61% accuracy vs ~ 39–44% for digital or film radiographs [3]. Such 3D information is clinically valuable for endodontic evaluation and treatment planning, allowing clinicians to assess the true extent of pulp chamber infections, periapical cysts, or granulomas and to plan surgical interventions accordingly. The broad adoption of dental CBCT reflects its utility in implantology, orthodontics, and oral surgery, as well as in baseline dental evaluations for oncology patients [2].

In patients with head and neck cancer, dental health management before and after radiation therapy (RT) is critical [4, 5]. Irradiation can compromise oral health by reducing salivary flow and blood supply to the jaws, leading to higher risk of dental caries, periodontal disease, and osteoradionecrosis (ORN) of the jaw [6]. ORN, a severe complication where irradiated bone fails to heal, has an incidence of roughly 1–9% in RT patients and occurs much more frequently in the mandible (~85% of cases) than the maxilla [6]. The risk of ORN is strongly dose-dependent, rising from $< 6\%$ at doses below 40 Gy to $\geq 20\%$ at doses above 60 Gy [6]. Clinical practice guidelines therefore recommend proactive dental management: for example, teeth anticipated to receive very high radiation doses may be extracted prophylactically (common thresholds are ≥ 70 Gy in the maxilla or ≥ 60 Gy in the mandible for considering extraction) to prevent ORN [7]. Even with such measures, post-RT dental extractions or infections can precipitate ORN, so accurately mapping radiation dose to each tooth is important in predicting risk. Per the classic Marx protocol, hyperbaric oxygen is used as an adjunct around dental surgery in irradiated jaws, typically ~ 20 pre-extraction and 10 post-extraction sessions at ~ 2.4 times atmospheric pressure for 90 min, and for established ORN as staged therapy beginning with ~30 sessions followed by limited debridement and ~10 additional dives to promote angiogenesis and wound healing [8].

In current practice, radiation oncologists and dental specialists collaborate to evaluate teeth in or near high-dose regions using CT imaging and clinical exam. However, this process is largely manual and qualitative. Automated tooth segmentation on planning CBCT scans could greatly enhance this workflow by providing precise tooth contours for dose-effect analysis [6]. Prior work by Thariat et al. introduced an atlas-based auto-segmentation of dental structures ("Dentalmaps"), demonstrating that using automatically segmented teeth to estimate per-tooth radiation dose was significantly more accurate (within 2 Gy in 75% of cases) than visual estimation without contours (within 2 Gy in only 30% of cases) [6]. Such tools improve communication between radiation oncologists and dentists and help identify teeth at highest risk for complications [6].

The MICCAI ToothFairy3 Challenge was organized to advance fully automated, multi-class segmentation of dental and maxillofacial structures in CBCT volumes [9–11]. The challenge dataset provides 3D CBCT scans with detailed annotations of 77 anatomical labels, including all teeth (with individual tooth identifiers), dental restorations, pulp canals, nerves, and surrounding tissues [9–12].

In this paper, we present our team's approach and results in the ToothFairy3 Challenge 2025. We aimed for a solution that is robust and computationally efficient, leveraging the MONAI Auto3DSeg framework to automatically configure a deep neural network for the task [13, 14]. We describe our data preparation (focusing on a subset of the training data with full dental field-of-view), model training with 5-fold cross-validation, Multi Label STAPLE ensemble fusion method, post-processing techniques, and cropping of an initial "Phase 1" prediction to perform a focused "Phase 2" inference for final predictions on the smaller nerve structures. We also discuss the clinical relevance of the results and how such automated segmentations can be integrated into radiation therapy planning to help reduce dental complications.

2 Methods

2.1 Dataset Selection

Phase 1 Dataset

We utilized the ToothFairy3 challenge training dataset, which consists of 532 CBCT scans annotated with 77 substructure classes [9–12]. Due to region of interest (ROI) and training time considerations, we restricted "Phase 1" training from the entire provided set to just the "Set B" subset, comprising 63 CBCT image-label pair cases as seen in Fig. 1A. This subset has a broader scanning range (head CBCT images capturing all teeth) compared to "Set A" (n = 417) and "Set C" (n = 52) from the full dataset, that were cropped and frequently missing challenge evaluated substructures. Each "Set B" image had an isotropic voxel size of approximately 0.3 mm^3, a median voxel volume of [168, 362, 371], and was provided with a corresponding segmentation label map for a subset of the 77 substructures. The 77 substructure classes in the challenge-provided dataset were consolidated into 46 substructures as described by the challenge organizers [12]. This full-sized dataset was used for initial training of a Phase 1 multi-class automated segmentation model.

Phase 2 Dataset

We cropped the full-sized Phase 1 dataset image and reference standard label pairs to an ROI around the mandible (label = 1). The ROI was determined based on the reference standard mandible label by identifying the point (x, y, z) representing the most anterior voxel for the mandible, then expanding laterally (x) by −110 and + 110 voxels (ensuring staying within boundaries of full-sized image); then expanding posteriorly (y) by + 100 voxels; then expanding superiorly from the most inferior mandibular point by 90 voxels. These expansion values were determined from preliminary analysis—not reported here—of the dataset to ensure inclusion of all of the relevant anatomy in Phase 2. The final result of this cropping is demonstrated in Fig. 1B. Note that this reduced the total Phase 2 image sizes by about 60 times compared to the full-sized Phase 1 images, dramatically reducing the image data needed to be evaluated during Phase 2 model training. Notably, Phase 2 was also restricted to training on the 63 "Set B" subset cases due to time constraints. Future studies should consider using all the available cases, especially since Phase 2 focuses on lower jawbone structures.

All image and label files were provided as de-identified and standardized Neuroimaging Informatics Technology Initiative (NIfTI) format.

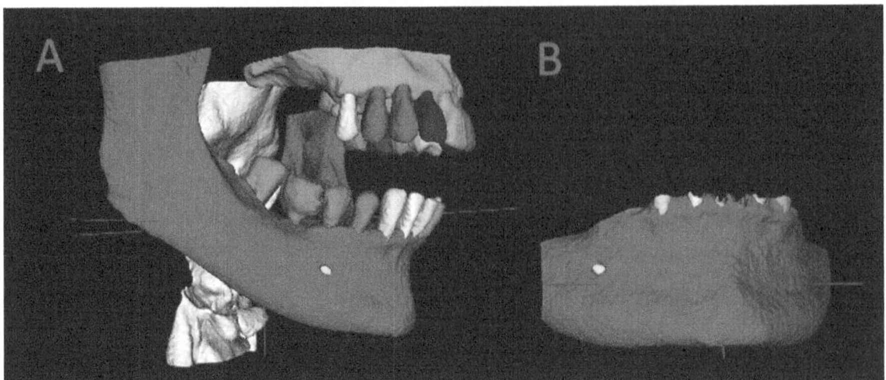

Fig. 1. Panel A demonstrates an example of an unaltered, ToothFairy3, "Set B", Phase 1 training set case 3D multi-label representation demonstrating the majority of challenge substructures. Note that the brown "Crown" structure in place of multiple teeth for this case. Panel B demonstrates an example of the corresponding cropped Phase 2 training set case 3D multi-label representation, which isolates the region of interest surrounding the Right Incisive Nerve, Left Incisive Nerve, and Lingual Nerve.

2.2 Preprocessing and Label Conversion

For Phase 1 alone, we resampled all CBCT images to a uniform resolution of [0.6, 0.6, 0.6] mm^3 isotropic spacing to standardize the input size for the network and to account for hardware memory and processing speed limitations for the larger image sizes seen with native resolution of [0.3, 0.3, 0.3] mm^3. Intensity values (in Hounsfield Units) were clipped to [–1000, 3800] for both Phase 1 and Phase 2, which encompasses the range from air to the highest densities of enamel/metal artifacts in the scans. We also applied systematic label remapping to simplify the segmentation task. In the original challenge labels, certain structures had high integer label values or were subdivided into many small categories (for example, each tooth's pulp cavity was labeled separately with IDs 111–148). We merged these into a consolidated label set for model training. Specifically, all pulp and periapical lesion labels were collapsed into a single "pulp" class, and the incisive and lingual canals (original labels 103–105) were re-indexed to fit within the 0–46 range (while preserving distinct labels for evaluation, background = 0). The remapping reduced sparsely represented classes and ensured that the network's output channel count did not skip any integer label values, to align with Auto3DSeg requirements. After conversion, the training label maps included: background, 32 individual tooth labels (upper and lower teeth 1–16), the mandibular and maxillary jawbone, dental restorations (implants, crowns, bridges; none included in challenge ranking metrics), bilateral inferior incisive nerves, alveolar canals, the lingual nerve, maxillary sinuses, pharynx, and a combined pulp category. Restoration-related classes (labels 8–10: bridge, crown, and implants) were not included in our model training and submission due to our interpretation of the Grand Challenge submission instructions. As a result, our reported metrics do not reflect performance on labels 8–10.

2.3 Model and Training

We adopted the Auto3DSeg automated segmentation pipeline implemented in MONAI, which streamlines model configuration and hyperparameter tuning [13, 14]. The chosen backbone model was SegResNet, a 3D residual UNet-like convolutional network known to perform well in medical image segmentation challenges [14, 15]. Auto3DSeg initialized a SegResNet with default encoder-decoder structure and optimized training settings based on our data. The encoder used five ResNet blocks with instance normalization, and the downsampling included five stages with 1, 2, 2, 4, and 4 convolutional blocks, respectively, similar to our prior experience [16]. We sectioned the training and inference into two phases.

Phase 1

We trained the Phase 1 model for 500 epochs on the 63 full-sized training images and associated reference standard multi-class labels, as seen in Fig. 1A, using a random 5-fold cross-validation (each fold held out ~20% of cases for validation). The training objective was a combined Dice + Cross-Entropy loss (implemented as DiceCELoss in MONAI, with equal weighting) computed over all foreground classes. Notably, we excluded background voxels from the Dice term to focus the loss on meaningful structures. We enabled automatic mixed precision (AMP) to accelerate training and used a batch size of 1 (one 3D volume per GPU iteration) and a region of interest (ROI) size of [192, 192, 128] due to memory and time constraints. Data augmentation included random intensity scaling and shifting, and slight rotations, as configured by Auto3DSeg's defaults, to improve generalization. Random flipping data augmentation was specifically disabled to prevent inaccurate training of contralateral dental substructures. We used a learning rate of 0.0003 and a weight decay of 0.00005 with the use of the AdamW optimizer. We were unable to use larger batch sizes, data caching or multiple workers because training repeatedly crashed due to VRAM, RAM, CPU, and I/O bottlenecks when increasing the usage of each of these parameters. All model training was conducted on a single NVIDIA RTX 4090 GPU (24 GB of VRAM available) but only utilized approximately 8 GB of VRAM during training. These decisions were made due to the longer training times and more frequent training crashes associated with using larger networks and ROIs associated with larger available VRAM utilization. Each fold's training took approximately 6–10 h. Our use of a single-GPU workstation contrasts with some recent Auto3DSeg challenge solutions that leveraged multi-GPU servers (8 × A40 GPUs) that performed more folds using different networks including Swin UNETR and DiNTS [15, 17, 18]. In our methodology, we focused on the single SegResNet model approach due to resource limitations; thereby accepting a longer training time, smaller ROI sizes, and smaller SegResNet network structures. This decision was made due to the superior performance of SegResNet compared to Swin UNETR and DiNTS as described by Myronenko et al. [15].

Phase 2

Phase 2 included training on the cropped version of the Phase 1 images and associated reference standard labels that focus on a small region of interest surrounding the difficult to infer lingual nerve as seen in Fig. 1B. These identical expansions were used during the Phase 2 inference stage. Phase 2 training was similar to Phase 1, except for an ROI of [221, 101, 91] voxels and no resampling to [0.6, 0.6, 0.6] mm^3. The VRAM used was limited to 3 GB. The purpose for retraining with the [0.3, 0.3, 0.3] mm^3 higher-resolution images was to try and segment the small nerve structures which have a very small tubular diameter.

2.4 Inference and Ensemble Fusion

First, we ran inference with each of the 5-fold SegResNet Phase 1 models on each test CBCT, yielding five candidate label maps as shown in Fig. 2. We then applied a label fusion algorithm to combine these outputs into one consensus segmentation. We used the Multi-Label Simultaneous Truth and Performance Level Estimation (STAPLE) implemented in SimpleITK to produce a fused label map [19]. STAPLE is an expectation-maximization algorithm that weighs each input segmentation by its estimated accuracy and computes a probabilistic "true" segmentation [19]. We chose STAPLE because it is well-suited for fusing multiple-label maps and can handle the multi-class nature of our problem (via an extension to Multi-Label STAPLE).

After STAPLE ensemble was performed, we converted any aberrant class predictions touching the pharynx (label = 7) to the pharynx We also removed any mandible instance lesions that had a volume less than 200,000 voxels, which would indicate false positive instance lesions. We then cropped the image for Phase 2, and Fig. 3 represents the cropped ROI for Phase 2 inference as described in Sect. 2.3. Phase 2 inference was conducted similarly to the steps seen in Phase 1 inference, except for the use of a set of five different cross-validation models that were trained on the cropped dataset as shown in Fig. 1B. Note that Figs. 1, 2 and 3 represent an in-sample case from Fold 1 and therefore give an artificially high inference performance appearance. Due to the small number of selected training set cases (n = 63), no "Set B" cases were left out-of-sample for internal testing for quantitative or qualitative analysis prior to challenge submission. This was done to try and create the most generalizable model possible from the largest training set possible.

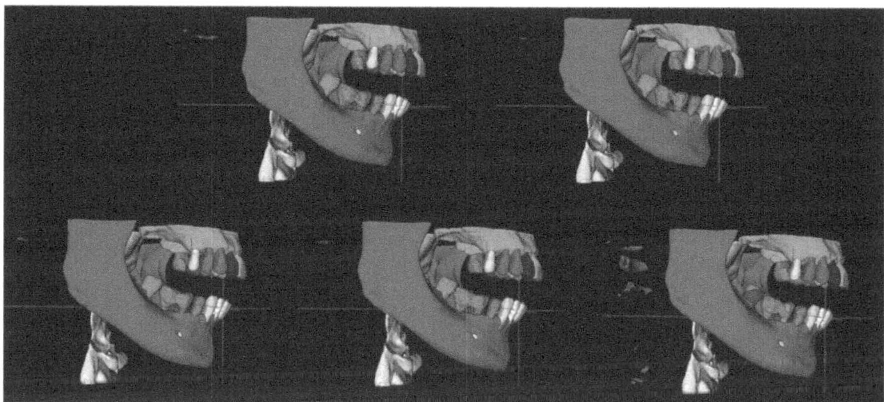

Fig. 2. For Phase 1 inference, we apply the trained SegResNet models to predict multi-class label maps (folds 1–5) and convert back to the native image resolution as seen in these 3D multi-label representations. Note that this is an in-sample validation case from training fold 1 (top left). Therefore folds 2–5 (top middle, top right, bottom left, bottom right) had this case in the training sets and had artificially high performance during this inference sanity check.

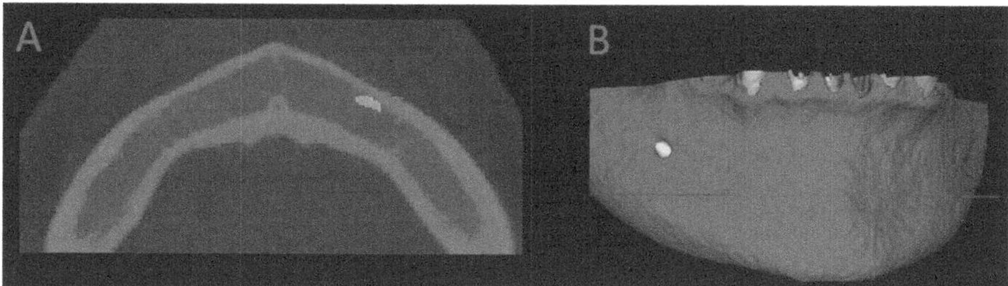

Fig. 3. Axial CBCT image (A) and a 3D (B) multi-label representation demonstrating cropping of the Phase 1 ensembled segmentation performed by identifying the point (x, y, z) representing the most anterior voxel for the easily segmented mandible, then expanding laterally (x) by –110 and + 110 voxels; then expanding posteriorly (y) by + 100 voxels; then expanding superiorly from the most inferior mandibular point by 90 voxels. This was used to predict the Left Incisive Nerve, Right Incisive Nerve, and Lingual Nerve during Phase 2 inference.

3 Results

We evaluated our approach through 5-fold cross-validation on the training set and on the held-out validation set of the ToothFairy3 Challenge [12]. Table 1 summarizes the 5-fold cross-validation performance for the challenge-evaluated structures for each fold.

Table 1. Cross-validation results and the training set's average volume for each substructure evaluated within the ToothFairy3 challenge dataset. Mean ± Std represents the mean and standard deviation Dice performance across the 5 training folds.

Class ID	Structure	Number of Cases Structure Present	Average Volume (mm3)	Mean ± Std
0	Background	—	—	—
1	Lower Jawbone	63	46822	0.977 ± 0.005
2	Upper Jawbone	61	12145	0.941 ± 0.008
3	Left Inferior Alveolar Canal	63	410	0.793 ± 0.018
4	Right Inferior Alveolar Canal	63	422	0.746 ± 0.052
5	Left Maxillary Sinus	44	1494	0.937 ± 0.022
6	Right Maxillary Sinus	42	1524	0.950 ± 0.018
7	Pharynx	63	22689	0.975 ± 0.030
11	Upper Right Central Incisor	59	486	0.960 ± 0.052
12	Upper Right Lateral Incisor	57	347	0.952 ± 0.049
13	Upper Right Canine	58	534	0.957 ± 0.039
14	Upper Right First Premolar	55	466	0.95 ± 0.072
15	Upper Right Second Premolar	50	452	0.839 ± 0.047
16	Upper Right First Molar	51	901	0.854 ± 0.053
17	Upper Right Second Molar	50	799	0.793 ± 0.069
18	Upper Right Third Molar (Wisdom Tooth)	26	637	0.844 ± 0.079
21	Upper Left Central Incisor	57	481	0.961 ± 0.032
22	Upper Left Lateral Incisor	59	340	0.948 ± 0.060

(continued)

Table 1. *(continued)*

Class ID	Structure	Number of Cases Structure Present	Average Volume (mm3)	Mean ± Std
23	Upper Left Canine	59	539	0.937 ± 0.034
24	Upper Left First Premolar	57	466	0.954 ± 0.055
25	Upper Left Second Premolar	53	444	0.908 ± 0.050
26	Upper Left First Molar	54	905	0.827 ± 0.047
27	Upper Left Second Molar	53	799	0.868 ± 0.02
28	Upper Left Third Molar (Wisdom Tooth)	29	608	0.886 ± 0.093
31	Lower Left Central Incisor	59	236	0.928 ± 0.010
32	Lower Left Lateral Incisor	61	282	0.937 ± 0.033
33	Lower Left Canine	60	475	0.948 ± 0.034
34	Lower Left First Premolar	59	389	0.842 ± 0.047
35	Lower Left Second Premolar	55	425	0.921 ± 0.0350
36	Lower Left First Molar	40	915	0.822 ± 0.0520
37	Lower Left Second Molar	50	869	0.820 ± 0.087
38	Lower Left Third Molar (Wisdom Tooth)	37	780	0.943 ± 0.010
41	Lower Right Central Incisor	60	237	0.941 ± 0.008
42	Lower Right Lateral Incisor	60	281	0.941 ± 0.033
43	Lower Right Canine	59	474	0.959 ± 0.045

(continued)

Table 1. *(continued)*

Class ID	Structure	Number of Cases Structure Present	Average Volume (mm3)	Mean ± Std
44	Lower Right First Premolar	59	381	0.945 ± 0.060
45	Lower Right Second Premolar	55	436	0.893 ± 0.078
46	Lower Right First Molar	45	809	0.780 ± 0.059
47	Lower Right Second Molar	44	857	0.728 ± 0.085
48	Lower Right Third Molar (Wisdom Tooth)	36	809	0.873 ± 0.060
50	Tooth Pulp	61	588	0.785 ± 0.014
51	Left Incisive Nerve	58	19	0.318 ± 0.208
52	Right Incisive Nerve	55	17	0.106 ± 0.205
53	Lingual Nerve	60	8	0 ± 0
Phase 1 Mean	All Phase 1 Substructures	63	—	0.850 ± 0.017
*51	Left Incisive Nerve Phase 2	58	19	0.688 ± 0.013
*52	Right Incisive Nerve Phase 2	55	17	0.665 ± 0.009
*53	Lingual Nerve Phase 2	60	8	0.681 ± 0.006
Combined Mean	Phase 1 Substructures Except Phase 2 Nerves	63	—	0.879 ± 0

Each fold's validation Dice was computed as the average Dice across all predicted structures in that fold's validation cases (averaging per-case Dice, weighted equally per class). The scores per fold were relatively consistent, in the range 0.822–0.867. The mean Dice over all folds was approximately 0.850 for these single-model approaches. We observed that larger structures (teeth and jaw) were segmented with higher accuracy (Dice ~ 0.977 for mandible), whereas smaller structures like incisive nerves and lingual nerves were more challenging (Dice 0.0–0.318) during Phase 1, lowering the overall

Phase 1 average. Table 1 shows the relationship between 5-fold cross-validation average Dice performance for Phase 1 and Phase 2 substructures vs the average volume of the substructures. Note that the Phase 2 inference successfully improved the performance of the Lingual Nerve Dice from 0.0 to 0.681, the Left Incisive Nerve Dice from 0.318 to 0.688 and the Right Incisive Nerve Dice from 0.106 to 0.665.

For the final evaluation of the challenge's out-of-sample validation set, our two-phase ensemble approach achieved an overall average Dice of 0.87. This aggregate performance is slightly higher than the cross-validation mean, which is expected due to the usage of the Multi Label STAPLE ensemble technique, post-processing to clean up the mandible and pharynx labels, and Phase 2's focus on improving the smaller nerve substructures. Qualitatively, the automated segmentations aligned well with the reference standard labels for most structures for in-sample validation cases, as illustrated in Fig. 3.

The model accurately delineated individual teeth, even in the presence of moderate metal artifacts from dental fillings on in-sample validation qualitative and quantitative analysis. Minor qualitative discrepancies were observed in areas of poor image quality, around metal implants or crowns causing streak artifacts, and the model occasionally missed small portions of a tooth or misclassified an artifact as part of a tooth.

4 Discussion

Our challenge submission demonstrates that a light-weight two-phase Auto3DSeg framework can produce competitive results for complex multi-class segmentation of dental CBCT scans. By leveraging MONAI's Auto3DSeg framework, we minimized the need for manual network design and hyperparameter tuning. This is particularly useful given the large number of classes (dozens of distinct structures) and the class imbalance inherent in the ToothFairy3 dataset. Larger structures (teeth, jaws) dominate the volume, whereas tiny structures (like canals and nerves) occupy far fewer voxels as shown in Table 1. The substructure results demonstrate performance correlating with structure volume, as shown in Table 1.

The lower Dice for very small classes (nerves) from single-phase models on lower resolution [0.6, 0.6, 0.6] mm^3 data suggests room for improvement. One possible extension would be additional phases cropping around specific dental substructures (nerves or pulp) relative to their position to confidently segmented structures (mandible or teeth), similar to our method for focusing on the nerves. This could refine the segmentation of additional fine structures (tooth-specific pulp) that a single-phase model might overlook. Notably, this study was successful in improving Lingual Nerve Dice from 0.0 to 0.681, the Left Incisive Nerve Dice from 0.318 to 0.688 and the Right Incisive Nerve Dice from 0.106 to 0.665 after utilizing this multi-phasic cropping-inference with higher resolution of [0.3, 0.3, 0.3] mm^3 approach. Due to time limitations, additional substructure-focused phases beyond our nerve-focused Phase 2 could not be conducted in the present study.

Another point of discussion is the benefit of ensemble fusion using STAPLE [19]. The STAPLE algorithm is advantageous in that it accounts for each model's reliability and is theoretically more robust than a simple majority vote or average in cases of systematic bias [19]. In our unreported qualitative analysis of the out-of-sample "Set A" and "Set C" test case's inference using STAPLE vs single fold model predictions,

STAPLE tended to produce cleaner segmentation borders, especially in areas of uncertainty (for instance, if one fold's model slightly over-segmented a tooth and another fold's model under-segmented it, STAPLE often found a middle ground). This resulted in fewer false positives like isolated tooth fragments. However, STAPLE also introduced a bit of smoothing; occasionally upon qualitative analysis, a tiny structure that only one model detected (e.g. a small root tip fragment) was dropped in the fused result if the other models missed it. In future work, a possible improvement could be to incorporate test-time augmentation or to weigh models differently for different subsets of structures (if one model is known to handle nerves better, for example).

An additional strategy to improve on the limited "Set B" dataset consisting of only 63 cases would be to double the size of this dataset by flipping the images and labels laterally along the y/z plane, then swapping all the label values for the left/right substructures. This differs from standard random flipping data augmentation, since this also modifies the reference standard labels themselves to their contralateral substructure label values. This was not performed in this study due to time and training time constraints.

From a clinical perspective, the relevance of accurate tooth segmentation in head and neck radiotherapy is significant. With automated segmentation, we can generate dose-volume metrics for each tooth in a patient's radiation plan, something that is impractical to do manually for dozens of teeth. These per-tooth dose metrics could facilitate communication between the oncology and dental team to best inform personalized dental management. For instance, if the model identifies that a particular molar is in a 70 Gy region, the care team might opt for an extraction or intensive prophylactic dental care prior to RT [7]. Alternatively, post-radiation, an oral surgeon may reconsider placing an implant into a heavily irradiated region of bone. Conversely, teeth receiving lower doses could be preserved and monitored, avoiding unnecessary extractions. In the long term, the data generated by automated segmentation across many patients could feed into predictive models for ORN or radiation-related dental caries. Previous studies have shown that pre-RT dental care, guided by imaging and dose considerations, can reduce complication rates [5]. Automation will make it easier to apply such guidelines consistently. Additionally, our segmentation includes not just the teeth, but also critical adjacent structures (mandible, maxilla, nerves, pulp). This could aid in detecting any anatomic variations, such as an aberrant mandibular canal course, or more refined dose-volume metrics that surgeons and radiation oncologists, respectively, should be aware of when planning interventions [1, 3].

One challenge worth noting is the image quality variability in CBCT. Dental CBCT scans often suffer from cone-beam artifacts and scatter, especially in the presence of metal. Our model was trained on the provided dataset, which included typical artifacts, and seemed to generalize across them to an extent. But in cases with extremely poor image quality (e.g., motion blurring or extensive metal streaks), performance may degrade. A potential mitigation strategy is to incorporate metal artifact reduction algorithms or to train the model on simulated artifact-augmented data. Another limitation is that our model did not explicitly differentiate between permanent teeth and dental implant, bridge, and crown structures as noted earlier due to our interpretation of the Grand Challenge submission instructions. Future studies should incorporate all of the available substructures in training datasets to generate more clinically relevant and useful models.

5 Conclusion

We have developed a two-phase 3D multi-class automated segmentation algorithm for dental CBCT images as part of the MICCAI ToothFairy3 Challenge 2025. Our method combined the ease-of-use of Auto3DSeg with a robust Multi Label STAPLE ensemble of a 3D SegResNet model, followed by tight cropping around small and hard to segment substructures. With relatively modest hardware (single GPU, RTX 4090, VRAM requirements <8 GB), we achieved accurate segmentation of 43 anatomical structures with an overall Dice of 0.87 on the challenge validation set. This performance approaches that of human expert contours for many structures and exceeds earlier atlas-based methods in this domain [5, 6]. The outcome demonstrates that modern deep learning models can handle the complexity of full-mouth dental segmentation in CBCT, provided that careful preprocessing and training strategies are employed.

Moving forward, we plan to refine the model to further boost accuracy on clinically important substructures, and to integrate the segmentation output into a pipeline for radiation dose analysis in patients with larger field of view head and neck cancer CT simulation scans. The ultimate goal is to deploy such technology in the clinical workflow for head and neck oncology, for example, generating automatic dental reports that flag high-dose teeth and quantify patient-specific risk factors for ORN. With continued improvements, automated tooth segmentation can become a valuable tool to personalize and improve supportive care for patients receiving radiotherapy.

Acknowledgments. This study was made possible by ToothFairy3 and its organizers. We would like to extend our sincere thanks to the organizers for hosting the challenge and for their continuous support.

Data Availability. Our code for all pre-processing, training, and post-processing is available as open-source at GitHub: dlabella29/ToothFairy25, to facilitate reproducibility and further research by the community. We hope that this work contributes to bridging the gap between computer-assisted dental imaging and practical clinical decision-making, enhancing outcomes in dental and radiation oncology.

Disclosures of Interests. The authors have no competing interests to declare that are relevant to the content of this article.

References

1. Kaasalainen, T., Ekholm, M., Siiskonen, T., Kortesniemi, M.: Dental cone beam CT: an updated review. Phys. Med. **88**, 193–217 (2021)
2. Tyndall, D.A., Price, J.B., Tetradis, S., Ganz, S.D., Hildebolt, C., Scarfe, W.C.: Position statement of the American academy of oral and maxillofacial radiology on selection criteria for the use of radiology in dental implantology with emphasis on cone beam computed tomography. Oral Surg Oral Med Oral Pathol Oral Radiol **113**(6), 817–826 (2012)

3. Jaju, P.P., Jaju, S.P.: Clinical utility of dental cone-beam computed tomography: current perspectives. Clin. Cosmet. Investig. Dent. **6**, 29–43 (2014)
4. Ozen, J., Dirican, B., Oysul, K., Beyzadeoglu, M., Ucok, O., Beydemir, B.: Dosimetric evaluation of the effect of dental implants in head and neck radiotherapy. Oral Surg. Oral Med. Oral Pathol. Oral Radiol. Endodontol. **99**(6), 743–747 (2005)
5. Thariat, J., De Mones, E., Darcourt, V., Poissonnet, G., Dassonville, O., Savoldelli, C., et al.: Dent et irradiation : denture et conséquences sur la denture de la radiothérapie des cancers de la tête et du cou. Cancer/Radiothérapie **14**(2), 128–136 (2010)
6. Thariat, J., Ramus, L., Maingon, P., Odin, G., Gregoire, V., Darcourt, V., et al.: Dentalmaps: automatic dental delineation for radiotherapy planning in head-and-neck cancer. Int. J. Radiat. Oncol. Biol Phys. **82**(5), 1858–1865 (2012)
7. Watson, E., Dorna Mojdami, Z., Oladega, A., Hope, A., Glogauer, M.: Clinical practice guidelines for dental management prior to radiation for head and neck cancer. Oral Oncol. **123**, 105604 (2021)
8. Marx, R.E.: A new concept in the treatment of osteoradionecrosis. J. Oral Maxillofac. Surg. **41**(6), 351–357 (1983)
9. Bolelli, F., Marchesini, K., Van Nistelrooij, N., Lumetti, L., Pipoli, V., Ficarra, E., et al.: Segmenting Maxillofacial Structures in CBCT Volumes [Internet]. Available from: https://toothfairy2.grand-challenge.org/
10. Bolelli, F., Lumetti, L., Vinayahalingam, S., Di Bartolomeo, M., Pellacani, A., Marchesini, K., et al.: Segmenting the inferior alveolar canal in CBCTs volumes: the toothfairy challenge. IEEE Trans. Med. Imaging **44**(4), 1890–1906 (2025)
11. Lumetti, L., Pipoli, V., Bolelli, F., Ficarra, E., Grana, C.: Enhancing patch-based learning for the segmentation of the mandibular canal. IEEE Access **12**, 79014–79024 (2024)
12. ToothFairy3 Challenge Homepage [Internet]. [cited 2025 Aug 8]. Available from: https://toothfairy3.grand-challenge.org/
13. Myronenko, A.: 3D MRI brain tumor segmentation using autoencoder regularization (2018). http://arxiv.org/abs/1810.11654
14. The MONAI Consortium: Project MONAI. Zenodo. 2020. https://doi.org/10.5281/zenodo.4323059
15. Myronenko, A., Yang, D., He, Y., Xu, D.: Automated 3D Segmentation of Kidneys and Tumors in MICCAI KiTS 2023 Challenge (2023)
16. LaBella, D.: Ensemble Deep Learning Models for Automated Segmentation of Tumor and Lymph Node Volumes in Head and Neck Cancer Using Pre- and Mid-Treatment MRI: Application of Auto3DSeg and SegResNet. p. 259–73 (2025)
17. He, Y., Yang, D., Roth, H., Zhao, C., Xu, D.: DiNTS: Differentiable Neural Network Topology Search for 3D Medical Image Segmentation (2021)
18. Hatamizadeh, A., Nath, V., Tang, Y., Yang, D., Roth, H., Xu, D.: Swin UNETR: Swin Transformers for Semantic Segmentation of Brain Tumors in MRI Images (2022)
19. Warfield, S.K., Zou, K.H., Wells, W.M.: Simultaneous truth and performance level estimation (STAPLE): an algorithm for the validation of image segmentation. IEEE Trans. Med. Imaging **23**(7), 903–921 (2004)

Morphology-Driven Deep Watershed Transform for 3D Tooth Segmentation

Tomasz Szczepański[1(✉)] and Szymon Płotka[2]

[1] Sano Centre for Computational Medicine, Cracow, Poland
t.szczepanski@sanoscience.org

[2] Jagiellonian University, Cracow, Poland

Abstract. Segmentation of dentomaxillofacial structures in Cone-Beam Computed Tomography (CBCT) remains challenging, particularly for fine details such as root apices and nerve canals, which are crucial for evaluating root resorption in digital dentistry or to make surgical planning more precise. We present an approach that unifies instance detection and multi-class dentomaxillofacial structure segmentation in CBCT scans, in the scope of the ToothFairy3 Challenge. We adapt a Deep Watershed method, modeling each anatomical structure as a continuous 3D energy basin encoding voxel distances to class boundaries. This instance-aware representation ensures accurate segmentation of narrow, complex dentomaxillofacial structures. We train and evaluate our solution on the ToothFairy3 dataset, comprising 532 CBCT scans with voxel-wise annotations. Our method achieved a mean Dice coefficient of 0.742 and HD95 of 111.13 on the test set. We provide implementation at https://github.com/tomek1911/TF3.

Keywords: CBCT segmentation · ToothFairy3 Challenge · Morphological inductive bias · Deep Watershed

1 Introduction

In this report, we describe our solution for Task 1, "Multi-class segmentation" of the ToothFairy3 challenge. Automatic tooth segmentation in dental CBCT volumes is a critical step for various clinical applications, including orthodontic planning, endodontics, and surgical guidance. Building upon previous efforts in the ToothFairy challenges, we present a method adapted to the increased complexity of ToothFairy3. Compared to ToothFairy2, the new dataset contains 52 additional CBCT volumes acquired with a different scanner, and annotations have been substantially expanded to include 35 new labels, covering pulpy cavities for all 32 teeth, left and right incisive canals, and the lingual canal. The quality of annotations has also been improved, offering a richer resource for developing robust segmentation algorithms.

The task requires accurate voxel-wise labeling of all tooth structures and internal anatomical features within high-resolution CBCT volumes. It presents

F. Bolelli et al. (Eds.): ODIN 2025, LNCS 16473, pp. 159–167, 2026.
https://doi.org/10.1007/978-3-032-20711-1_15

several challenges: the small size and variability of pulp cavities, the complex shape of incisive and lingual canals, and the presence of noise and artifacts in CBCT scans. Furthermore, inter-patient anatomical variations and differences in scanner acquisition parameters increase the difficulty of generalizing segmentation models.

Several methods have been proposed for tooth segmentation in previous challenges and research field [1,4]. Classical approaches include atlas-based registration, graph-based techniques, or multi-stage approaches but the common part is that all recent advances leverage deep learning for volumetric segmentation. Notably, approaches such as SGANET [5], TSG-GCN [6], ToothSeg [3] and GEPAR3D [9] have demonstrated the effectiveness of combining volumetric convolutional networks with morphology-aware guidance. What is more, incorporating geometry-related features has been shown to enhance the model's generalization to external datasets [8].

Our approach extends the methodology proposed in GEPAR3D, incorporating a 3D Deep Watershed Transform guided by a direction map to enable morphology-aware learning of more than 32 teeth classes. This design allows the network to leverage both volumetric context and fine-grained morphological cues, leading to precise delineation of teeth and internal structures such as pulp cavities or nerve canals. To accommodate the high-resolution CBCT volumes within challenge memory constraints, we adapt a sliding window inference strategy, improving upon the MONAI-based sliding window used in the original GEPAR3D implementation. By combining morphology-guided learning with efficient volumetric inference, our solution effectively addresses the increased label complexity, variability, and inherent challenges of ToothFairy3.

2 Methods

An overview of our pipeline is presented in Fig. 1. The proposed solution builds upon the GEPAR3D method [9], extending it to the multi-class setting required by ToothFairy3. Our model jointly addresses multi-class semantic segmentation and instance-level regression, enabling it to separate individual teeth while also capturing their internal anatomical structures. To support both multi-class and binary segmentation objectives, we integrate strategies such as majority voting across classes and pulp fusion to ensure consistent labeling of internal cavities. During training, we introduce auxiliary objectives to enhance morphological awareness: an Energy Direction loss to model complex apex geometries and elongated nerve canals (see Fig. 2), and an instance regression task to generate energy maps that guide the 3D Deep Watershed Transform. These components together encourage the network to learn both local morphological details and global structural consistency.

Deep Watershed Instance Regression. To produce the inputs required by the Deep Watershed algorithm we train the network to solve two complementary volumetric regression tasks: (i) a continuous energy-basin regression that

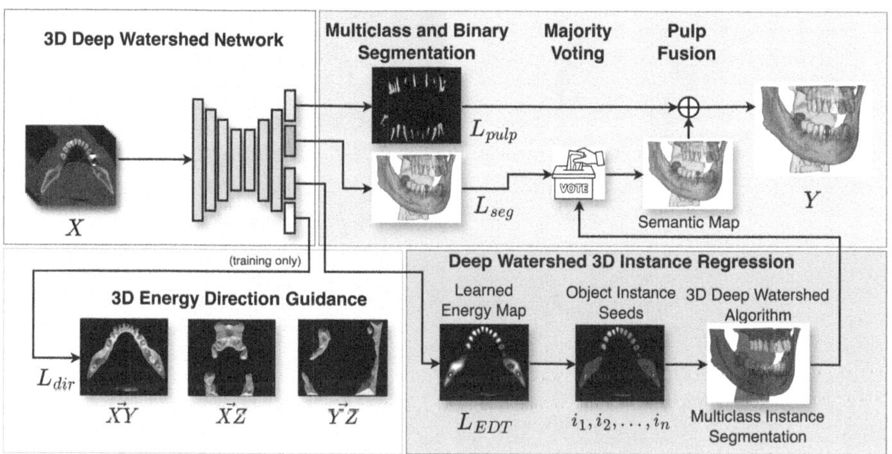

Fig. 1. An overview of the proposed solution, which unifies instance detection and multi-class segmentation for dentomaxillofacial structures in CBCT scans. Our model simultaneously performs multi-class segmentation and instance regression (gray). It also handles both multi-class and binary segmentation, incorporating techniques like majority voting and pulp fusion (blue). During training, we capture complex apex geometries via an Energy Direction loss (yellow) and use an instance regression task to generate energy maps for the Deep Watershed Algorithm (red). (Color figure online)

encodes each *pulp-free* tooth instance as a smooth scalar field and (ii) a per-voxel direction (descent) estimate that refines boundary localization, especially in regions with steep gradients such as root apices and elongated nerve canals (see Fig. 3). We first create a secondary set of instance labels in which all pulp voxels have been removed from tooth instances (this guarantees that tooth instances are disjoint and suitable for watershed processing). Ground-truth energy basins $E_{GT}(\mathbf{r})$ are computed on these pulp-free instances using the Euclidean Distance Transform (EDT) to the each instance boundary separately (based on semantic classes of GT) and then normalized to $[0, 1]$ for numerical stability. The network regresses a continuous energy map $\widehat{E}(\mathbf{r})$ (single-channel) using a mean squared error objective:

$$L_{EDT} = \frac{1}{N} \sum_{\mathbf{r}} \left(E_{GT}(\mathbf{r}) - \widehat{E}(\mathbf{r}) \right)^2.$$

For directional supervision we compute the gradient field of the ground truth energy $\nabla E_{GT}(\mathbf{r})$ (implemented via a 3D Sobel-Feldman operator along x, y, z) and form unit direction vectors

$$\mathbf{u}_{GT}(\mathbf{r}) = \frac{\nabla E_{GT}(\mathbf{r})}{\max\{\|\nabla E_{GT}(\mathbf{r})\|_2, \varepsilon\}},$$

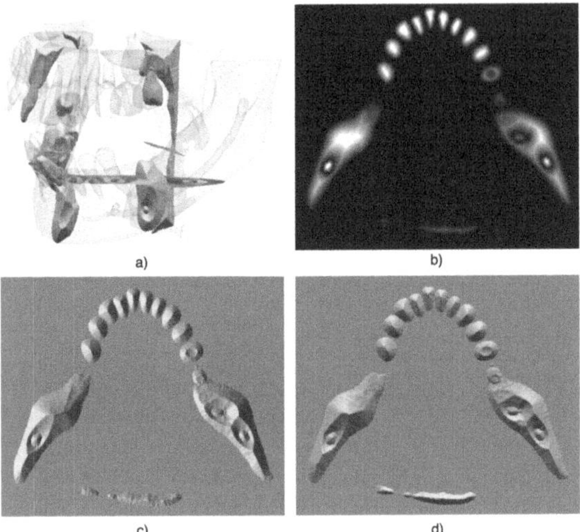

Fig. 2. We provide slices of the 3D Energy Direction Map (a) overlaid with semi-transparent (opacity 0.5) segmentation labels, enabling visualization of structural boundaries within spatial context. The direction map, derived by applying a 3D Sobel kernel to the distance map, assists the model in segmenting elongated and thin structures. While the distance map (b) approaches zero at the nerve canalâĂŞbone boundary, the direction map shows contrasting values, highlighting regions that are difficult to segment. Boundary regions between individual teeth (c, d) are similarly marked by abrupt vector changes, where regression errors are heavily penalized through the angular loss L_{dir}, enforcing directional consistency.

with a small ε to avoid division by zero. The model predicts a 3-channel direction vector $\widehat{\mathbf{u}}(\mathbf{r})$ which we normalize voxelwise. We supervise the directions with an angular loss:

$$L_{\text{dir}} = \frac{1}{N} \sum_{i=1}^{N} \left(\frac{\cos^{-1}\left(\langle \mathbf{u}_{GT}^{(i)}, \widehat{\mathbf{u}}^{(i)} \rangle\right)}{\pi} \right)^2,$$

where N is the total number of voxels. We clip $\cos^{-1}$ inputs to $[-1, 1]$ for stability and divide by π to scale the angular error to $[0, 1]$. To focus the direction learning on anatomically relevant boundaries we mask N, see Fig. 2c to include voxels belonging to tooth instances and to thin/elongated semantic classes (e.g. nerve canals) but exclude pulp voxels.

Deep Watershed Instance Classification via Majority Voting. At inference, we first obtain voxel-wise semantic predictions for all classes (i.a. teeth without pulp, nerve canals, pulp binary map, jaw/skull bones) and the predicted continuous energy map $\widehat{E}$. To isolate found instances we binarize the semantic outputs into a *objects mask*. Seed points for watershed are extracted from predicted Energy Map basins by thresholding basin depth (empirically $\beta = 0.5$).

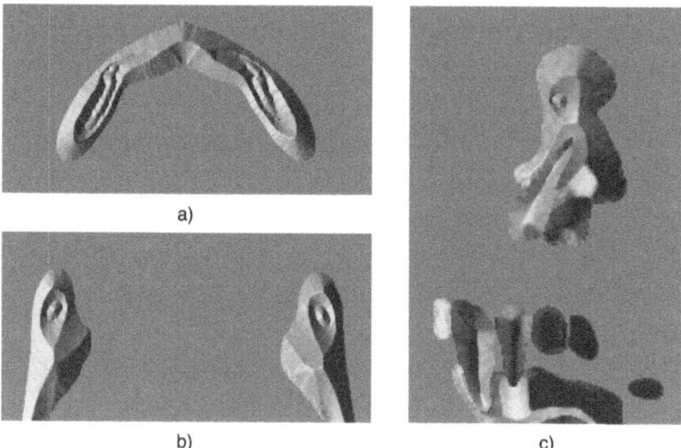

Fig. 3. Slices of the 3D Energy Direction Map with the inferior alveolar nerve visualized (a, b) show that the map clearly delineates the boundary between nerve and bone, both in perpendicular cross-sections and along the canal. In (c), the nerve canal and root apices are visible, with rapid angular transitions in the vector field highlighting anatomically complex regions. These transitions are particularly pronounced at the root apices, where fine, tapering structures curve sharply and diverge from surrounding bone.

The Watershed Transform is then run on $\widehat{E}$ constrained to *objects mask* and using the extracted seeds. This yields disjoint 3D objects instances V_j.

Each resulting instance is assigned a semantic class by majority voting on the multi-class semantic branch:

$$\text{class}(V_j) \; = \; \arg\max_c \sum_{\mathbf{r} \in V_j} \mathbf{1}\{S(\mathbf{r}) = c\},$$

where $S(\mathbf{r})$ is the per-voxel semantic prediction and $\mathbf{1}\{\cdot\}$ is the indicator function.

Pulp Fusion. During training, pulp voxels are optimized independently through L_{pulp}. Pulp segmentation is trained separately as a binary segmentation problem. We optimize a composite loss $L_{pulp} = L_{BCE}^{(w)} + L_{Dice}$, where $w_p = 5$ is for positive voxels to counteract severe imbalance. Since ToothFairy3 provides pulp annotations for all 32 teeth, but evaluation metrics treat pulp as a single aggregated class, we collapse these labels into one fused pulp mask. The final prediction is obtained by first running instance segmentation via deep watershed and majority voting for tooth and canal classes, followed by assigning pulp voxels on top of the corresponding multi-class predictions. This ensures consistency with the challenge evaluation protocol while still leveraging detailed pulp annotations during learning.

Overall Training Objective. The final loss function combines the contributions from semantic segmentation, pulp segmentation, and instance regression. Specifically, we use a weighted sum of four components: (i) multi-class semantic segmentation loss L_{seg}, implemented as a combination of cross-entropy and Dice; (ii) binary pulp segmentation loss L_{pulp}, formulated as weighted BCE plus

Dice to address strong class imbalance; (iii) energy basin regression loss L_{EDT}, which drives accurate continuous energy map prediction for watershed separation; and (iv) direction field loss L_{dir}, which regularizes geometric consistency by enforcing alignment between predicted and ground-truth descent directions. This design balances voxel-level classification with morphology-aware instance regression, ensuring robust segmentation of both large structures (e.g., jaw bones) and fine-scale anatomy (nerve canals, root apices).

Memory-Efficient Sliding-Window Inference. Large 3D volumes exceed GPU memory limits during dense prediction, so inference is typically performed with a sliding-window approach with overlapping patches. The default MONAI implementation accumulates intermediate patch predictions in lists before merging, which leads to high memory consumption proportional to the number of overlapping patches. To address this, we implemented a memory-efficient variant that directly accumulates predictions into preallocated output tensors, avoiding intermediate storage.

For each patch, we apply the model to obtain multi-class logits, energy distance maps, and pulp probabilities. Predictions are weighted by an importance map (constant or Gaussian blending) and accumulated on the fly into global tensors: voxel-wise probability sums on the CPU for multi-class segmentation, and GPU-accumulated maps for distance and pulp outputs. A separate weight accumulator ensures correct normalization. This design prevents redundant storage of overlapping patches while retaining smooth blending across patch boundaries. The memory-efficient approach reduces inference RAM memory usage substantially while preserving identical prediction quality to the original MONAI sliding window inferer.

3 Experimental Design

3.1 Dataset

We train and evaluate our method on the novel ToothFairy3 dataset [1,2,7], which consists of multi-center data from centers A, B, and C, comprising 417, 63, and 52 cases, respectively. For training, we randomly selected 10 cases from each center for validation (30 in total), while the remaining 502 cases were used for training.

3.2 Implementation Details

All scans are resampled to an isotropic resolution of $0.3 \times 0.3 \times 0.3\,\text{mm}^3$, with Hounsfield Unit intensities clipped to $[0, 3000]$ and normalized to $[0, 1]$. During training, we randomly crop $288 \times 200 \times 160$ patches and pad with zeros if necessary. The model is trained for 400 epochs with AdamW, batch size of 2, and a cosine annealing scheduler. The loss function is defined as:

$$L = \Lambda_1 L_{EDT} + \Lambda_2 L_{seg} + \Lambda_3 L_{dir} + \Lambda_4 L_{pulp}, \quad (1)$$

Table 1. Official top 8 leaderboard test phase results for Task 1 - Multi-class segmentation of ToothFairy3 challenge.

Position	Team	mDSC (%)	mHD95 (mm)
1.	Black_Myth	79.81 ± 6.4	88.72 ± 32.33
2.	TAIR Lab	79.20 ± 6.5	93.18 ± 30.43
3.	sjtu_eiee	77.05 ± 7.5	104.59 ± 37.21
4.	ring821	76.84 ± 9.7	104.40 ± 47.98
5.	DLaBella29	73.86 ± 7.1	97.71 ± 33.20
6.	SMIR (ours)	74.22 ± 8.1	111.13 ± 39.40
7.	LAVIA Lab	69.70 ± 9.4	144.97 ± 48.90
8.	gagaha	55.1 ± 17.6	172.49 ± 63.60

with empirically set weights $\Lambda_1 = 10$, $\Lambda_2 = 0.1$, $\Lambda_3 = 1.0$, $\Lambda_4 = 1.0$ for balance. The initial learning rate and weight decay are set to $1e^{-3}$ and $1e^{-4}$, respectively.

Our implementation was developed with PyTorch 2.4.0 and MONAI 1.4.0. Training was performed on a single NVIDIA A100 GPU (80 GB) using float32 precision, while inference employed mixed precision (float16) and was executed on an NVIDIA T4 GPU (16 GB).

3.3 Evaluation Metrics

The segmentation performance was quantitatively evaluated using two metrics: the Dice Similarity Coefficient (DSC, %) to measure volumetric overlap and the 95th percentile Hausdorff Distance (HD95, mm) to assess boundary accuracy. A third evaluation criterion, segmentation time, will be reported by the organizers following publication of the final ranking board.

4 Results

This section presents the quantitative and qualitative results from the official test phase leaderboard for "Task 1 - Multi-class Segmentation".

Quantitative Results. Our solution participated in the "Task 1 - Multi-class Segmentation" challenge. Table 1 shows the official test phase leaderboard of the best eight submissions. Overall, we achieved a mDSC of 74.22±8.1% and a mHD95 of 111.13±39.40 mm across all 50 test cases. In the final leaderboard, we ranked 6th overall, and 5th in terms of mDSC among the 12 teams.

Qualitative Results. As shown in Fig. 4, our method produces generally accurate segmentations. Some errors remain, primarily undersegmentation of jaw bone structures or omission of the lingual nerve. Nonetheless, the method successfully delineated most of the challenging inferior alveolar nerve canal and correctly classified individual tooth instances.

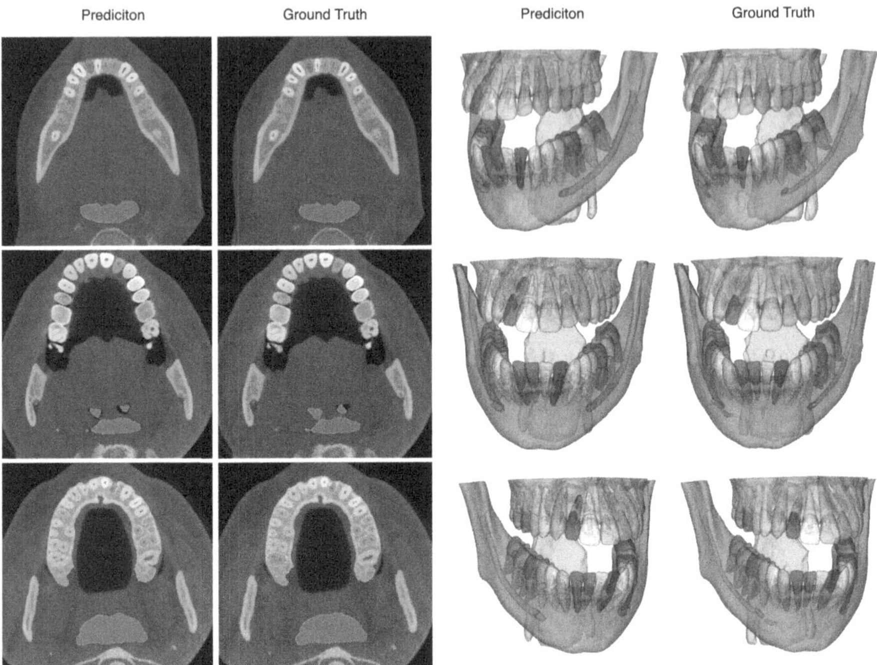

Fig. 4. Qualitative results of our method, proposed as a solution to the ToothFairy3 challenge. We visualize sample from validation set, center A. Ground truth is shown on the right, with both a 3D rendering and a representative 2D slices, while corresponding predictions are shown on the left. Our method yields precise nerve canal segmentation, as shown in the top-row slices and 3D transparent volumes, but shows reduced accuracy in matching the ground truth upper and lower jaw bone.

5 Conclusions

In this work, we presented our solution for the ToothFairy3 challenge, addressing multi-class segmentation of CBCT scans including tooth instances, pulp cavities, nerve canals, and jaw structures. Our method extends the GEPAR3D framework with a 3D deep watershed transform guided by direction maps, enabling morphology-aware learning and robust instance separation adapted to 45 dentomaxillofacial classes. Handling pulp as a separate binary task allowed effective fusion with Deep Watershed-based instances while avoiding label overlap.

We further introduced a memory-efficient sliding-window inference to process large CBCT volumes and optimized a combined loss comprising multi-class, pulp, and instance regression components to balance geometric precision with fine-structure accuracy. This design improved delineation of challenging anatomical features, such as root apices, narrow nerve canals, and pulp cavities.

Unfortunately, our method achieved results inferior to those reported in GEPAR3D. Unlike that approach, we did not leverage a geometrical prior to regularize the loss function, as a Statistical Shape Model was not available for the ToothFairy3 dentomaxillofacial labels. Furthermore, after submission we discovered that our Direction Map labels had been discretized, which substantially reduced the information they carried. We plan to address this issue in future iterations.

Future work will integrate pulp directly into the multi-class segmentation branch and refine the direction-map auxiliary task to better capture narrow pulp fragments and fine canal structures, aiming to further enhance segmentation accuracy and anatomical fidelity.

Acknowledgements. Tomasz Szczepański is supported by the EU's Horizon 2020 programme (grant no. 857533, Sano) and the Foundation for Polish Science's International Research Agendas programme (MAB PLUS/2019/13), co-financed by the EU under the European Regional Development Fund and the Polish Ministry of Science and Higher Education (contract no. MEiN/2023/DIR/3796).

Disclosure Of Interests. The authors have no competing interests to declare.

References

1. Bolelli, F., Lumetti, L., Vinayahalingam, S., et al.: Segmenting the inferior alveolar canal in CBCT volumes: the toothfairy challenge. IEEE Trans. Med. Imaging (2024)
2. Bolelli, F., et al.: Segmenting maxillofacial structures in CBCT volumes. In: Proceedings of the Computer Vision and Pattern Recognition Conference, pp. 5238–5248 (2025)
3. Cui, Z., Zhang, B., Lian, C., et al.: Hierarchical morphology-guided tooth instance segmentation from CBCT images. In: Feragen, A., Sommer, S., Schnabel, J., Nielsen, M. (eds.) Information Processing in Medical Imaging - IPMI 2021. Lecture Notes in Computer Science, vol. 12729, pp. 150–162. Springer, Cham (2021). https://doi.org/10.1007/978-3-030-78191-0_12
4. Isensee, F., Kirchhoff, Y., Kraemer, L., Rokuss, M., Ulrich, C., Maier-Hein, K.H.: Scaling NNU-net for CBCT segmentation. In: Wang, Y., et al. (eds.) MICCAI 2024. LNCS, vol. 15571, pp. 13–20. Springer, Cham (2024). https://doi.org/10.1007/978-3-031-88977-6_2
5. Li, P., Liu, Y., Cui, Z., et al.: Semantic graph attention with explicit anatomical association modeling for tooth segmentation from CBCT images. IEEE Trans. Med. Imaging **41**(11), 3116–3127 (2022)
6. Liu, Y., Zhang, S., Wu, X., et al.: Individual graph representation learning for pediatric tooth segmentation from dental CBCT. IEEE Trans. Med. Imaging (2024)
7. Lumetti, L., Pipoli, V., Bolelli, F., Ficarra, E., Grana, C.: Enhancing patch-based learning for the segmentation of the mandibular canal. IEEE Access **12**, 79014–79024 (2024)
8. Szczepański, T., Grzeszczyk, M.K., Płotka, S., et al.: Let me DeCode you: decoder conditioning with tabular data. In: Linguraru, M.G., et al. (eds.) MICCAI 2024. LNCS, vol. 15003, pp. 228–238. Springer, Cham (2024). https://doi.org/10.1007/978-3-031-72384-1_22
9. Szczepański, T., et al.: Gepar3D: geometry prior-assisted learning for 3D tooth segmentation. In: Gee, J.C., et al. (eds.) MICCAI 2025. LNCS, vol. 15961, pp. 218–228. Springer, Cham (2025). https://doi.org/10.1007/978-3-032-04937-7_21

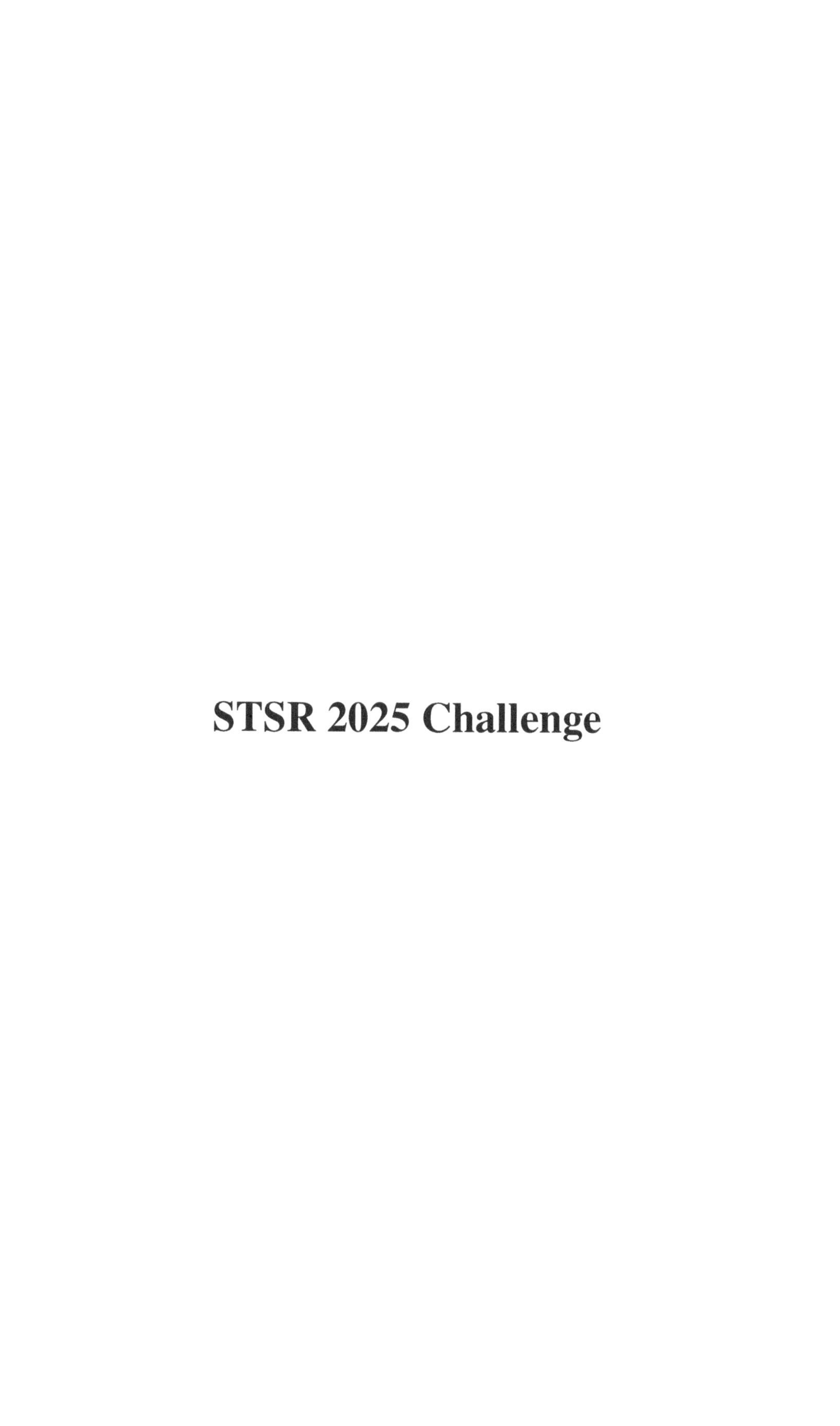

STSR 2025 Challenge

Efficient nnU-Net for Tooth and Root Canal Segmentation in CBCT

Changkai Ji, Yusheng Liu, Yuxian Jiang, and Lisheng Wang(✉)

School of Automation and Intelligent Sensing, Shanghai Jiao Tong University, Shanghai 200240, People's Republic of China
{changkaiji,lswang}@sjtu.edu.cn

Abstract. Accurate segmentation of teeth and root pulp canals from cone-beam computed tomography (CBCT) images is essential for clinical applications such as treatment planning, root canal therapy, and prosthetics. Manual segmentation is time-consuming, subjective, and impractical for routine use, motivating the need for automated approaches. In this work, we propose a solution based on nnU-Net for multi-class dental structure segmentation. Our pipeline incorporates customized preprocessing, efficient training, and lightweight post-processing. Furthermore, we introduce inference acceleration strategies, including the removal of redundant augmentations and optimized interpolation, which reduce inference time by nearly fourfold with only marginal performance degradation. Experimental results on the MICCAI STSR 2025 Challenge Task 1 demonstrate that our approach achieves competitive segmentation accuracy across multiple metrics, achieving a top-three ranking in the competition. These findings highlight the effectiveness of nnU-Net and our acceleration strategies in achieving a favorable balance between accuracy and efficiency, underscoring the potential of our method for clinical deployment. Our codes are available at: https://github.com/duola-wa/MICCAI-2025-STSR-Task-1.

Keywords: CBCT segmentation · nnU-Net · Root canal segmentation · Inference acceleration

1 Introduction

The MICCAI STSR 2025 Challenge Task 1 focuses on the segmentation of teeth and root pulp canals from cone-beam computed tomography (CBCT) images. CBCT is a widely used imaging modality in dental diagnostics, providing high-resolution 3D reconstructions of hard tissues with relatively low radiation doses [2]. The task involves accurately segmenting teeth and their corresponding root pulp canals from a set of labeled and unlabeled CBCT images. The challenge aims to push the boundaries of automated segmentation for dental structures, which are critical for clinical applications such as treatment planning, root canal therapy, and dental prosthetics [8,12]. The competition is designed to evaluate

F. Bolelli et al. (Eds.): ODIN 2025, LNCS 16473, pp. 171–180, 2026.
https://doi.org/10.1007/978-3-032-20711-1_16

both segmentation accuracy and efficiency, with the goal of developing robust methods suitable for clinical settings.

Manual segmentation of dental structures in CBCT images is a labor-intensive and highly specialized task that relies heavily on the expertise of experienced radiologists and dental professionals [5,15]. This process requires meticulous attention to detail and considerable time, as the accurate delineation of complex anatomical structures like teeth and root pulp canals can be challenging. Furthermore, manual segmentation is inherently subjective, with variations in results between different practitioners, which can lead to inconsistencies and affect the reliability of clinical decision-making. The time-consuming nature of manual segmentation also makes it impractical for routine clinical workflows, where rapid and reliable decisions are crucial.

In response to these limitations, deep learning approaches have gained considerable attention in recent years for automating medical image segmentation tasks [1,6,7,9–11,13,19]. These methods have shown remarkable promise in reducing the time and effort involved in manual segmentation, while maintaining or even surpassing the accuracy of junior clinicians. Deep learning models are capable of learning complex patterns from large-scale datasets, enabling them to automatically identify and segment anatomical structures with high consistency and precision [14]. This has made them particularly attractive for dental and maxillofacial imaging, where accurate segmentation is critical for diagnosis and treatment planning.

Despite the successes of deep learning methods, challenges remain in applying these techniques to CBCT images. The segmentation of fine structures such as teeth and their root pulp canals requires a high level of detail and precision [3]. Additionally, the high computational cost associated with deep learning models can pose a challenge, especially in clinical settings where real-time processing and low resource consumption are crucial [20]. Balancing the trade-off between segmentation accuracy and computational efficiency is therefore a key challenge in the development of practical solutions for dental image segmentation.

To address these challenges, we propose a solution based on nnU-Net [4], a deep learning framework that has shown robust performance in medical image segmentation tasks. nnU-Net automatically adapts to the specific characteristics of a given dataset, making it a strong choice for multi-class segmentation problems such as this one. In our approach, we incorporate a variety of strategies to optimize the trade-off between segmentation quality and computational efficiency. The performance of our method was validated by achieving top-three results in the MICCAI STSR 2025 Challenge Task 1, demonstrating its effectiveness and potential for real-world applications.

- Our method achieved satisfactory segmentation accuracy, effectively identifying both teeth and root pulp canals across various validation cases.
- We optimized and accelerated the inference runtime, ensuring that the model could perform efficiently even with large-scale datasets.

- Our approach secured a top-three finish in the MICCAI STSR 2025 Challenge Task 1, demonstrating the effectiveness and competitiveness of our solution in the field of dental image segmentation.

2 Proposed Method

2.1 Framework Overview

As shown in Fig. 1, we propose a solution based on the nnU-Net framework. The overall architecture of our model is specifically designed to handle the segmentation of teeth and root pulp canals in CBCT images effectively.

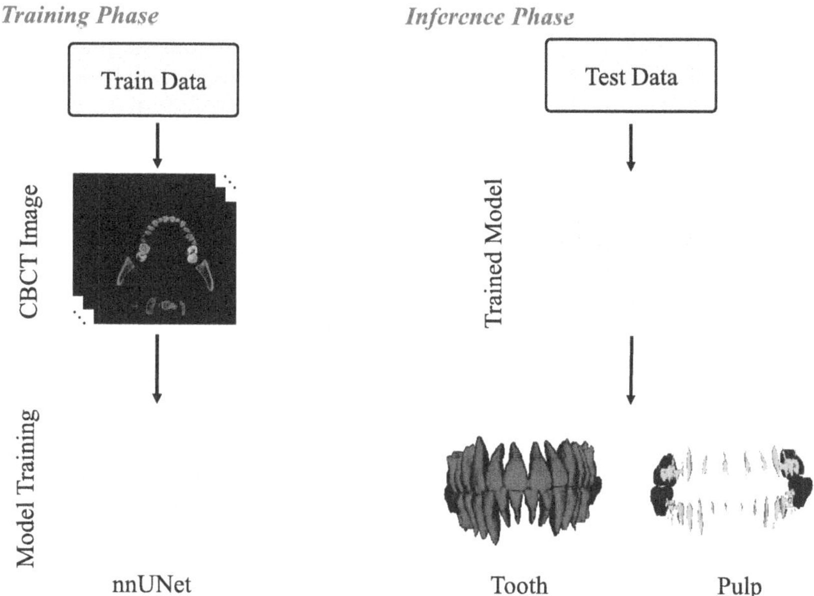

Fig. 1. The overall structure of our nnU-Net-based model for teeth and root pulp canal segmentation.

2.2 Data Preprocessing

In our approach, we perform a series of preprocessing steps to ensure the integrity and consistency of the dataset before training the model. After confirming the integrity of the dataset, we normalize the images to a consistent scale and intensity range. This step helps to standardize the data, making it easier for the model to learn meaningful features. Additionally, we apply necessary transformations, such as resampling the images to a uniform resolution, ensuring that the data is suitable for the nnU-Net framework. These preprocessing steps allow the model to efficiently process the CBCT images and perform accurate segmentations of the teeth and root pulp canals.

2.3 Model Training

For training the model, we utilize the nnU-Net framework, which is specifically designed to handle a variety of medical image segmentation tasks. The training process begins by using a 3D full-resolution approach, allowing the model to learn spatially rich features from the original high-resolution data. We leverage the entire training dataset, ensuring that the model learns from a comprehensive set of images representing a diverse range of cases. During training, the nnU-Net model adapts to the specific characteristics of the dataset, automatically adjusting its architecture to achieve optimal segmentation performance.

2.4 Post-processing

During the post-processing phase, we address the label mapping required by the nnU-Net framework, which expects labels to be sequentially incremented starting from 1. Specifically, we map the segmentation output label values, which are sequentially incremented to meet nnU-Net's requirements, back to their original label values. The label mapping is applied through a lookup table, which is constructed to accommodate all possible label values in the dataset, with the specific labels being mapped according to the predefined mapping dictionary. This approach provides a fast and effective method for label mapping, reducing computational overhead by directly modifying the label values within the image data without additional redundant processing steps.

3 Experiments and Results

3.1 Dataset and Assessment Metrics

The dataset consists of both labeled and unlabeled CBCT images. The training set includes 30 labeled images with segmentation masks for teeth and root canal structures, alongside 300 unlabeled images for model development. The validation set contains 40 images [16–18].

The evaluation of segmentation algorithms considers both segmentation accuracy and computational efficiency. For accuracy, the following metrics are used: Dice Similarity Coefficient (DSC) for overlap evaluation, Normalized Surface Distance (NSD) for surface proximity, mean Intersection-over-Union (mIoU) for region overlap, and Identification Accuracy (IA) for correct identification of anatomical structures. In terms of efficiency, the algorithm's running time and GPU memory consumption are assessed during inference.

3.2 Implementation Details

Environments and Requirements. The specific details of the computational environment and dependencies are provided in Table 1. Our model was trained for 1000 epochs.

Table 1. System Configuration

Ubuntu version	Ubuntu 24.04 LTS
CPU	Intel(R) Xeon(R) Platinum 8352S CPU @ 2.20 GHz
RAM	503 GB
GPU	1 NVIDIA GeForce RTX 4090 (24G)
CUDA version	12.4
Programming language	Python 3.9.19
Deep learning framework	PyTorch (torch 1.12.1, torchvision 0.19.1)
Codes available at	https://github.com/duola-wa/MICCAI-2025-STSR-Task-1

Inference Acceleration. To improve the inference speed of our model, we implemented two key optimizations.

Firstly, we simplified the inference pipeline by disabling certain computationally expensive operations. Specifically, we omitted the use of applying multiple augmentations (e.g., rotations, flips) during inference and averaging the results. While this operation can improve segmentation accuracy, it significantly increases inference time due to the additional computations required for each augmentation.

Secondly, we refined the interpolation step in handling multi-class predictions. Rather than using traditional, computationally expensive integer-based resampling techniques, we opted for a more efficient method utilizing floating-point tensors and the interpolate function from PyTorch. This approach maintains the precision of the predictions while enhancing throughput. Together, these optimizations allowed for faster and more efficient inference across the test set.

3.3 Results and Analysis

Quantitative Performance. The segmentation results are summarized in Table 2. The results indicate that the model with speed-up achieved slightly lower accuracy metrics across all evaluation criteria, such as Dice, mIoU, and NSD. However, the time required for inference in the speed-up version was significantly reduced, with the total time for inference dropping from 3257 s to 852 s.

Table 2. Segmentation Results with and without Speed-Up

Model	Dice		mIoU		NSD		IA	Time (s)
	Instance	Image	Instance	Image	Instance	Image		
w/ Speed-Up	0.6691	0.9659	0.5535	0.9343	0.8655	0.9979	0.6910	852
w/o Speed-Up	0.6738	0.9671	0.5593	0.9365	0.8672	0.9980	0.6953	3257

Although there was a slight drop in segmentation performance, the substantial improvement in processing time makes the accelerated model particularly advantageous for clinical scenarios where rapid results are essential. In situations where time-sensitive decisions are needed, such as in real-time diagnostic systems, this speed-up could provide significant benefits. For the final test submission, we chose the accelerated version of the model, prioritizing efficiency while maintaining segmentation accuracy.

We further designed a two-stage segmentation framework in addition to the one-stage nnU-Net baseline. In the first stage, a tooth instance segmentation model was trained using external data, enabling simultaneous delineation of individual teeth and assignment of their FDI indices. This model was then applied to the 300 unlabeled cases to generate pseudo-labels. Unreliable labels were filtered out before using the remaining labels to retrain and enhance the tooth instance segmentation network. After obtaining a refined tooth-level segmentation model, we applied it to the labeled pulp dataset to extract accurate regions of interest (ROIs) for each tooth, thereby providing localized inputs for the second stage.

In the second stage, we introduced task-specific segmentation networks for different tooth categories. A binary segmentation model was trained to handle impacted teeth, while a six-class model was designed for other teeth, incorporating five rootpulp-related classes and one tooth-level class. This hierarchical design aimed to leverage tooth-level localization in the first stage to support finer anatomical segmentation in the second stage. Moreover, by decomposing each case into multiple tooth-level ROIs, the framework effectively transformed a single annotated scan into dozens of tooth-specific training samples. This substantially alleviated the data scarcity problem, as the original per-case annotations were expanded into a richer set of per-tooth instances for supervision. The quantitative performance of this two-stage framework is reported in Table 3, along with the results of the one-stage baseline model.

Table 3. Comparison of one-stage and two-stage segmentation models

Model	Dice		mIoU		NSD		IA
	Instance	Image	Instance	Image	Instance	Image	
One-stage nnU-Net	0.6738	0.9671	0.5593	0.9365	0.8672	0.9980	0.6953
Two-stage nnU-Net	0.626	0.9207	0.511	0.8682	0.8354	0.9753	0.5896

Although the two-stage segmentation framework was conceptually designed to leverage hierarchical localization and fine-grained classification, its performance lagged behind the one-stage nnU-Net baseline. A key limitation lies in the dependency of the second stage on the quality of the first-stage predictions. If the tooth instance segmentation is inaccurate or fails to properly delineate certain teeth, the subsequent ROI extraction becomes unreliable, thereby compromising the downstream segmentation of roots and pulp canals. In contrast, the one-stage model avoids this error propagation by directly performing holistic multi-class segmentation. Nevertheless, we believe that with more robust tooth-level segmentation in the first stage, the two-stage framework has the potential to achieve competitive performance, as the modular design is inherently well-suited for capturing both global and localized anatomical structures.

Qualitative Results. As shown in Fig. 2, our model effectively segments teeth and root canals across various cases. For (a) normal cases, (b) cases with multiple missing teeth, and (c) cases with a small field of view, the model consistently produces accurate segmentation results.

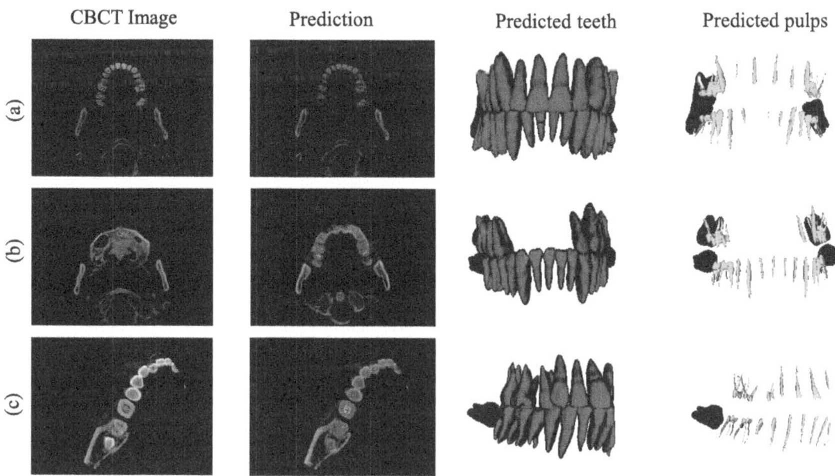

Fig. 2. Qualitative results of our model on different test cases: (a) normal case, (b) case with multiple missing teeth, and (c) case with a small field of view.

As shown in Fig. 3, we compare the segmentation results with and without inference acceleration. The results using the speed-up method still maintain high quality, demonstrating that the acceleration does not significantly compromise accuracy. The visual comparison highlights that, despite a slight drop in precision during testing, the accelerated model maintains satisfactory segmentation performance for both teeth and root canals. This suggests that the trade-off between speed and accuracy is favorable for real-time clinical applications.

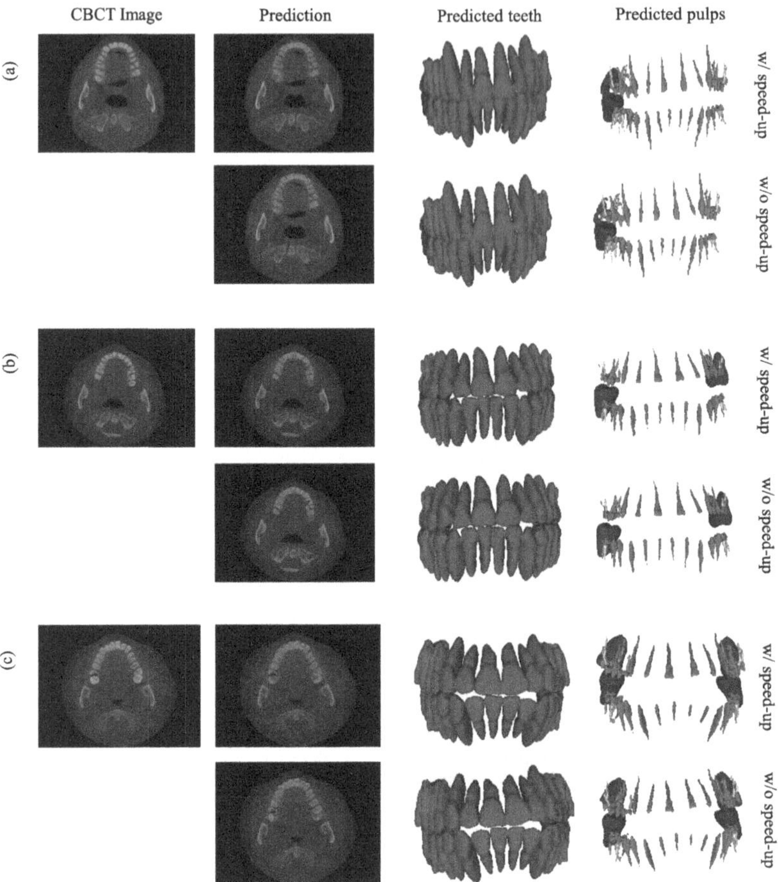

Fig. 3. Comparison of segmentation results with and without acceleration. Each case shows the segmentation performance before and after applying the inference speed-up.

4 Conclusion

In this paper, we presented an nnU-Net-based framework for the segmentation of teeth and root pulp canals from CBCT images. Our method integrates effective preprocessing, robust training using nnU-Net, and efficient post-processing to perform accurate multi-class segmentation. To address the challenge of high computational costs during inference, we designed acceleration strategies that simplified the inference pipeline and optimized interpolation operations. The proposed optimizations reduced inference time by nearly fourfold while maintaining comparable segmentation accuracy. Both quantitative and qualitative results confirm that the method provides reliable and efficient segmentation, making it suitable for clinical scenarios where rapid decision-making is crucial.

References

1. Bolelli, F., et al.: Segmenting the inferior alveolar canal in CBCTs volumes: the toothfairy challenge. IEEE Trans. Med. Imaging (2024)
2. De Vos, W., Casselman, J., Swennen, G.: Cone-beam computerized tomography (CBCT) imaging of the oral and maxillofacial region: a systematic review of the literature. Int. J. Oral Maxillofac. Surg. **38**(6), 609–625 (2009)
3. Duan, W., Chen, Y., Zhang, Q., Lin, X., Yang, X.: Refined tooth and pulp segmentation using U-net in CBCT image. Dentomaxillofacial Radiol. **50**(6), 20200251 (2021)
4. Isensee, F., et al.: nnu-net: Self-adapting framework for u-net-based medical image segmentation. arXiv preprint arXiv:1809.10486 (2018)
5. Ji, C., et al.: Mammo net: integrating gaze supervision and interactive information in multi-view mammogram classification. In: Greenspan, H., et al. (eds.) MICCAI 2023. LNCS, vol. 14226, pp. 68–78. Springer, Cham (2023). https://doi.org/10.1007/978-3-031-43990-2_7
6. Ji, C., Liu, Y., He, L., Jiang, Y., Huang, C., Wang, L.: Two-stage semi-supervised nnU-net framework for tooth segmentation in CBCT images. In: Wang, Y., et al. (eds.) MICCAI 2024. LNCS, vol. 15571, pp. 100–109. Springer, Cham (2024a). https://doi.org/10.1007/978-3-031-88977-6_10
7. Ji, C., Liu, Y., He, L., Jiang, Y., Huang, C., Wang, L.: A two-stage semi-supervised nnU-net model for automated tooth segmentation in panoramic x-ray images. In: Wang, Y., et al. (eds.) MICCAI 2024. LNCS, vol. 15571, pp. 91–99. Springer, Cham (2024b). https://doi.org/10.1007/978-3-031-88977-6_9
8. Jiang, Y., Liu, Y., Ji, C., Wang, L.: Enhanced multi-structure segmentation in CBCT images with adaptive structure optimization. In: Wang, Y., et al. (eds.) MICCAI 2024. LNCS, vol. 15571, pp. 30–40. Springer, Cham (2024). https://doi.org/10.1007/978-3-031-88977-6_4
9. Jiang, Y., et al.: Morphology prior enhanced teeth segmentation for high-resolution oral scans. IEEE J. Biomed. Health Inform. (2025)
10. Lin, Z., Liu, Y., Wu, J., Wang, D.H., Zhang, X.Y., Zhu, S.: Multi-modal pre-post treatment consistency learning for automatic segmentation and evaluation of the circle of willis. Comput. Med. Imaging Graph. **122**, 102521 (2025)
11. Liu, Y., Xin, R., Yang, T., Wang, L.: Inferior alveolar nerve segmentation in CBCT images using connectivity-based selective re-training. In: Wang, Y., et al. (eds.) MICCAI 2024. LNCS, vol. 15571, pp. 3–12. Springer, Cham (2024). https://doi.org/10.1007/978-3-031-88977-6_1
12. Liu, Y., et al.: Individual graph representation learning for pediatric tooth segmentation from dental CBCT. IEEE Trans. Med. Imaging (2024)
13. Ronneberger, O., Fischer, P., Brox, T.: U-net: convolutional networks for biomedical image segmentation. In: Navab, N., Hornegger, J., Wells, W., Frangi, A. (eds.) MICCAI 2015. LNCS, vol. 9351, pp. 234–241. Springer, Cham (2015). https://doi.org/10.1007/978-3-319-24574-4_28
14. Shen, D., Wu, G., Suk, H.I.: Deep learning in medical image analysis. Annu. Rev. Biomed. Eng. **19**(1), 221–248 (2017)
15. Wang, S., Ouyang, X., Liu, T., Wang, Q., Shen, D.: Follow my eye: using gaze to supervise computer-aided diagnosis. IEEE Trans. Med. Imaging **41**(7), 1688–1698 (2022)

16. Wang, Y., Chen, X., Qian, D., Ye, F., Wang, S., Zhang, H.: Semi-supervised Tooth Segmentation: First MICCAI Challenge, SemiToothSeg 2023, Held in Conjunction with MICCAI 2023, Vancouver, BC, Canada, 8 October 2023, Proceedings, vol. 14623. Springer, Cham (2024)
17. Wang, Y., et al.: MICCAI 2023 STS challenge: a retrospective study of semi-supervised approaches for teeth segmentation. Pattern Recogn. **170**, 112049 (2026)
18. Wang, Y., et al.: STS MICCAI 2023 challenge: grand challenge on 2D and 3D semi-supervised tooth segmentation. arXiv preprint arXiv:2407.13246 (2024)
19. Zhang, Y., et al.: Children's dental panoramic radiographs dataset for caries segmentation and dental disease detection. Sci. Data **10**(1), 380 (2023)
20. Zhong, T., et al.: Tips: tooth instance and pulp segmentation based on hierarchical extraction and fusion of anatomical priors from cone-beam CT. Artif. Intell. Med. 103247 (2025)

Learning-Based CBCT–IOS Registration with PointNet++ and SVD

Changkai Ji, Yusheng Liu, Yuxian Jiang, and Lisheng Wang(✉)

School of Automation and Intelligent Sensing, Shanghai Jiao Tong University, Shanghai 200240, People's Republic of China
{changkaiji,lswang}@sjtu.edu.cn

Abstract. Accurate registration of intraoral scans (IOS) and cone-beam computed tomography (CBCT) is a critical prerequisite for precise diagnosis and treatment planning in dentistry. However, large modality discrepancies and dense point clouds make this task challenging in practice. In this work, we propose a learning-based framework for CBCT–IOS registration, developed in the context of the MICCAI STSR Task 2 2025 Challenge. Our method leverages dual PointNet++ encoders to extract modality-specific features, followed by a differentiable SVD head that execute rigid-body constraints in the predicted transformation. To enhance robustness, we design geometric data augmentation strategies, while point cloud sampling and simplification are employed to accelerate inference. Ablation studies demonstrate that augmentation substantially reduces registration errors, while relaxing CBCT filtering thresholds further improves alignment by preserving richer anatomical cues. Overall, our approach achieves competitive performance, ranking second on the validation leaderboard, and provides a practical balance between accuracy and efficiency.

Keywords: CBCT-IOS registration · PointNet++ · Rigid transformation · Data augmentation · Inference acceleration

1 Introduction

Three-dimensional registration of dental data plays a crucial role in computer-aided diagnosis, treatment planning, and surgical guidance [3,10]. In clinical practice, intraoral scans (IOS) provide high-resolution crown geometry, while cone-beam computed tomography (CBCT) offers comprehensive information on both crowns and roots [15]. Accurate alignment of these heterogeneous modalities is essential for integrating complementary anatomical details, thereby enhancing the precision and reliability of dental treatment [13]. To promote the development of robust registration algorithms, the MICCAI STSR 2025 Challenge Task 2 was organized to benchmark algorithms that can effectively handle multi-modal data discrepancies and to encourage practical solutions that may translate into real-world clinical applications.

F. Bolelli et al. (Eds.): ODIN 2025, LNCS 16473, pp. 181–190, 2026.
https://doi.org/10.1007/978-3-032-20711-1_17

Despite its importance, CBCT–IOS registration remains a challenging task. The two modalities differ substantially in terms of resolution, field of view, and information content [9]. IOS captures only the visible crowns with fine detail but lacks root structures, whereas CBCT provides full jaw coverage but contains significant noise and redundant information. These discrepancies introduce difficulties in establishing reliable correspondences and estimating robust transformations. Moreover, limited availability of paired ground-truth annotations further complicates the training of data-driven approaches.

Recent advances in deep learning have achieved remarkable success across imaging tasks [2,7,8,11,12,20]. Researchers have increasingly applied deep learning methods to multi-modal 3D registration problems [9]. Such methods alleviate the need for handcrafted descriptors and have achieved promising results in various medical imaging domains. However, deep learning-based approaches often require large annotated datasets [4,16], and their inference pipelines may still suffer from inefficiency due to the high dimensionality of volumetric data and dense point clouds. Therefore, it remains an open question how to design a framework that is both accurate and computationally efficient [5,6].

In this work, we propose a learning-based registration framework specifically designed for CBCT–IOS alignment in the MICCAI STSR 2025 Challenge. Our method employs PointNet++ encoders to extract modality-specific features from IOS and CBCT point clouds [14], followed by a transformation head based on singular value decomposition (SVD) that enforces rigid-body constraints in the predicted matrix [19]. To enhance robustness, we incorporate extensive data augmentation during training, enabling the model to generalize well across diverse clinical cases. Additionally, we use point cloud sampling and simplification to accelerate inference, reducing computational overhead and enabling fast inference without compromising accuracy. As a result, we achieve competitive performance on the validation leaderboard. Our contributions can be summarized as follows:

- We design data augmentation strategies to improve model robustness and registration accuracy under diverse clinical conditions.
- We adopt point cloud sampling and simplification techniques to accelerate inference while maintaining accuracy.
- Our method achieves second place on the validation leaderboard of the STSR 2025 Task 2, demonstrating both effectiveness and efficiency.

2 Method

2.1 Framework Overview

Figure 1 illustrates the overall architecture of our proposed framework for CBCT-IOS registration. The framework follows a learning-based paradigm that takes as input two point clouds: one sampled from the IOS mesh and the other from the CBCT volume. Both point clouds are independently encoded by two PointNet++ encoders, which are responsible for extracting hierarchical geometric features. The extracted features are subsequently aligned through a feature matching module, followed by a SVD head that estimates the rigid transformation matrix between the two modalities. This transformation is then used to map the IOS points into the CBCT coordinate system. During training, multiple loss terms are employed to jointly supervise the transformation prediction, including point-based losses, Chamfer distance, and penalties on rotation and translation. This design ensures that the model captures both global and local geometric correspondences in a computationally efficient manner.

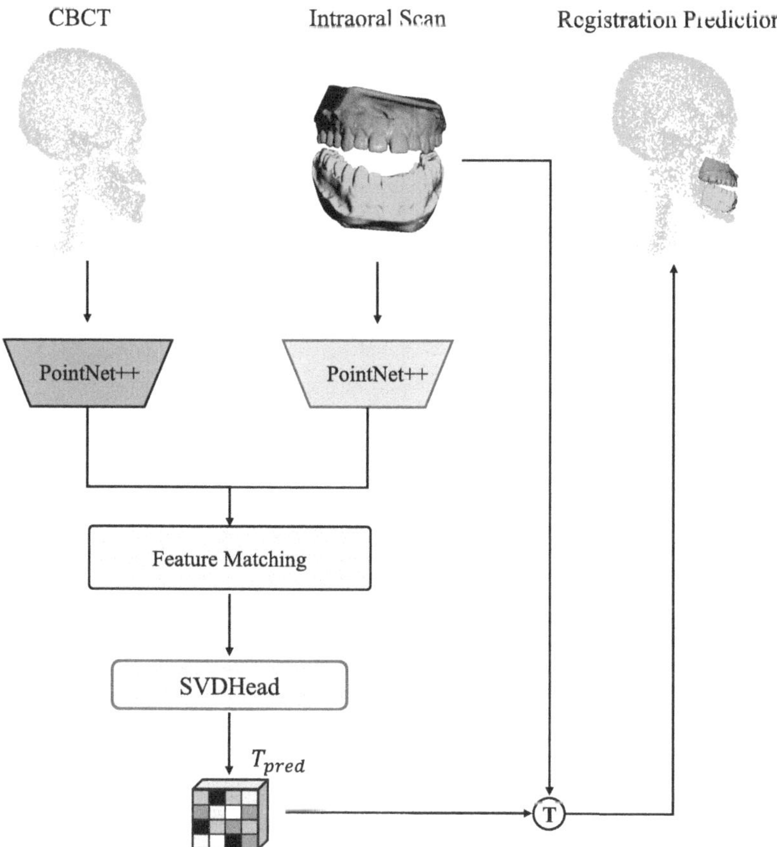

Fig. 1. Overview of our registration model. CBCT scans and intraoral scans are separately processed by PointNet++, followed by feature matching and rigid transformation estimation using SVD. The predicted transformation is applied to align the intraoral scans with CBCT data.

2.2 Data Augmentation

To enhance the robustness and generalization of the proposed model, we employed a series of data augmentation strategies tailored to 3D point clouds. Specifically, random rigid transformations, including rotations and translations, were applied independently to both the IOS-derived point sets. These augmentation techniques enrich the diversity of the training dataset and mitigate the risk of overfitting, particularly in scenarios where annotated data is limited.

To better illustrate the effectiveness of our augmentation strategies, Fig. 2 provides a visual example. The first column presents the original CBCT and IOS pairs prior to augmentation, while the subsequent three columns demonstrate augmented versions of the same case. These examples highlight how the applied transformations produce diverse yet clinically plausible variations, enabling the model to learn invariances that are essential for accurate and robust registration.

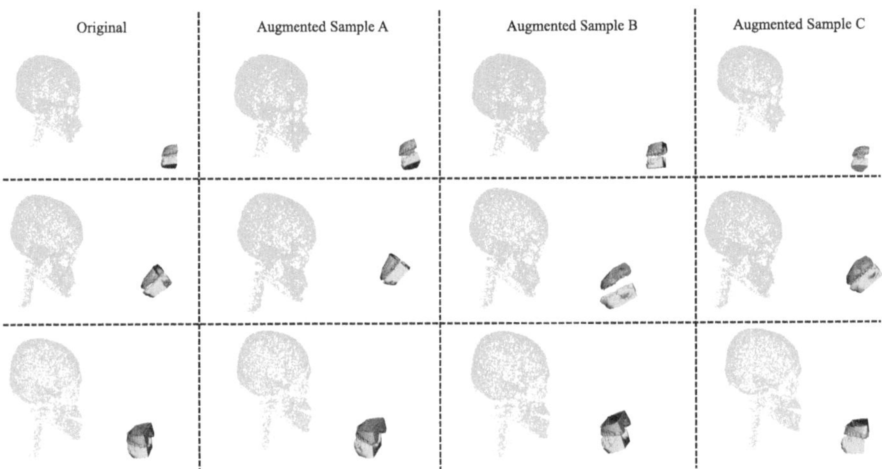

Fig. 2. The visualization of data augmentation strategies. The first column shows the original CBCT and IOS pairs, while the subsequent columns display augmented versions of the same case, demonstrating the diverse and clinically plausible variations produced by the applied transformations.

2.3 Model Training

The training of our framework follows a fully supervised paradigm, where the objective is to learn accurate rigid transformations between CBCT and IOS point clouds. A central component of the architecture is the feature extraction stage, implemented via PointNet++ encoders. PointNet++ extends the original PointNet architecture by introducing hierarchical feature learning, where local neighborhood information is progressively aggregated at multiple scales. This design allows the network to capture both fine-grained geometric details and global structural context, which is essential for modeling complex dental anatomy. In our framework, two independent PointNet++ encoders are employed, one for the CBCT point cloud and the other for the IOS point cloud. These dual encoders extract modality-specific features while preserving their geometric consistency.

The extracted feature representations are then passed to the transformation estimation module, referred to as the SVDHead. This module aligns the latent embeddings of the two modalities by constructing a correspondence matrix and applying a differentiable SVD. The SVDHead directly estimates the optimal rigid transformation matrix, decomposed into a rotation matrix and a translation vector, which maps the IOS point cloud onto the CBCT reference. Compared with regression-based alternatives, the SVD-based formulation offers improved stability and guarantees the orthogonality of the predicted rotation matrix.

Optimization is performed using the Adam optimizer. During training, the network parameters are updated to minimize a composite loss function that jointly enforces geometric alignment and transformation accuracy, which will be detailed in the following subsection. This training strategy enables the network to converge reliably and generalize well to unseen test data.

2.4 Loss Function

To achieve robust and accurate registration, we adopt a composite loss function that integrates multiple complementary objectives. Each component of the loss is designed to address a specific aspect of the alignment problem, ensuring both local geometric consistency and global rigid transformation accuracy.

Point Loss. This term enforces point-wise consistency between the transformed source point cloud $\hat{\mathbf{P}}_{src}$ and the ground truth aligned point cloud $\mathbf{P}_{gt}$. It is formulated as a mean squared error (MSE), directly penalizing local misalignments:

$$\mathcal{L}_{point} = \frac{1}{N} \sum_{i=1}^{N} \left\| \hat{\mathbf{p}}_{src}^{(i)} - \mathbf{p}_{gt}^{(i)} \right\|^2 .$$

Chamfer Distance. To capture global shape similarity, we compute the bidirectional Chamfer distance between the predicted source $\hat{\mathbf{P}}_{src}$ and the target CBCT $\mathbf{P}_{tgt}$:

$$\mathcal{L}_{chamfer} = \sum_{p \in \hat{\mathbf{P}}_{src}} \min_{q \in \mathbf{P}_{tgt}} \|p - q\|^2 + \sum_{q \in \mathbf{P}_{tgt}} \min_{p \in \hat{\mathbf{P}}_{src}} \|q - p\|^2 .$$

This term encourages the transformed point sets to occupy the same geometric space.

Rotation Loss. We explicitly constrain the predicted rotation $\hat{R}$ to be consistent with the ground truth R_{gt}. The rotation loss $\mathcal{L}_{rot}$ is defined as:

$$\mathcal{L}_{rot} = \arccos \left(\frac{\mathrm{Tr}(\hat{R} R_{gt}^{\top}) - 1}{2} \right) .$$

Translation Loss. As translation misalignment often dominates registration error in clinical practice, we emphasize translation accuracy by computing the Euclidean distance between the predicted $\hat{t}$ and ground truth t_{gt} translation vectors:

$$\mathcal{L}_{trans} = \left\|\hat{t} - t_{gt}\right\|_2^2.$$

Matrix Regularization. To ensure the predicted transformation matrix remains a valid rigid body transformation, we introduce a regularization term that penalizes deviations from orthogonality and unit determinant:

$$\mathcal{L}_{mat} = \left\|\hat{R}^\top \hat{R} - I\right\|_F^2.$$

Overall Loss. The total loss integrates all components in a weighted sum:

$$\mathcal{L} = \lambda_p \cdot \mathcal{L}_{point} + \lambda_c \cdot \mathcal{L}_{chamfer} + \lambda_r \cdot \mathcal{L}_{rot} + \lambda_t \cdot \mathcal{L}_{trans} + \lambda_m \cdot \mathcal{L}_{mat},$$

where, the weighting coefficients $\lambda_p = 0.5$, $\lambda_c = 1.0$, $\lambda_r = 1.0$, $\lambda_t = 3.0$, and $\lambda_m = 0.3$ are employed. The relatively higher weight assigned to the translation loss reflects its critical importance for achieving clinically meaningful registration accuracy.

2.5 Inference Acceleration

To ensure computational efficiency and enable practical deployment, we implemented a point cloud sampling and simplification strategy. During inference, the original CBCT scans often produce dense point sets. The density of these sets substantially increases computational cost without proportionally improving accuracy. To address this, we uniformly subsampled the CBCT point clouds to a fixed number of points, while IOS meshes were converted to point clouds with a comparable resolution. This design ensures balanced complexity between modalities, reduces GPU memory consumption, and accelerates inference speed.

Importantly, this balance between efficiency and precision makes the framework more applicable in real-world clinical scenarios, where both accuracy and time efficiency are crucial.

3 Experiments and Results

3.1 Dataset and Assessment Metrics

The dataset provided by the STSR 2025 challenge comprises paired CBCT volumes and IOS meshes [17,18]. In the training phase, two subsets are available: a labeled set, where each CBCT-IOS pair is annotated with an affine transformation matrix aligning the upper and lower dentition, and an unlabeled set containing paired CBCT volumes and IOS meshes. In addition, a validation set is released without annotations, serving as the benchmark for leaderboard evaluation.

For quantitative evaluation, two complementary metrics are used: the mean translation error, which measures the Euclidean distance between predicted and ground-truth translation vectors, and the mean rotation error, computed as the geodesic distance between the predicted and reference rotation matrices. These metrics directly reflect the fidelity of the registration outcome, with lower values indicating higher accuracy. Although computational efficiency, such as inference time and GPU memory usage, is not explicitly scored in the validation phase due to the limitations of the challenge platform, it remains a practical consideration when deploying the methods in real clinical workflows.

3.2 Implementation Details

Environments and Requirements. All experiments were conducted on a workstation, and the details of the hardware and software configuration are summarized in Table 1. The model was trained using the PyTorch framework for a total of 200 epochs.

Table 1. System Configuration

Ubuntu version	Ubuntu 24.04 LTS
CPU	Intel(R) Xeon(R) Platinum 8352S CPU @ 2.20GHz
RAM	503 GB
GPU	1 NVIDIA GeForce RTX 4090 (24G)
CUDA version	12.4
Programming language	Python 3.9.19
Deep learning framework	PyTorch (torch 1.12.1, torchvision 0.19.1)
Codes available at	https://github.com/duola-wa/MICCAI-2025-STSR-Task-2

3.3 Results and Analysis

To evaluate the effectiveness of our method, we present a series of ablation studies focusing on different design choices. As shown in Table 2, applying data augmentation substantially improves registration accuracy. Both translation and rotation errors are reduced, highlighting the importance of introducing geometric variability during training. By exposing the model to diverse transformations, augmentation enhances robustness to unseen cases and prevents overfitting, leading to a more generalizable registration framework.

As shown in Table 3, incorporating Iterative Closest Point (ICP) refinement reduces the mean translation error relative to the baseline prediction [1]. However, given the limited overall gain and additional computational cost, ICP was not included in our final pipeline.

Table 4 further compares the performance under different CBCT filtering thresholds. The threshold refers to the intensity cutoff applied to CBCT voxels

Table 2. Effect of data augmentation on registration accuracy.

Setting	Mean Translation Error (mm)	Mean Rotation Error (°)
w/o Augmentation	230.80	37.54
w/ Augmentation	165.57	24.00

Table 3. Effect of ICP refinement on registration accuracy.

Method	Mean Translation Error (mm)	Mean Rotation Error (°)
w/o ICP	165.57	24.00
w/ ICP	157.68	43.56

when extracting point clouds. A higher threshold retains densest regions such as enamel and cortical bone, while a lower threshold preserves a larger portion of anatomical structures, including lower-density bone. Relaxing the criterion from 800 to 600 therefore increases the number of target points available for alignment, which leads to a modest improvement in both translation and rotation accuracy. This suggests that incorporating a richer set of structural cues benefits the registration process.

Table 4. Effect of CBCT filtering threshold on registration accuracy (w/o ICP).

Filtering Condition	Mean Translation Error (mm)	Mean Rotation Error (°)
CBCT > 800	165.57	24.00
CBCT > 600	164.46	23.71

4 Conclusion

In this paper, we present a learning-based framework for CBCT–IOS registration, tailored to the MICCAI STSR Task 2 2025 Challenge. The framework integrates dual PointNet++ encoders with a differentiable SVD head to estimate rigid transformations under orthogonality constraints. By leveraging tailored data augmentation and efficient point cloud sampling, our approach seeks to balance accuracy and inference speed. Experimental results demonstrate the effectiveness of the proposed augmentation strategies. Ultimately, our method achieved second place on the validation leaderboard. These results highlight the potential of our framework for clinical applications that demand rapid and reliable responses. In future work, we plan to further explore semi-supervised strategies to better leverage unlabeled data and to investigate lightweight architectures that further reduce computational overhead for deployment in clinical settings.

References

1. Besl, P.J., McKay, N.D.: Method for registration of 3-D shapes. In: Sensor fusion IV: control paradigms and data structures. vol. 1611, pp. 586–606. Spie (1992)
2. Bolelli, F., et al.: Segmenting the inferior alveolar canal in CBCTS volumes: the toothfairy challenge. IEEE Trans. Med. Imaging (2024)
3. Flügge, T., Derksen, W., Te Poel, J., Hassan, B., Nelson, K., Wismeijer, D.: Registration of cone beam computed tomography data and intraoral surface scans-a prerequisite for guided implant surgery with cad/cam drilling guides. Clin. Oral Implant Res. **28**(9), 1113–1118 (2017)
4. Ji, C., et al.: Mammo-net: integrating gaze supervision and interactive information in multi-view mammogram classification. In: International Conference on Medical Image Computing and Computer-Assisted Intervention, pp. 68–78. Springer (2023)
5. Ji, C., Liu, Y., He, L., Jiang, Y., Huang, C., Wang, L.: Two-stage semi-supervised NNU-net framework for tooth segmentation in CBCT images. In: International Conference on Medical Image Computing and Computer-Assisted Intervention, pp. 100–109. Springer (2024)
6. Ji, C., Liu, Y., He, L., Jiang, Y., Huang, C., Wang, L.: A two-stage semi-supervised NNU-net model for automated tooth segmentation in panoramic x-ray images. In: International Conference on Medical Image Computing and Computer-Assisted Intervention, pp. 91–99. Springer (2024)
7. Jiang, Y., Liu, Y., Ji, C., Wang, L.: Enhanced multi-structure segmentation in CBCT images with adaptive structure optimization. In: International Conference on Medical Image Computing and Computer-Assisted Intervention, pp. 30–40. Springer (2024)
8. Jiang, Y., et al.: Morphology prior enhanced teeth segmentation for high-resolution oral scans. IEEE J. Biomed. Health Inform. (2025)
9. Kim, S., et al.: Best of both modalities: Fusing CBCT and intraoral scan data into a single tooth image. In: International Conference on Medical Image Computing and Computer-Assisted Intervention, pp. 553–563. Springer (2024)
10. Lim, S.W., Hwang, H.S., Cho, I.S., Baek, S.H., Cho, J.H.: Registration accuracy between intraoral-scanned and cone-beam computed tomography-scanned crowns in various registration methods. Am. J. Orthod. Dentofac. Orthop. **157**(3), 348–356 (2020)
11. Liu, Y., Xin, R., Yang, T., Wang, L.: Inferior alveolar nerve segmentation in CBCT images using connectivity-based selective re-training. In: International Conference on Medical Image Computing and Computer-Assisted Intervention, pp. 3–12. Springer (2024)
12. Liu, Y., et al.: Individual graph representation learning for pediatric tooth segmentation from dental CBCT. IEEE Trans. Med. Imaging (2024)
13. Olczyk, A., Malicka, B., Skośkiewicz-Malinowska, K.: Retrospective study of the morphology of third maxillary molars among the population of lower Silesia based on analysis of cone beam computed tomography. PLoS ONE **19**(2), e0299123 (2024)
14. Qi, C.R., Yi, L., Su, H., Guibas, L.J.: Pointnet++: Deep hierarchical feature learning on point sets in a metric space. Adv. Neural Inf. Process. Syst. **30** (2017)
15. Su, S., et al.: Evaluation of the accuracy of cone-beam computed tomography image segmentation of isolated tooth roots based on the dynamic threshold method. BMC Oral Health **23**(1), 752 (2023)

16. Wang, S., Ouyang, X., Liu, T., Wang, Q., Shen, D.: Follow my eye: using gaze to supervise computer-aided diagnosis. IEEE Trans. Med. Imaging **41**(7), 1688–1698 (2022)
17. Wang, Y., Chen, X., Qian, D., Ye, F., Wang, S., Zhang, H.: Semi-supervised Tooth Segmentation: First MICCAI Challenge, SemiToothSeg 2023, Held in Conjunction with MICCAI 2023, Vancouver, BC, Canada, October 8, 2023, Proceedings, vol. 14623. Springer Nature (2024)
18. Wang, Y., et al.: Sts miccai 2023 challenge: grand challenge on 2D and 3D semi-supervised tooth segmentation. arXiv preprint arXiv:2407.13246 (2024)
19. Wang, Y., Solomon, J.M.: Deep closest point: Learning representations for point cloud registration. In: Proceedings of the IEEE/CVF International Conference on Computer Vision, pp. 3523–3532 (2019)
20. Zhang, Y., et al.: Children's dental panoramic radiographs dataset for caries segmentation and dental disease detection. Scientific Data **10**(1), 380 (2023)

U-Mamba2-SSL for Semi-supervised Tooth and Pulp Segmentation in CBCT

Zhi Qin Tan[1(✉)], Xiatian Zhu[2], Owen Addison[1], and Yunpeng Li[1]

[1] Centre for Oral, Clinical and Translational Sciences, King's College London, London, UK
{zhi_qin.tan,owen.addison,yunpeng.li}@kcl.ac.uk

[2] Surrey Institute for People-Centred AI, University of Surrey, Surrey, UK
xiatian.zhu@surrey.ac.uk

Abstract. Accurate segmentation of teeth and pulp in Cone-Beam Computed Tomography (CBCT) is vital for clinical applications like treatment planning and diagnosis. However, manual segmentation requires extensive expertise and is exceptionally time-consuming, highlighting the critical need for automated semi-supervised segmentation algorithms that can utilize unlabeled data. In this paper, we propose **U-Mamba2-SSL**, a novel semi-supervised learning framework that builds on the U-Mamba2 model and employs a multi-stage training strategy. The framework first pre-trains U-Mamba2 in a self-supervised manner using a disruptive autoencoder. It then leverages unlabeled data through consistency regularization, where we introduce input and feature perturbations to ensure stable model outputs. Finally, a pseudo-labeling strategy is implemented with a reduced loss weighting to minimize the impact of potential errors. U-Mamba2-SSL obtained 0.917 DSC and 0.948 mIoU on the hidden test set, achieving first place in Task 1 of the STSR 2025 challenge. The code is available at https://github.com/zhiqin1998/UMamba2.

Keywords: Semi-supervised learning · U-Mamba2-SSL · CBCT Imaging · Tooth and Pulp Segmentation · STSR 2025 Challenge

1 Introduction

Cone-Beam Computed Tomography (CBCT) provides comprehensive 3D information of the oral region and is an important imaging tool in dentistry, as shown by its rapid adoption in dental clinics [10]. Precision segmentation of the tooth and pulp structures is vital to various applications such as dental conditions diagnosis, orthodontic procedures, treatment and surgery planning [14,20]. However, manual segmentation of CBCT scans requires specialized training and is extremely time-consuming due to its high resolution containing a massive number of voxels and the high variability across scans, making it impractical

Supplementary Information The online version contains supplementary material available at https://doi.org/10.1007/978-3-032-20711-1_18.

F. Bolelli et al. (Eds.): ODIN 2025, LNCS 16473, pp. 191–200, 2026.
https://doi.org/10.1007/978-3-032-20711-1_18

to scale up in practice. This highlights the significance of developing effective semi-supervised approaches with only limited labeled data while leveraging a large amount of unlabeled CBCT scans [2,23,24].

Semi-supervised learning (SSL) incorporates elements from both supervised and unsupervised learning [4,26], utilizing both labeled and unlabeled data to improve the performance on the supervised task by exploring the latent knowledge from unlabeled data. This alleviates the need for a significant amount of labels, which can require considerable resources to obtain. We focus on three categories of SSL: 1) Knowledge transfer with pre-training refers to the transfer of knowledge from one task to another via pre-training, where autoencoders [8,21,22] are trained to reconstruct corrupted input from a large amount of unlabeled data to guide the randomly initialized model weights towards potentially better regions; 2) Consistency regularization training [5,13,15] based on the smoothness assumption, enforces the model to produce similar output after perturbing the input, internal features, or model weights, pushing the model towards better generalization capability; and 3) Pseudo labeling method [12], one of the most common approaches in SSL due to its simplicity and model-agnostic nature. It is a form of entropy regularization [6] with unlabeled data, reducing the overlap of class probability distribution and favoring a low-density class separation.

In this paper, we present U-Mamba2-SSL, a multi-stage semi-supervised learning framework for tooth and pulp segmentation in 3D CBCT images, developed in the scope of the STSR 2025 Task 1 Challenge [1]. To exploit the vast amount of unlabeled CBCT data, we first pre-train U-Mamba2 [17] with the disruptive autoencoder on all provided data. Then, the second training stage involves using the labeled data for supervised learning and the unlabeled data for unsupervised learning via consistency regularization techniques in the input and feature spaces. Lastly, the final stage introduces the pseudo labeling method to the training procedure of the previous stage, with a lower loss weight to further optimize the model weights. The extensive experiments demonstrate the superior performance of our method, outperforming other alternatives and achieving first place with an average score of 0.789 in the STSR 2025 hidden test set.

2 Method

Figure 1 shows the overall process of the U-Mamba2-SSL framework, consisting of three training stages where we first pre-train the U-Mamba2 [17] model with reconstruction objectives, then combine supervised loss for the labeled data and unsupervised loss with consistency regularization for the unlabeled data. The final third stage introduces pseudo labeling to the training objectives.

U-Mamba2 integrates Mamba2 [3] state space models into the U-Net architecture at the bottleneck region to enhance its ability to capture long-range dependencies. Mamba2 improves upon Mamba [7] by enforcing stronger constraints on the hidden space structure, leading to higher efficiency without compromising its performance compared to transformer-based alternatives. We present the details of the three training stages: pre-training, consistency regularization training, and pseudo labeling, in the following subsections. Note that the final checkpoint of each training stage is used to initialize the model of the subsequent stage.

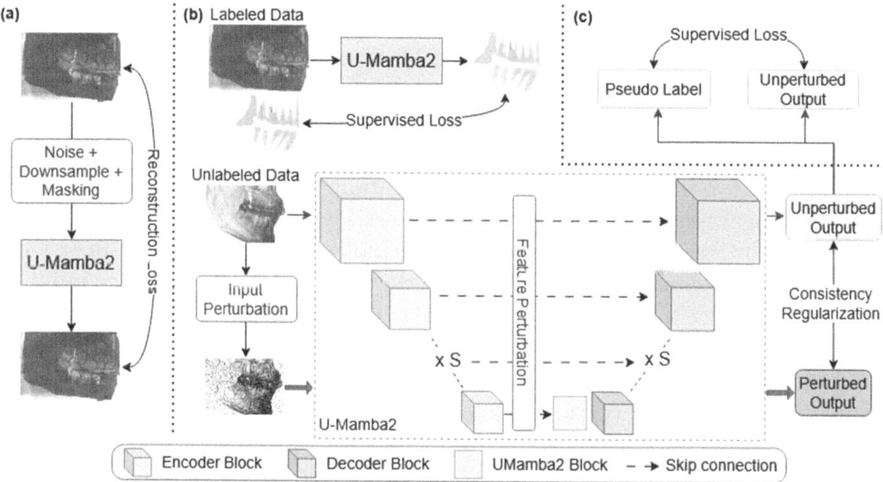

Fig. 1. Overall diagram of the proposed U-Mamba2-SSL framework. (a) The first pre-training stage; (b) The second consistency regularization training stage; (c) The third pseudo labeling training stage.

Problem Formulation. Let $\mathcal{D}_l = \{(x_1^l, y_1), ..., (x_n^l, y_n)\}$ represent the n labeled samples and $\mathcal{D}_u = \{x_1^u, ..., x_m^u\}$ represent the m unlabeled samples, where $x_i^l \in \mathbb{R}^{H \times W \times D}$ is the i-th labeled input image, $y_i \in \mathbb{R}^{C \times H \times W \times D}$ is its corresponding voxel-level label, and x_i^u is the i-th unlabeled input image. Here, C is the number of classes while H, W, D are the spatial dimensions. Our goal is to exploit the larger number of unlabeled samples (*i.e.* $m \gg n$) to train a 3D segmentation model.

2.1 First Stage: Pre-training with Disruptive Autoencoder

In the medical image domain, data scarcity due to various factors such as complex ethical regulations for accessing and releasing datasets publicly, presents challenges to model pre-training. Therefore, unlike in computer vision tasks of natural images, models for medical image applications are often trained from scratch with random initialization of model weights. However, recent works [18,21] have shown that pre-training deep learning models for medical image tasks can lead to better models that can extract meaningful feature representations to enhance the performance of downstream segmentation tasks, particularly when there is limited labeled data to train from scratch effectively.

In the first stage of our proposed SSL framework, we utilize all training data (*i.e.* $\mathcal{D}_l \cup \mathcal{D}_u$) to pre-train U-Mamba2 via the disruptive autoencoder (DAE) [21] method. The DAE method combines three low-level reconstruction tasks for pre-training, namely denoising, super-resolution, and recovering masked information.

Denoising refers to the task of restoring the original input from its noisy version, obtained by introducing random additive Gaussian noise to the original input. The model must learn to restore all local details in images, such as edges and textures, to output a good denoised image. Besides that, super-resolution is the task of increasing the resolution of a low-resolution image, created artificially by downsampling the original input with linear interpolation. To obtain a good upsampled image, the model must be able to recover the fine details of the image with both local and global information. Lastly, we apply masking to random cubical regions in the input image, setting the voxel values to zero. As most of the information in medical images is not global but is in the finer local details, we use a small cube size relative to the spatial dimensions of the input to prevent discarding too much local information. The model is directed to recover the masked regions, leading to the ability to extract meaningful global context. After applying the three input disruptions, U-Mamba2 learns to reconstruct the original image from the corrupted input with an L1 loss function.

2.2 Second Stage: Consistency Regularization Training

We exploit the smoothness assumption and employ consistency regularization training in the second training stage, enforcing the invariance of predictions on the model. In this training stage, we use a combination of supervised loss and unsupervised loss to learn the model parameters. For a labeled training sample, x_i^l, and its voxel-level class label, y_i, the model is trained in a supervised fashion based on the combination of Dice loss and cross-entropy loss, $\mathcal{L}_S$. For an unlabeled training sample, x_i^u, it is first passed through the model to obtain an unperturbed output, $\hat{y}_i^u$. Then, we introduce input and feature perturbations [13] to x_i^u and obtain the perturbed output, $\tilde{y}_i^u$, by passing the perturbed input through the model. The semi-supervised consistency regularization loss, $\mathcal{L}_{CR}$, is computed as the $\mathcal{L}_1$ loss between $\hat{y}_i^u$ and $\tilde{y}_i^u$. We describe the perturbation details in the following paragraphs.

Input Perturbations. We apply strong data augmentation to the unlabeled data to obtain a perturbed input. It is crucial not to apply spatial (*e.g.* mirroring or rotation) augmentations, as in the context of segmentation, these transformations are non-local and violate the smoothness assumption. Specifically, in this stage, we apply median filter, Gaussian blur, Gaussian noise, random brightness, random contrast, low-resolution simulation, and image sharpening filter.

Feature Perturbations. The perturbed inputs are passed through the encoder blocks in U-Mamba2 to obtain multi-scale 3D feature maps. Before the encoder feature maps are connected to the decoder blocks via skip connections, we apply random perturbations in the feature space to encourage the model to learn more robust and generalizable feature representations. The feature perturbations consist of dropping activations or injecting noise in the encoder feature maps:

- Random Spatial Dropout [19]: We apply random channel-wise dropout with a probability of 0.5. In contrast to i.i.d. dropout, this promotes channel-wise independence in the encoder feature maps.
- Random Activation Dropout [16]: Activations with high values are randomly dropped to enforce the model to focus on inactive regions in the feature map. We randomly sample a threshold, $\gamma_{drop} \sim \mathcal{U}(0.7, 0.9)$, then set all activations above the γ_{drop} percentile to zero. As a result, the top $10\% - 30\%$ highly activated regions in the feature map are dropped.
- Noise Injection: A noise tensor with the same shape as the feature map is first sampled from a uniform distribution, $N \sim \mathcal{U}(-0.3, 0.3)$. As the activations in the feature maps vary, we ensure that the noise tensor is proportional to the feature map by first multiplying the noise tensor with the feature map before adding it as $Z + (Z \odot N)$, where $Z \in \mathbb{R}^{F \times H \times W \times D}$ is the feature map, $\odot$ is element-wise multiplication, and F is the number of channels.

Semi-supervised Learning Schedule. In practice, we utilize both labeled and unlabeled data during each training epoch. The overall loss signal from both labeled and unlabeled data is computed as

$$\mathcal{L} = \mathcal{L}_S + \omega_{CR}\mathcal{L}_{CR} \ , \tag{1}$$

where ω_{CR} is the unsupervised loss weight function. ω_{CR} ramps up exponentially [11] from zero to a fixed weight, W_{CR}, at the $0.2T_{ep}$ epoch where T_{ep} is the total number of training epochs. Additionally, we linearly increase the proportion of unlabeled data in each epoch from 10% to 50% at the $0.4T_{ep}$ epoch, allowing the model to focus on learning the main segmentation task in the early phase.

2.3 Third Stage: Pseudo Labeling

After the second training stage, we obtain a good U-Mamba2 segmentation model that can maintain local smoothness around its predictions. We capitalize on this feature by further training the model with the pseudo labeling [12] strategy. Specifically, the model's predictions on unlabeled samples are considered pseudo labels and used for model training in a supervised manner. For the predicted class of each voxel, if the class confidence is above a given confidence threshold, λ_{conf}, then we use the predicted class as ground truth; otherwise, the voxel is set to the background class and is ignored in the loss calculation.

In this stage, the loss function from Eq. 1 becomes:

$$\mathcal{L} = \mathcal{L}_S + \omega_{CR}\mathcal{L}_{CR} + W_{PL}\mathcal{L}_{PL} \ , \tag{2}$$

where $\mathcal{L}_{PL}$ is the supervised loss computed with the pseudo labels and ignores the background class, and W_{PL} is the loss weight for $\mathcal{L}_{PL}$ to balance the loss terms. Similar to the second stage, we linearly increase the proportion of unlabeled samples in each training epoch from 30% to 50% at the $0.2T_{ep}$ epoch.

Table 1. Development environments and requirements.

System	Ubuntu 24.04
CPU	Intel(R) Core(TM) Ultra 9 285K
RAM	2 × 32GB; 6400 MHz
GPU	NVIDIA RTX 5090 32 GB
CUDA version	12.9
Programming language	Python 3.11
Deep learning framework	PyTorch 2.7.1, nnU-Net 2.6.2

3 Experiments

3.1 Dataset and Evaluation Metrics

The evaluation metrics include Dice Similarity Coefficient (DSC), Normalized Surface Distance (NSD), Mean Intersection over Union (mIoU), and Identification Accuracy (IA) to evaluate the segmentation region overlap and boundary distance. In addition, the algorithm runtime and memory consumption are also evaluated and ranked.

3.2 Implementation Details

Preprocessing. We resize all inputs to the median voxel spacing of all training data, $(0.3, 0.25, 0.25)$, resulting in a median input size of $(337, 640, 640)$. Then, we clip the input data to the 0.5th and 99.5th percentiles, followed by data normalization based on the mean and standard deviation of the voxel values.

Environment Settings. The development environments and requirements are presented in Table 1.

Training Protocols. We implement U-Mamba2-SSL with the nnU-Net [9] framework, using a patch-size training and sliding window inference strategy. During training, we randomly apply rotation, scaling, Gaussian noise, Gaussian blur, brightness and contrast transform, low resolution simulation, and mirroring as data augmentation. We randomly crop input patches so that at least 33% of the voxels contain a foreground label. W_{CR}, W_{PL}, and λ_{conf} are set to 50, 0.1, and 0.75, respectively. All models have 7 encoder-decoder stages and follow the model configuration in Table 2. The provided 30 labeled training samples are split into 20 training and 10 internal validation splits, where the internal validation split is used to monitor training progress and offline evaluation. We select the checkpoint with the highest DSC on our internal validation set and report the performance metrics on the hidden validation set.

Table 2. Training configuration.

Pre-trained Model	See Sect. 2.1
Batch size	2
Patch size	$128 \times 256 \times 256$
Total epochs	500
Optimizer	SGD with 0.99 momentum
Initial learning rate	0.01
Lr decay schedule	Polynomial LR decay
Training time	13 h
Loss function	See Eq. (1) and (2)
Number of model parameters	156M
Number of flops	6.22T

4 Results and Discussion

4.1 Quantitative Results

Table 3 presents the results of our proposed method compared with two baselines, nnU-Net and U-Mamba2. We observe that all methods achieved high DSC, NSD, and mIoU metrics, which measure overall image-level performance. However, U-Mamba2-SSL outperforms others significantly in IA, which calculates the average percentage of classes with IoU > 0.5 across all images. The bottom three rows of Table 3 also report the ablation study of our proposed method. Notably, pre-training leads to the largest leap in IA, from 0.464 to 0.731, while incorporating consistency regularization and pseudo labeling further increases IA to 0.738.

Table 3. Evaluation results on the validation set. CR denotes consistency regularization; PL denotes pseudo label. Our ablation study is reported in the bottom three rows, with the last row referring to the final U-Mamba2-SSL.

Methods	Pre-train	CR	PL	DSC	NSD	mIoU	IA	Average
nnU-Net [9]	-	-	-	0.963	0.997	0.928	0.286	0.794
U-Mamba2 [17]	-	-	-	0.965	0.998	0.930	0.464	0.839
U-Mamba2-SSL	✓	×	×	0.967	0.998	0.937	0.731	0.908
	✓	✓	×	0.967	0.999	0.935	0.736	**0.910**
	✓	✓	✓	0.967	0.999	0.935	0.738	**0.910**

4.2 Qualitative Results

Figure 2 shows the qualitative comparison between the ground truth and our model's predictions of the scans with the highest and lowest DSC in our internal

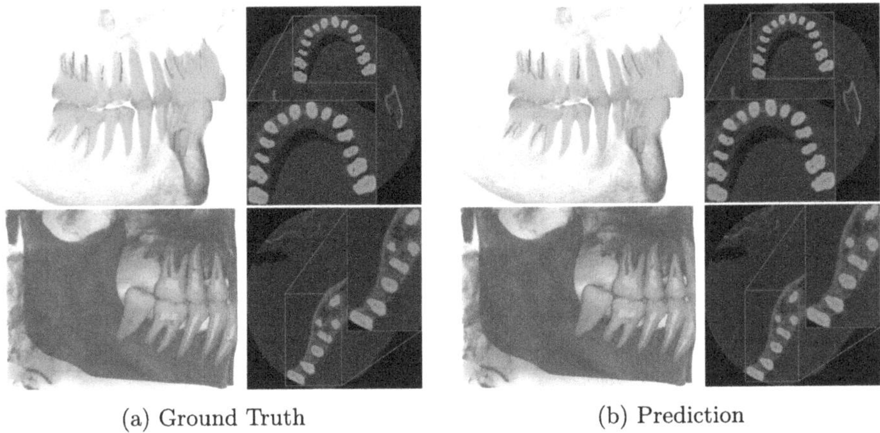

(a) Ground Truth (b) Prediction

Fig. 2. Qualitative results of U-Mamba2-SSL on the internal validation set. The 3D render and a representative 2D slice are shown for: (Top) the best scoring case and (Bottom) the worst scoring case.

validation set, in the top and bottom rows, respectively. Generally, we observe that our method can accurately differentiate between the tooth and different classes of pulp and root canal. The failure cases of our method typically stem from the inability to precisely predict the thickness and the length or extent of the pulp. Moreover, our model also struggles with limited field of view (LFOV) CBCTs where it predicts more false positives around the image edges.

4.3 Final Challenge Submission

We scale up our training procedure by training on all available data for 1000 epochs and increasing the input patch size to 160x256x256. For inference, we use a sliding window inference with a tile size of 0.9, and enable mirroring in the anterior/posterior and left/right axes during test-time augmentation (See Appendix A for the speed optimization). Our method achieved a 0.969 DSC, 0.998 NSD, 0.940 mIoU, and 0.806 IA on the validation set, while obtaining a DSC, NSD, mIoU, and IA of 0.917, 0.882, 0.948, and 0.577, respectively, on the final hidden test set, securing first place in Task 1 of the STSR 2025 challenge.

4.4 Limitation and Future Work

Our work, while successful, is not without limitations. First, the dataset consists of full and LFOV CBCTs, which differ in content and image properties. Next, the IA metric drops significantly on the final hidden test set, signifying possible overfitting or domain shift. Future work should design data processing and augmentation techniques tailored to the different types of CBCTs to leverage their differences and improve model generalizability. Lastly, as only a small region of interest (ROI) in the CBCT image contains the foreground classes, future research can exploit this to prevent wasting computation on non-foreground regions, allowing the model to focus on the true ROI.

5 Conclusion

We presented U-Mamba2-SSL, a novel multi-stage semi-supervised learning framework for tooth and pulp segmentation in CBCT scans, in the scope of the STSR 2025 challenge. The framework consists of first pre-training U-Mamba2 with the disruptive autoencoder, utilizing unlabeled data for consistency regularization, and a pseudo labeling strategy in the final stage. Our results demonstrate that the proposed framework can substantially enhance model performance, achieving first place with an average score of 0.789 on the hidden test set in Task 1 of the STSR 2025 challenge.

Acknowledgements. We thank all the data owners for making the medical images publicly available and Codabench [25] for hosting the challenge platform.

Disclosure of Interests. The authors have no competing interests to declare that are relevant to the content of this article.

References

1. MICCAI STSR 2025 Challenge Task 1: Semi-supervised Teeth and Plup Root Canal Segmentation in 3D CBCT Scans. https://www.codabench.org/competitions/6468. Accessed: 25th August 2025
2. Cui, W., et al.: Ctooth+: a large-scale dental cone beam computed tomography dataset and benchmark for tooth volume segmentation. In: MICCAI Workshop on Data Augmentation, Labelling, and Imperfections, pp. 64–73 (2022)
3. Dao, T., Gu, A.: Transformers are SSMs: Generalized models and efficient algorithms through structured state space duality. In: Proceeding International Conference Machine Learning (ICML). Vienna, Austria (2024)
4. van Engelen, J.E., Hoos, H.H.: A survey on semi-supervised learning. Mach. Learn. **109**(2), 373–440 (2020)
5. Fan, Y., Kukleva, A., Dai, D., Schiele, B.: Revisiting consistency regularization for semi-supervised learning. Int. J. Comput. Vis. (IJCV) **131**(3), 626–643 (2023)
6. Grandvalet, Y., Bengio, Y.: Semi-supervised learning by entropy minimization. In: Proceeding Advance Neural Information Processing System (NeurIPS) (2004)
7. Gu, A., Dao, T.: Mamba: Linear-time sequence modeling with selective state spaces. arXiv:2312.00752 (2023)
8. He, K., Chen, X., Xie, S., Li, Y., Dollár, P., Girshick, R.: Masked autoencoders are scalable vision learners. In: Proceeding IEEE Conference Computer Visualization Pattern Recog. (CVPR), pp. 16000–16009 (2022)
9. Isensee, F., Jaeger, P.F., Kohl, S.A.A., Petersen, J., Maier-Hein, K.H.: nnu-net: a self-configuring method for deep learning-based biomedical image segmentation. Nat. Methods **18**(2), 203–211 (2021)

10. Jaju, P.P., Jaju, S.P.: Clinical utility of dental cone-beam computed tomography: current perspectives. Clin. Cosmet. Investig. Dent. **6**, 29–43 (2014)
11. Laine, S., Aila, T.: Temporal ensembling for semi-supervised learning. arXiv:1610.02242 (2016)
12. Lee, D.H.: Pseudo-label: The simple and efficient semi-supervised learning method for deep neural networks. In: International Conference Machine Learning (ICML) Workshop: Challenges in Representation Learning (WREPL) (2013)
13. Ouali, Y., Hudelot, C., Tami, M.: Semi-supervised semantic segmentation with cross-consistency training. In: Proceeding IEEE Conference Computer Visualization Pattern Recognition (CVPR) (2020)
14. Patel, S., Durack, C., Abella, F., Shemesh, H., Roig, M., Lemberg, K.: Cone beam computed tomography in endodontics – a review. Int. Endod. J. **48**(1), 3–15 (2015)
15. Sinha, S., Dieng, A.B.: Consistency regularization for variational auto-encoders. In: Proceeding Advance Neural Information Processing System (NeurIPS), pp. 12943–12954 (2021)
16. Srivastava, N., Hinton, G., Krizhevsky, A., Sutskever, I., Salakhutdinov, R.: Dropout: a simple way to prevent neural networks from overfitting. J. Mach. Learn. Res. (JMLR) **15**(56), 1929–1958 (2014)
17. Tan, Z.Q., Zhu, X., Addison, O., Li, Y.: U-mamba2: scaling state space models for dental anatomy segmentation in CBCT. arXiv:2509.12069 (2025)
18. Tang, Y., et al.: Self-supervised pre-training of Swin transformers for 3D medical image analysis. In: Proceeding IEEE Conference Computer Visualization Pattern Recognition (CVPR), pp. 20698–20708. New Orleans, LA, USA (2022)
19. Tompson, J., Goroshin, R., Jain, A., LeCun, Y., Bregler, C.: Efficient object localization using convolutional networks. In: Proceeding IEEE Conference Computer Visualization Pattern Recognition (CVPR), pp. 648–656 (2015)
20. Tyndall, D.A., Price, J.B., Tetradis, S., Ganz, S.D., Hildebolt, C., Scarfe, W.C.: Position statement of the American academy of oral and maxillofacial radiology on selection criteria for the use of radiology in dental implantology with emphasis on cone beam computed tomography. Oral Surg Oral Med Oral Pathol Oral Radiol **113**(6), 817–826 (2012)
21. Valanarasu, J.M.J., et al.: Disruptive autoencoders: leveraging low-level features for 3D medical image pre-training. In: Proceeding International Conference on Medical Imaging with Deep Learning. vol. 250, pp. 1553–1570 (2024)
22. Vincent, P., Larochelle, H., Lajoie, I., Bengio, Y., Manzagol, P.A.: Stacked denoising autoencoders: learning useful representations in a deep network with a local denoising criterion. J. Mach. Learn. Res. (JMLR) **11**(110), 3371–3408 (2010)
23. Wang, Y., et al.: A multi-modal dental dataset for semi-supervised deep learning image segmentation. Sci. Data **12**(1), 117 (2025)
24. Wang, Y., et al.: MICCAI 2023 STS challenge: a retrospective study of semi-supervised approaches for teeth segmentation. Pattern Recogn. **170**, 112049 (2026)
25. Xu, Z., et al.: Codabench: flexible, easy-to-use, and reproducible meta-benchmark platform. Patterns **3**(7), 100543 (2022)
26. Yang, X., Song, Z., King, I., Xu, Z.: A survey on deep semi-supervised learning. IEEE Trans. Knowl. Data Eng. **35**(9), 8934–8954 (2023)

nnUNet for Semi-supervised Tooth and Pulp Root Canal Segmentation in CBCT

Ajo Babu George[1](✉) and Sadhvik Bathini[2]

[1] DiceMed, Odisha, India
drajo_george@dicemed.in
[2] Indian Institute of Technology Kharagpur, Kharagpur, West Bengal, India

Abstract. A solution for the Semi-supervised Teeth Segmentation and Registration (STSR) 2025 Challenge, which focused on the precise segmentation of teeth and pulp root canals in 3D Cone Beam Computed Tomography (CBCT) scans is presented in this paper. Accurate segmentation of the pulp root canal is crucial for clinical visualization and treatment planning, but manual annotation is extremely labor-intensive. The presented approach uses a semi-supervised framework powered by nnU-Net, leveraging a small labeled dataset of 30 scans alongside a much larger unlabeled dataset of 300 scans. To effectively utilize the unlabeled data, pseudo-labeling was employed to generate annotations, and the model was subsequently trained. The results for both tooth and pulp structures yield a Dice score of 0.8088 and an mIoU of 0.9638 in the all-data track, while the Dice score in the coreset track is 0.69. These metrics highlight the model's ability to accurately identify and delineate the target structures.

Keywords: Teeth Segmentation · Semi-supervised learning · nnUNet · CBCT · Pulp · Root canals

1 Introduction

The field of dentistry is increasingly benefiting from computer-aided diagnosis tools, particularly for treatment planning and prognosis evaluation. Precise segmentation of teeth and especially the root pulp canal from 3D Cone-Beam Computed Tomography (CBCT) scans is a crucial pre-processing step for many of these applications. This enables clearer visualization of dental anatomy, which in turn helps in developing more refined treatment strategies. However, manual annotation of these regions is an extremely labor-intensive task, requiring a substantial investment of time and human resources. This makes acquiring large, labeled datasets a significant challenge for training robust deep learning models.

Recent developments in deep learning have shown great promise in dental image analysis, with models capable of high-accuracy segmentation and disease classification [2,4]. Networks like U-Net and its derivatives, including nnU-Net,

F. Bolelli et al. (Eds.): ODIN 2025, LNCS 16473, pp. 201–210, 2026.
https://doi.org/10.1007/978-3-032-20711-1_19

have become standard for medical image segmentation tasks [1]. nnU-Net, in particular, stands out for its ability to automatically adapt to various 3D and 2D medical imaging tasks without extensive manual tuning of hyperparameters [7].

Despite these advances, a major limitation common to all deep learning-based methods is their reliance on a large quantity of high-quality training data, which is difficult and expensive to obtain for medical imaging. The manual annotation of 3D volume data, for example, requires experts to label each 2D slice, making the process even more challenging. To address this, semi-supervised learning has emerged as a highly practical approach, allowing models to benefit from a large quantity of readily available unlabeled data alongside a small set of labeled data [5].

This is the very purpose behind the Semi-supervised Teeth Segmentation (STS) Challenge. The challenge, a pioneering event in tooth segmentation, aimed to stimulate the development of effective semi-supervised algorithms for both 2D PXI and 3D CBCT volumes. The STS 2023 Challenge [8–10] focused on tooth instance segmentation. A significant research gap remains in the precise, automated segmentation of the intricate pulp root canal. This task is more complex due to the high variability in pulp canal morphology and the need for fine-grained annotation consistency.

A primary motivation is to advance the field of dental image analysis by developing a robust methodology for segmenting both teeth and pulp root canals using a semi-supervised learning strategy. Public dental imaging resources primarily focus on 2D panoramic radiographs rather than volumetric CBCT, especially for pediatric and mixed-dentition cohorts, highlighting the scarcity of large annotated 3D datasets and motivating semi-supervised learning for this task [12]. This approach is essential because the manual annotation of pulp canals is particularly labor-intensive due to their complex and variable morphology. The challenge dataset provided a scenario typical of real clinical settings: a limited number of labeled scans (30) and a large pool of unlabeled data (300). The following are the contibutions:

- A pseudo-labeling technique using the nnU-Net framework was adopted to leverage the large-scale unlabeled dataset. This approach allows a model to learn from a much larger volume of data, improving its robustness and generalization capabilities.
- The pipeline includes comprehensive pre-processing steps, such as resampling, cropping, and normalization.
- By combining these techniques, a model achieved robust performance across both teeth and pulp segmentation tasks, demonstrating its scalability and potential for real-world clinical applications where annotated data is scarce.

2 Method

The methodology employs a semi-supervised learning strategy to address the challenge of limited labeled data. Figure 1 describes the overall pipeline involves pre-processing the 3D CBCT scans, followed by a pseudo-labeling technique and extensive model training.

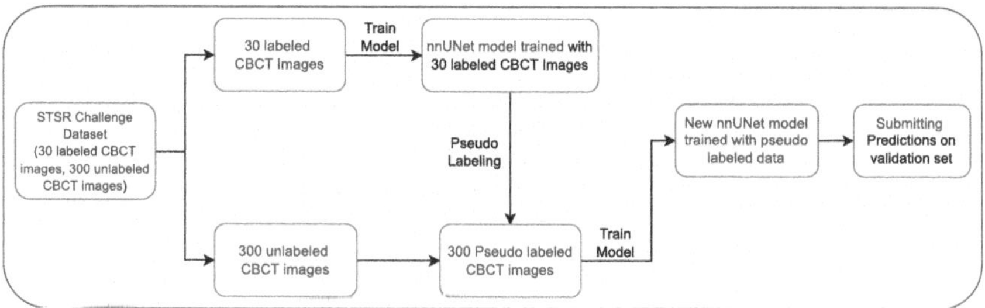

Fig. 1. Overall Pipeline of the proposed methodology.

2.1 nnU-Net Architecture

The nnU-Net framework [6] is employed for the network architecture, a self-contained python package that automatically optimizes network structure and training strategies for medical image segmentation. The architecture has a characteristic U-shape, where 3D arrays representing each input image undergo a series of convolutions, maximum pooling, up-convolutions, and concatenation steps. The initial half of the network is responsible for feature extraction, while the second half synthesizes the segmentation output. The design includes horizontal concatenation steps that pass early network information to later stages, a key feature of U-Net-based architectures.

3 Experiments

3.1 Dataset and Evaluation Metrics

The dataset for this task consists of 3D CBCT images for semi-supervised segmentation of teeth and pulp root canals. The training dataset consists of two parts: a labeled set of 30 images with fine-grained segmentation masks for teeth, wisdom teeth, and various root canal structures, and a much larger unlabeled set of 300 images. For public validation, 40 labeled images are provided, with segmentation results submitted to the Codabench platform for evaluation.

3.2 Implementation Details

Preprocessing. The images are first resampled and cropped to a default size that the nnUNet model configures while maintaining key anatomical features. A per-scan z-score normalization is applied to each image, standardizing the data with a mean of 0 and a standard deviation of 1 across the non-zero voxels.

Table 1. Development environments and requirements.

System	CentOS 7.6
CPU	Intel Xeon SKL G-6148 CPU@2.4GHz
RAM	384 GB
GPU (number and type)	NVIDIA V100
CUDA version	11.0
Programming language	Python 3.20
Deep learning framework	torch 2.0, torchvision 0.2.2

Environment Settings. The development environments and requirements are presented in Table 1.

3.3 Semi-supervised Pseudo-Labeling Scheme

A core component of the methodology is the use of a pseudo-labeling technique to leverage the large amount of unlabeled data. An initial nnU-Net model is trained for 750 epochs on the 30 available labeled scans. This trained model is then used to generate pseudo-labels for the 300 unlabeled scans. The pseudo-labeled data is then used to retrain the model for an extended period of 500 epochs. This approach effectively expands the training set, allowing the model to learn from a much larger volume of data than the labeled set alone. Extensive training improves the model's ability to accurately segment variable pulp canal morphology.

Table 2. Training protocols of the nnUNet model trained with 30 labeled scans

Pre-trained Model	None (training from scratch)
Batch size	2
Patch size	128 × 128 × 128
Total epochs	750
Optimizer	SGD with Nesterov momentum (0.99)
Initial learning rate (lr)	0.01
Lr decay schedule	Polynomial decay ($lr = lr_0(1 - \frac{epoch}{max\_epoch})^{0.9}$)
Training time	∼12 h
Loss function	Cross-entropy + Dice loss (sum)
Number of model parameters	∼30–35M[a]
Number of flops	∼250–300G[b]

Table 3. Training protocols of the nnUNet model trained with 300 pseudo labeled scans

Pre-trained Model	None (training from scratch)
Batch size	2
Patch size	128 × 128 × 128
Total epochs	500
Optimizer	SGD with Nesterov momentum (0.99)
Initial learning rate (lr)	0.01
Lr decay schedule	Polynomial decay ($lr = lr_0(1 - \frac{epoch}{max\_epoch})^{0.9}$)
Training time	~36 h
Loss function	Cross-entropy + Dice loss (sum)
Number of model parameters	~30–35M[c]
Number of flops	~250–300G[d]

4 Results and Discussion

The proposed methodology demonstrates robust performance in both teeth and pulp segmentation, successfully addressing the challenges of a limited labeled dataset. The semi-supervised approach, which combines pseudo-labeling with the nnU-Net framework, proved to be scalable to large CBCT datasets.

Figure 2 and Table 2 detail the training curves and protocols, respectively, for the initial model utilizing the limited dataset of 30 labeled images. Another nnUNet model trained on the 300 pseudo-labeled images is illustrated by the training curves and protocols presented in Fig. 3 and Table 3. These figures provide a comprehensive overview of the training progression and the impact of the semi-supervised approach on the model's final performance.

Table 4. Mean Dice and IoU Scores for Valid Dental Anatomy Labels.

Label ID	Anatomical Structure	Mean Dice	Mean IoU
1	Dental Hard Tissues	0.9591	0.9215
2	Pulp Chamber	0.8298	0.7100
4	Palatal Root	0.7449	0.5971
5	Mesial Root Canal	0.4976	0.3730
6	Distal Root Canal	0.6700	0.5116
7	Mesiobuccal Root Canal	0.6986	0.5390
8	Mesiolingual Root Canal	0.5978	0.4366
9	Distobuccal Root Canal	0.7150	0.5583
12	Impacted Tooth	0.9565	0.9173

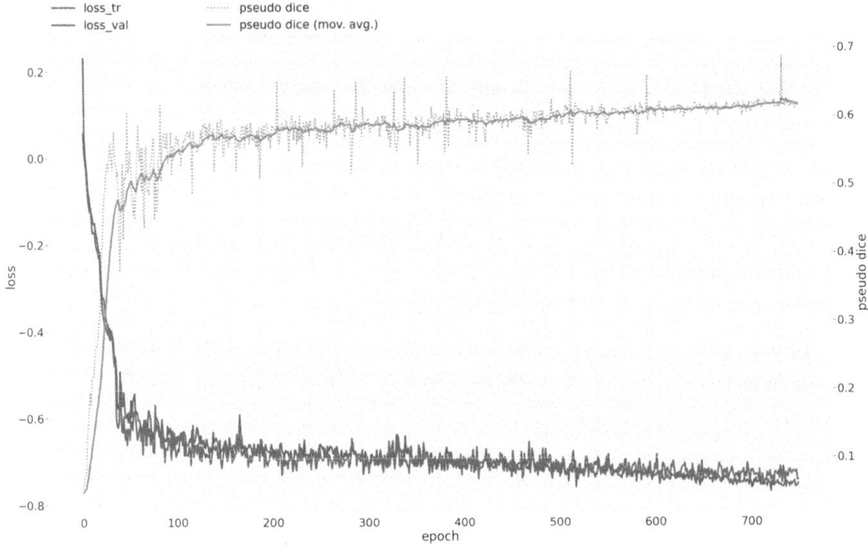

Fig. 2. Training and validation curves from nnUNet with 30 labeled scans.

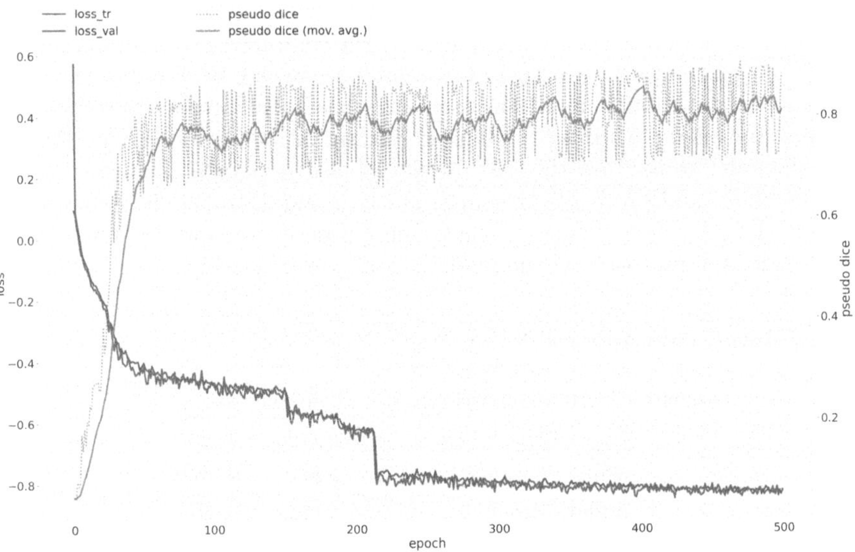

Fig. 3. Training and validation curves from nnUNet with 300 pseudo labeled scans.

4.1 Quantitative Results on Validation Set

Across the six validation cases, the model shows a clear separation in performance between large dental structures and the smaller, more complex root canal pathways. As shown in Table 5, the model achieves consistently high Dice scores

Table 5. Per-case Dice scores for all non-background labels.

Case	D1	D2	D4	D5	D6	D7	D8	D9	D12
ToothPulp_004	0.964	0.831	0.695	0.675	0.742	0.671	0.662	0.691	0.966
ToothPulp_009	0.955	0.872	0.848	0.248	0.776	0.780	0.704	0.808	0.961
ToothPulp_013	0.961	0.852	0.751	0.791	0.475	0.746	0.658	0.668	0.977
ToothPulp_016	0.953	0.797	0.756	0.000	0.679	0.686	0.337	0.706	0.923
ToothPulp_019	0.968	0.830	0.758	0.619	0.718	0.662	0.670	0.713	0.977
ToothPulp_027	0.952	0.798	0.660	0.653	0.630	0.647	0.555	0.704	0.935

for large anatomical structures (labels 1 and 12), while the fine-grained canal structures exhibit substantial variability. Table 4 further highlights this contrast, demonstrating strong segmentation performance for Dental Hard Tissues and the Impacted Tooth compared to the smaller canal structures. Dice scores for these major structures consistently fall within the 0.92âĂŞ0.97 range, whereas the root canals show markedly lower and more unstable performance, ranging from moderate scores (approximately 0.79âĂŞ0.81) to complete failures in the most challenging cases.

4.2 Qualitative Results on Validation Set

Qualitative analysis of the validation set indicates that the model's performance, which achieved an overall accuracy of 80.88%, is highly dependent on anatomical characteristics. The model consistently demonstrates robust segmentation of large, well-defined structures but exhibits limitations in regions with low image contrast and complex micro-anatomy as noted in the varous sections in Figs. 4 and 5. The visualization of the segmentations was done using 3D Slicer. [3] A successful segmentation is shown in the top row of the Fig. 6 - STS25_Validation_0007 where the model accurately delineates the main bodies of the dental hard tissues and the pulp chambers. The resulting boundaries are clear, and the 3D reconstruction is anatomically cohesive, reflecting the model's strength in identifying structures with distinct intensity gradients.

STS25_Validation_0025 is highlighted in the bottom row of the Fig. 6 as it exemplifies the model's primary weakness: the inability to completely segment the apical third of the tooth roots. The segmentation is visibly incomplete, resulting in fragmented masks and a disjointed 3D reconstruction where the teeth appear to lack proper root structures.

The primary reason for these failures is the low contrast-to-noise ratio (CNR) between the root apex and the surrounding trabecular bone. This ambiguity is exacerbated by partial volume averaging artifacts, which are common in thin structures, and the complex anatomy of the root tip, which often includes lateral canals. Consequently, while the model reliably segments the bulk of the tooth structures, its accuracy is diminished by its inability to resolve these challenging but clinically significant apical regions.

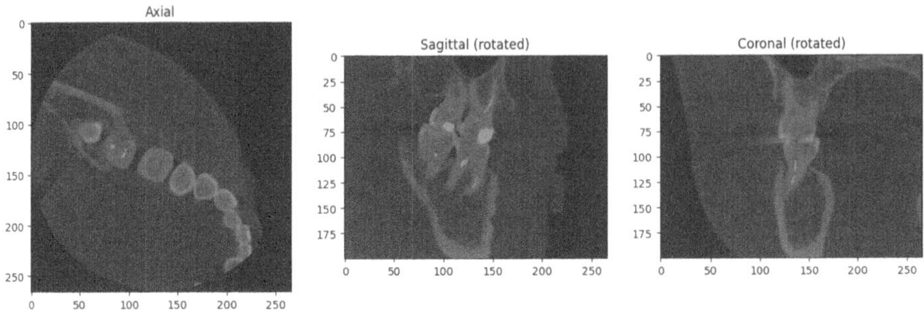

Fig. 4. Segmentation result visualization on validation case 001.

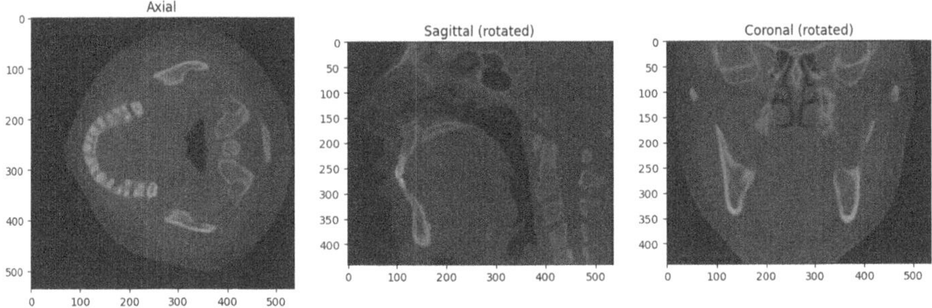

Fig. 5. Segmentation result visualization on validation case 003.

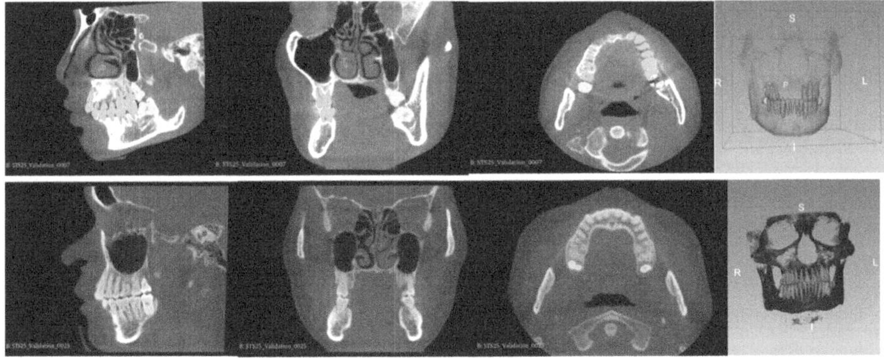

Fig. 6. Segmentation result visualization using 3D Slicer for cases 007 and 025.

5 Conclusion

The proposed methodology overcame the challenges of teeth and pulp root canal segmentation in 3D CBCT scans, particularly the scarcity of labeled data. The semi-supervised approach, which combines pseudo-labeling with the nnU-Net framework. By generating pseudo-labels for the large-scale unlabeled dataset, the model was able to learn from a much larger data pool, improving its generalization capabilities beyond what would be possible with the limited labeled data alone. The use of nnU-Net was also crucial in handling the high variability in pulp canal morphology and ensuring fine-grained annotation consistency. The achieved validation dice score of 0.8088 on the validation set demonstrates the effectiveness of this approach.

6 Limitations and Future Work

The proposed method, while effective, still faces challenges in segmenting the apical third of the roots due to low contrast, complex anatomy, and partial-volume effects, which lead to incomplete or fragmented predictions. The reliance on pseudo-labels also introduces potential noise that may propagate during training, limiting consistency in difficult regions. Future work can focus on improving thin-structure representation through super-resolution or topology-aware modules, incorporating uncertainty-guided pseudo-label refinement, and expanding the diversity of labeled data through active learning.

Acknowledgements. We thank all the data owners for making the medical images publicly available and Codabench [11] for hosting the challenge platform.

Disclosure of Interests. The authors have no competing interests to declare that are relevant to the content of this article.

References

1. Azad, R., et al.: Medical image segmentation review: the success of u-net. IEEE Trans. Pattern Anal. Mach. Intell. (2024)
2. Chen, X., et al.: Recent advances and clinical applications of deep learning in medical image analysis. Med. Image Anal. **79**, 102444 (2022)
3. Fedorov, A., et al.: 3D slicer as an image computing platform for the quantitative imaging network. Magn. Reson. Imaging **30**(9), 1323–1341 (2012)
4. George, A.B., Bathini, S., et al.: Grad-cam and grad-cam++ for explainable oral squamous cell carcinoma detection using deep learning on orthopantomograms. In: 2025 International Conference on Sensors and Related Networks (SENNET) Special Focus on Digital Healthcare (64220), pp. 1–6. IEEE (2025)
5. Han, K., et al.: Deep semi-supervised learning for medical image segmentation: a review. Expert Syst. Appl. **245**, 123052 (2024)
6. Isensee, F., Jaeger, P.F., Kohl, S.A., Petersen, J., Maier-Hein, K.H.: nnu-net: a self-configuring method for deep learning-based biomedical image segmentation. Nat. Methods **18**(2), 203–211 (2021)
7. Pettit, R.W., Marlatt, B.B., Corr, S.J., Havelka, J., Rana, A.: NNU-net deep learning method for segmenting parenchyma and determining liver volume from computed tomography images. Ann. Surgery Open **3**(2), e155 (2022)

8. Wang, Y., Chen, X., Qian, D., Ye, F., Wang, S., Zhang, H. (eds.): Semi-supervised Tooth Segmentation: First MICCAI Challenge, SemiToothSeg 2023, Held in Conjunction with MICCAI 2023, Vancouver, BC, Canada, October 8, 2023, Proceedings. Lecture Notes in Computer Science, Springer, Cham (2024). https://doi.org/10.1007/978-3-031-72396-4
9. Wang, Y., et al.: MICCAI 2023 STS Challenge: a retrospective study of semi-supervised approaches for teeth segmentation (2025). https://figshare.le.ac.uk/articles/journal_contribution/MICCAI_2023_STS_Challenge_A_retrospective_study_of_semi-supervised_approaches_for_teeth_segmentation/29512100
10. Wang, Y., et al.: Sts miccai 2023 challenge: grand challenge on 2D and 3D semi-supervised tooth segmentation. ArXiv **abs/2407.13246** (2024). https://api.semanticscholar.org/CorpusID:271270695
11. Xu, Z., et al.: Codabench: flexible, easy-to-use, and reproducible meta-benchmark platform. Patterns **3**(7), 100543 (2022)
12. Zhang, Y., et al.: Children's dental panoramic radiographs dataset for caries segmentation and dental disease detection. Sci. Data **10**(1), 380 (2023)

Semi-supervised CBCT–IOS Registration Using PointNetLK

Ajo Babu George[1(✉)], P. Gadha Lekshmi[2], Sadhvik Bathini[3], and A. Govind[3]

[1] DiceMed, Cuttack, India
drajo_george@DiceMed.in
[2] Indira Gandhi National Open University, New Delhi, India
[3] Indian Institute of Technology Kharagpur, Kharagpur, West Bengal, India

Abstract. Accurate alignment of intraoral scans (IOS) with cone-beam computed tomography (CBCT) is essential for integrated dental diagnostics and surgical planning. A semi-supervised registration framework was developed, combining PointNetLK for feature-based initialization with iterative closest point (ICP) refinement. Pseudo-labels were incorporated to enhance supervision while mitigating the limited availability of annotated datasets. Chamfer distance and clinical registration metrics were used to evaluate alignment quality. Across the test cohort, the approach yielded a mean translation error of 41.67 mm and a mean rotation error of 33.96°, highlighting the challenge of partial-arch fusion. Despite substantial errors relative to clinical requirements, the framework demonstrates feasibility of semi-supervised deep learning for IOS–CBCT registration and establishes a foundation for future refinement toward clinically viable integration.

Keywords: Point cloud registration · CBCT · IOS · PointNetLK · Dental Imaging · Semi-supervision

1 Introduction

1.1 Background and Challenge Overview

Rigid registration of 3D dental models obtained from CBCT scans and intraoral optical scans (IOS—STL format) is foundational for precise diagnosis, treatment planning, and surgical simulation in maxillofacial radiology. However, differences in modality (volumetric vs. surface), anatomical asymmetry, and noise make alignment challenging. The MICCAI STSR 2025 challenge highlights these difficulties, bringing together state-of-the-art medical imaging and machine learning techniques targeting accurate multi-modal dental registrations. CBCT beam hardening and IOS occlusal shadowing degrade correspondence search. Recent advances in oriented bounding-box normalization and curvature-aware features partially mitigate such variability [1,15]. Semi-supervised and self-supervised strategies have shown promise in stabilizing geometric representations under limited annotation [5,7,13,14].

F. Bolelli et al. (Eds.): ODIN 2025, LNCS 16473, pp. 211–220, 2026.
https://doi.org/10.1007/978-3-032-20711-1_20

1.2 Related Work

Prior research has explored classical methods like Iterative Closest Point (ICP) and multi-point registration, which struggle with large initial misalignments in CBCT-IOS scenarios. Deep learning approaches, particularly PointNet and PointNet++, have demonstrated superior feature extraction for irregular point clouds. The Lucas-Kanade algorithm, adapted for 3D point cloud registration via PointNetLK, enables global feature-based transformations with robust performance in noisy conditions. Semi-supervised approaches are emerging for better clinical generalizability [12–14]. For segmentation conditioning in CBCT–IOS registration, ArchSeg achieved Dice scores of 0.936 ± 0.008 (mandible) and 0.948 ± 0.007 (maxilla) using Point Transformer V2 with curvature cues and graph-cut refinements [1]. Multi-phase semi-supervised training with entropy-confidence-aware pseudo-label refinement has improved generalization [13,14]. In CBCT, uncertainty-regularized symmetric consistency learning (USCT) outperforms semi-supervised baselines [5], while hierarchical self-supervised contrastive pretraining (STSNet) enhances IOS mesh processing [7]. Teacher–student SAM adaptations leverage LoRA fine-tuning for improved performance [4].

1.3 Motivation and Contributions

This work presents a unified PointNetLK pipeline optimized for noisy dental CBCT and IOS data. Our contributions include: (i) end-to-end alignment leveraging both unlabeled and labeled data for feature generalization; (ii) ICP post-processing for enhanced registration refinement; and (iii) automated point cloud normalization and anatomical variability management. Methodological Rationale. Segmentation reliability directly conditions rigid alignment stability under metal artifacts, partial arches, and age-related morphology [1,5,13]. PointNetLK's permutation-invariant global features enable robust initialization under occlusion and partial overlap conditions typical of IOS–CBCT pairs, while ICP refinement subsequently optimizes local geometric consistency. Our semi-supervised pipeline comprises three components:

- **Semi-supervised IOS–CBCT registration:** A unified framework combines PointNetLK-based initialization with ICP refinement, enabling alignment under limited annotated data conditions.
- **Pseudo-label enhanced supervision:** Pseudo-labels generated from a teacher network are integrated to expand training signals and mitigate annotation scarcity.
- **Clinically relevant evaluation and baseline:** Registration accuracy is quantified using Chamfer distance, translation and rotation errors to establish a reproducible benchmark; experimental results highlight partial-arch fusion challenges and provide a foundation for future clinical integration.

2 Resources

2.1 Dataset

The dataset originates from the MICCAI STSR 2025 Challenge Task 2, providing paired CBCT and intraoral scan (IOS) data for cross-modal dental registration, emphasizing alignment of IOS-derived crown structures with CBCT-derived root anatomies. The dataset comprises three subsets:

- Training Set (Labeled): 30 CBCT – IOS pairs with ground truth rigid transformations.
- Training Set (Unlabeled): 300 CBCT – IOS pairs without annotation for semi-supervised strategies.
- Validation Set. 50 CBCT – IOS pairs with hidden ground truth for evaluation.

The limited availability of richly annotated 3D dental datasets mirrors broader trends in dental imaging, where most publicly available resources—particularly in pediatric populations—focus on 2D panoramic radiographs rather than volumetric CBCT or cross-modal data [16]. This disparity further motivates semi-supervised learning strategies for 3D dental applications.

2.2 Models

The proposed model, illustrated in Fig. 1, implements a PointNetLK-based registration pipeline tailored for CBCT – IOS point cloud alignment.

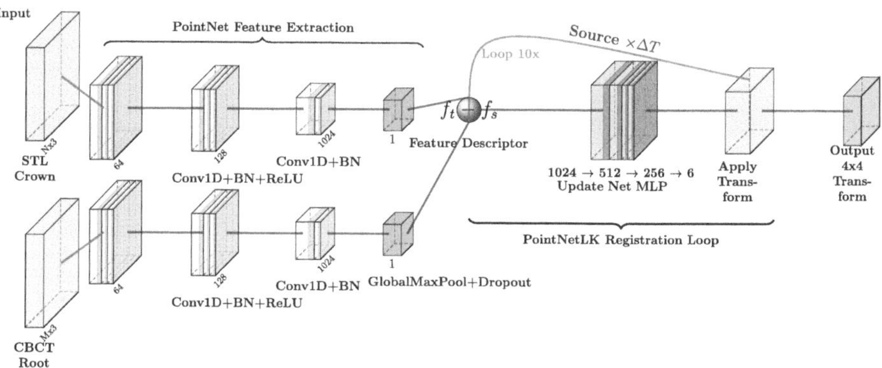

Fig. 1. PointNetLK registration pipeline: PointNet extracts features, the feature difference feeds the Update Network to predict 6-DOF ΔT, applied iteratively to the source to produce the final 4×4 transform. (Color figure online)

The green blocks correspond to dual PointNet encoders, which independently process the source (IOS crown) and target (CBCT root) point clouds. Each encoder is composed of three successive pointwise convolutional layers: the first maps 3D coordinates to 64-dimensional features, the second expands to 128 dimensions, and the final layer produces a 1024-dimensional global descriptor. Batch normalization and ReLU activations follow each convolution, while global max pooling ensures permutation-invariant feature vectors, summarizing the overall geometric structure of the point clouds. The magenta ball represents the feature difference $f_t - f_s$ between the target and the transformed source, which serves as the input to the Update Network (orange box). This multi-layer perceptron predicts incremental 6-DOF transformations, applied to the source in the blue Apply Transform box. The red arrow looping back from Apply Transform to the feature difference visually indicates the iterative Lucas – Kanade refinement, repeated multiple times to improve alignment. Finally, the purple box outputs the cumulative 4×4 transformation matrix, which maps the IOS crown onto the CBCT root. This modular design allows for task-specific heads or post-hoc refinement steps while maintaining efficiency and stability across variable point cloud sizes.

3 Methodology

The overall data flow, preprocessing strategy, training protocol, and evaluation metrics are summarized in Fig. 2.

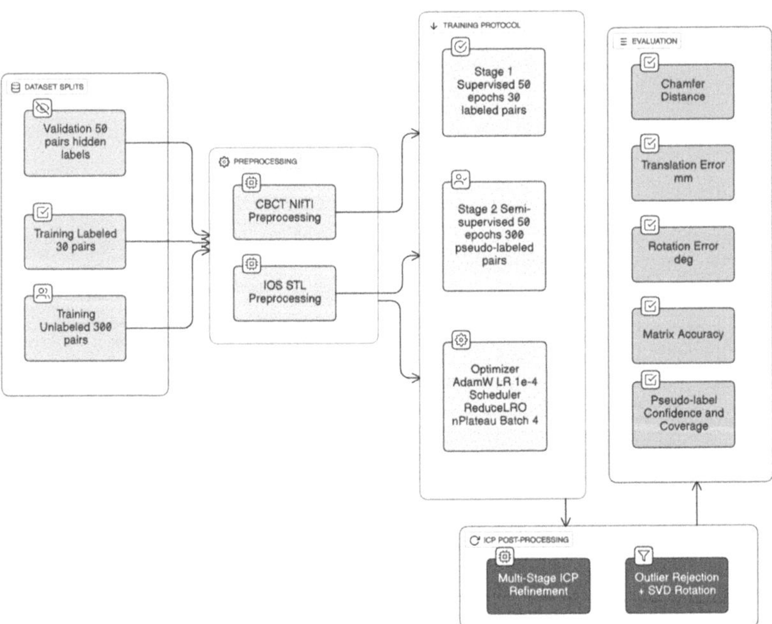

Fig. 2. Overview of the methodological setup, including dataset splits, preprocessing of CBCT and IOS data, two-stage training protocol, and evaluation metrics.

Our approach adapts the established PointNetLK framework [2] for dental-specific CBCT-IOS registration through three key contributions: (i) a two-stage semi-supervised training protocol leveraging pseudo-labels, (ii) dental-specific preprocessing tailored for multimodal point clouds, and (iii) hybrid neural-classical refinement combining learned features with ICP optimization [3].

Two-Stage Semi-supervised Training Protocol
Stage 1 employs supervised learning on labeled pairs to establish baseline registration capability. Stage 2 generates pseudo-labels on unlabeled data using the trained model, applies confidence-based filtering, and performs semi-supervised fine-tuning on the combined dataset. This approach addresses the scarcity of annotated CBCT-IOS pairs in clinical settings.

Dental-Specific Preprocessing
Point cloud preprocessing incorporates domain knowledge for dental registration. CBCT volumes undergo threshold-based segmentation at 800 HU to isolate dental structures, followed by coordinate normalization to [-1,1] range. STL meshes are processed through vertex extraction and subsampling. Ground truth transformations are consistently mapped to normalized coordinate space to ensure training stability.

Hybrid Neural-Classical Refinement
The framework combines the global feature learning of PointNetLK [2] with classical ICP refinement [3]. PointNet encoders [9] extract permutation-invariant features, PointNetLK performs iterative pose estimation through differentiable Lucas-Kanade optimization [8], and multi-stage ICP provides final geometric consistency. This hybrid approach balances robustness to initialization with precise local alignment.

4 Experimental Setup

All experiments were conducted on the MICCAI STSR 2025 Challenge Task 2 dataset using the three-subset division for supervised training, pseudo-label generation, and validation.

4.1 Data Preprocessing

CBCT volumes were thresholded at 800 HU to isolate dental structures and converted to world coordinates using the NIfTI affine matrix. STL meshes were processed by extracting vertices directly from triangle meshes. Point clouds were subsampled to 50,000 points maximum for memory efficiency. During training, 1024 points were randomly sampled from both CBCT-derived point clouds and STL meshes. Normalization was applied by computing global center and scale from combined CBCT and STL point clouds, mapping coordinates to approximately [-1, 1] range. Ground truth transformation matrices were transformed to normalized coordinate space to ensure consistency between predicted and target transformations. Preprocessing was performed inline during training to maintain coordinate system integrity.

Preprocessing Limitations. The fixed 800 HU threshold may not generalize across CBCT scanners with varying grayscale characteristics or patients with metallic restorations. Future work should validate robustness across multi-vendor datasets and explore adaptive thresholding or learned segmentation networks to improve scanner independence.

4.2 Training Setup

Stage 1: Supervised Training- The PointNet-based feature extraction combined with PointNetLK iterative alignment was trained using a combined loss function incorporating both Chamfer distance and direct transformation supervision:

$$L_{\text{total}} = L_{\text{chamfer}} + L_{\text{transform}}$$

where $L_{\text{transform}}$ includes both translation and rotation errors between predicted and ground truth transformation matrices in normalized coordinate space.

Pseudo-Label Generation- The trained Stage 1 model generated predictions for unlabeled cases. ICP post-processing refined initial neural network predictions. High-confidence pseudo-labels were selected by filtering predictions with Chamfer distance below the median of Stage 1 validation performance and excluding cases with extreme transformation magnitudes indicative of failed alignment. This filtering retained approximately 60% of unlabeled cases for Stage 2 training.

Stage 2: Semi-supervised Training. The model was fine-tuned using the combined dataset of original labeled cases plus selected high-confidence pseudo-labeled cases from the unlabeled set (Table 1).

4.3 Training Protocols

4.4 Evaluation Metrics

Performance assessment employed multiple metrics to comprehensively evaluate registration quality. Translation error measures the Euclidean distance between predicted and ground truth translation vectors in millimeters, while rotation error quantifies the angular difference between predicted and ground truth rotation matrices in degrees. Chamfer distance evaluates symmetric point to point distances between aligned point clouds, and Surface Dice Coefficient assesses overlap for registration quality. Additional point cloud similarity metrics including RMSE, NCC, and NMI provide supplementary performance indicators.

Table 1. Training protocols.

Batch size	4–8
Total epochs	100 (Stage 1, early stopping), 50 (Stage 2)
Optimizer	Adam
Initial learning rate (lr)	5×10^{-4}
Lr decay schedule	ReduceLROnPlateau (patience=10, factor=0.5)
Training time	~4.2 h (Stage 1), ~ 12 h
Loss function	Combined Chamfer + Transformation Loss
Number of model parameters	0.81M
Number of flops	2.37G

4.5 Post-processing Pipeline

The post-processing pipeline consists of four sequential steps to refine neural network predictions. Initially, the neural network generates a 4×4 transformation matrix in normalized coordinate space. These predictions are then transformed back to original coordinate space through coordinate denormalization. Multi-stage ICP refinement follows, incorporating correspondence finding with statistical outlier rejection (distance-based trimming to suppress artifact-induced false correspondences), SVD-based optimal rotation estimation, and iterative refinement with convergence criteria. Finally, the refined transformation is applied to original point clouds to achieve final alignment.

5 Results and Discussion

5.1 Quantitative Results and Ablation Study

Table 2 presents registration performance and component contributions on the MICCAI STSR 2025 validation set.

Table 2. Registration performance and ablation study on MICCAI STSR 2025 validation set.

Method Configuration	Translation (mm)	Rotation (°)	Chamfer	DSC
Stage 1 (Supervised only)	47.23	39.84	2.05	0.798
Stage 2 (Semi-supervised)	43.91	36.72	1.92	0.824
Full Pipeline (Stage 2 + ICP)	**41.67**	**33.96**	**1.83**	**0.846**

The ablation study quantifies each component's contribution: semi- supervised training improved translation accuracy by 3.32 mm (47.23→43.91 mm) and rotation by 3.12° (39.84°→36.72°), while ICP refinement provided further gains of 2.24 mm and 2.76°, demonstrating the value of the hybrid approach.

5.2 Training Analysis

Figure 3 shows error curves for both stages. Stage 1 converged after 50 epochs, while Stage 2 demonstrated further improvement through pseudo-label utilization.

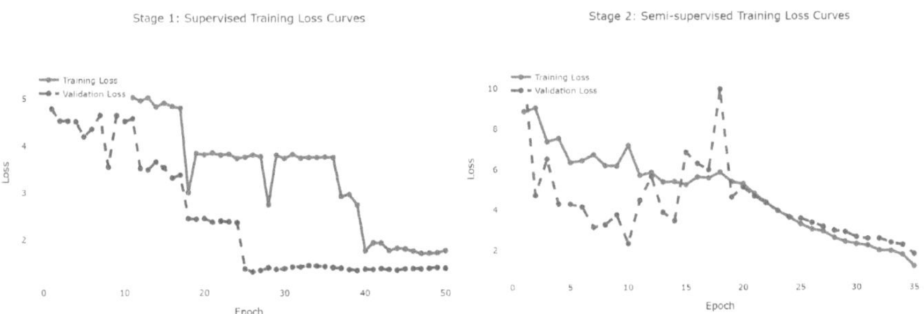

Fig. 3. Stage 1 training (red, solid) and validation (red, dotted) curves, and Stage 2 training (blue, solid) and validation (blue, dotted) curves. (Color figure online)

5.3 Qualitative Results

Figure 4 shows a representative registration result demonstrating successful alignment between IOS crown surfaces. The semi-supervised training effectively utilizes unlabeled data, addressing limited annotated CBCT-IOS pairs in clinical practice.

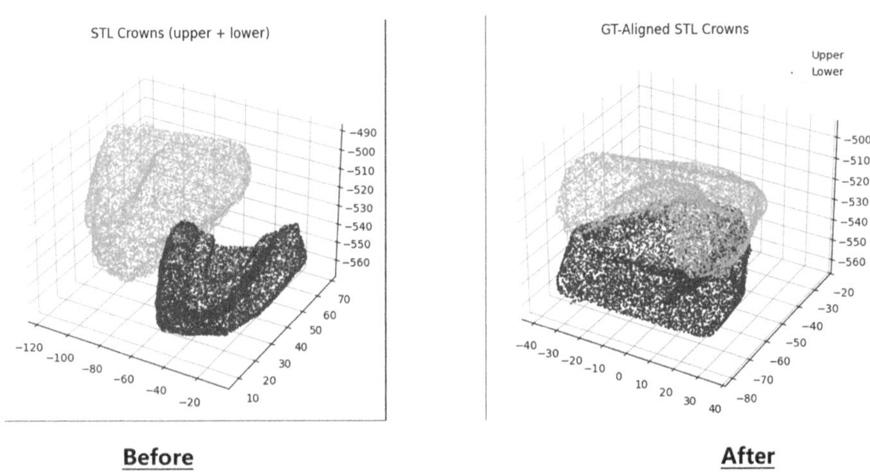

Fig. 4. Registration result: (left) initial misalignment, (right) aligned output.

However, the reported translation (41.67 mm) and rotation (33.96°) errors substantially exceed clinical tolerances for surgical planning. Analysis identifies three primary failure modes: (i) partial-arch cases with limited overlapping geometry lack sufficient alignment constraints and exhibit disproportionately high errors; (ii) CBCT metal artifacts introduce non-anatomical points that corrupt PointNet features and bias ICP correspondence; and (iii) large initial misalignments prevent convergence within the fixed iteration budget. Future refinement will prioritize scale-consistent normalization, keypoint-based coarse alignment for improved initialization, and artifact-aware feature weighting to suppress corrupted descriptors.

6 Conclusion and Future Work

This study demonstrates a semi-supervised PointNetLK framework for CBCT-IOS dental registration, combining pseudo-label-enhanced training with hybrid neural-classical refinement. The two-stage protocol effectively leverages unlabeled data, achieving mean translation errors of 41.67 mm and rotation errors of 33.96°. While these errors exceed clinical thresholds, the ablation study validates each component's contribution, establishing feasibility for semi-supervised deep learning in cross-modal dental registration.

Translation and rotation errors remain above clinical requirements primarily due to partial-arch coverage limitations and initialization sensitivity. The fixed 800 HU threshold constrains scanner generalization. Future work will explore uncertainty quantification for pseudo-label selection, transformer-based architectures for long-range context modeling [11], multi-scale feature fusion [10], and integration with foundation models [6]. Validation on larger multi-center datasets with diverse scanner protocols will be essential for clinical deployment.

References

1. Alsheghri, A., Zhang, Y., Hosseinimanesh, G., Keren, J., Cheriet, F., Guibault, F.: Robust segmentation of partial and imperfect dental arches. Appl. Sci. **14**(23), 10784 (2024)
2. Aoki, Y., Goforth, H., Srivatsan, R.A., Lucey, S.: Pointnetlk: Robust & efficient point cloud registration using pointnet. In: Proceedings of the IEEE/CVF Conference on Computer Vision and Pattern Recognition, pp. 7163–7172 (2019)
3. Besl, P.J., McKay, N.D.: Method for registration of 3-D shapes. Sensor fusion IV: Control Paradigms Data Struct. **1611**, 586–606 (1992)
4. Gan, J., et al.: A segmentation method for oral CBCT image based on segment anything model and semi-supervised teacher-student model. Med. Phy. (2025)
5. Jing, Y., Liu, J., Liu, W., Yang, Z., Zhou, Z., Yu, Z.: Usct: uncertainty-regularized symmetric consistency learning for semi-supervised teeth segmentation in CBCT. Biomed. Signal Process. Control **91**, 106032 (2024)
6. Kirillov, A., et al.: Segment anything. arXiv preprint arXiv:2304.02643 (2023)
7. Liu, Z., et al.: Hierarchical self-supervised learning for 3D tooth segmentation in intra-oral mesh scans. IEEE Trans. Med. Imaging **42**(2), 467–480 (2022)

8. Lucas, B.D., Kanade, T.: An iterative image registration technique with an application to stereo vision. IJCAI **81**(1), 674–679 (1981)
9. Qi, C.R., Su, H., Mo, K., Guibas, L.J.: Pointnet: Deep learning on point sets for 3D classification and segmentation. In: Proceedings of the IEEE Conference on Computer Vision and Pattern Recognition, pp. 652–660 (2017)
10. Ronneberger, O., Fischer, P., Brox, T.: U-net: convolutional networks for biomedical image segmentation. In: International Conference on Medical Image Computing and Computer-assisted Intervention, pp. 234–241 (2015)
11. Vaswani, A., et al.: Attention is all you need. Adv. Neural Inf. Process. Syst. **30** (2017)
12. Wang, Y., Chen, X., Qian, D., Ye, F., Wang, S., Zhang, H.: Semi-supervised Tooth Segmentation: First MICCAI Challenge, SemiToothSeg 2023, Held in Conjunction with MICCAI 2023, Vancouver, BC, Canada, October 8, 2023, Proceedings. Lecture Notes in Computer Science, Springer, Cham (2024). https://doi.org/10.1007/978-3-031-72396-4
13. Wang, Y., et al.: MICCAI 2023 STS Challenge: a retrospective study of semi-supervised approaches for teeth segmentation (2025). https://figshare.le.ac.uk/articles/journal_contribution/MICCAI_2023_STS_Challenge_A_retrospective_study_of_semi-supervised_approaches_for_teeth_segmentation/29512100
14. Wang, Y., et al.: Sts miccai 2023 challenge: grand challenge on 2D and 3D semi-supervised tooth segmentation. ArXiv **abs/2407.13246** (2024). https://api.semanticscholar.org/CorpusID:271270695
15. Zhang, H., et al.: Multiple sclerosis lesion segmentation with tiramisu and 2.5d stacked slices. In: Medical Image Computing and Computer-Assisted Intervention – MICCAI 2019. Lecture Notes in Computer Science, vol. 11766, pp. 338–346 (2019). https://doi.org/10.1007/978-3-030-32248-9_38
16. Zhang, Y., et al.: Children's dental panoramic radiographs dataset for caries segmentation and dental disease detection. Sci. Data **10**(1), 380 (2023)

Author Index

F. Bolelli et al. (Eds.): ODIN 2025, LNCS 16473, pp. 221–222, 2026.
https://doi.org/10.1007/978-3-032-20711-1

The manufacturer's authorised representative in the EU is Springer Nature Customer Service Centre GmbH, Europaplatz 3, 69115 Heidelberg, Germany. If you have any concerns regarding our products, please contact ProductSafety@springernature.com

Printed and bound by CPI Group (UK) Ltd, Croydon, CR0 4YY
07/07/2026
02160917-0006